59.99

369 0289888

This book is due for return on or before the last date shown below.

Urology for the Pediatrician

Guest Editors

PASQUALE CASALE, MD
WALID A. FARHAT, MD

PEDIATRIC CLINICS
OF NORTH AMERICA

www.pediatric.theclinics.com

August 2012 • Volume 59 • Number 4

SAUNDERS an imprint of ELSEVIER, Inc.

W.B. SAUNDERS COMPANY
A Division of Elsevier Inc.

1600 John F. Kennedy Boulevard • Suite 1800 • Philadelphia, Pennsylvania 19103-2899

http://www.theclinics.com

THE PEDIATRIC CLINICS OF NORTH AMERICA Volume 59, Number 4
August 2012 ISSN 0031-3955, ISBN-13: 978-1-4557-3910-3

Editor: Kerry Holland
Developmental Editor: Donald Mumford

The Pediatric Clinics of North America (ISSN 0031-3955) is published bimonthly by Elsevier Inc., 360 Park Avenue South, New York, NY 10010-1710. Months of issue are February, April, June, August, October, and December. Periodicals postage paid at New York, NY and additional mailing offices. Subscription prices are $191.00 per year (US individuals), $444.00 per year (US institutions), $259.00 per year (Canadian individuals), $591.00 per year (Canadian institutions), $308.00 per year (international individuals), $591.00 per year (international institutions), $93.00 per year (US students and residents), and $159.00 per year (international and Canadian residents and students). To receive students/resident rare, orders must be accompanied by name of affiliated institution, date of term, and the signature of program/residency coordinator on institution letterhead. Orders will be billed at individual rate until proof of status is received. Foreign air speed delivery is included in all *Clinics* subscription prices. All prices are subject to change without notice. **POSTMASTER:** Send address changes to *The Pediatric Clinics of North America*, Elsevier Health Sciences Division, Subscription Customer Service, 3251 Riverport Lane, Maryland Heights, MO 63043. **Customer Service: 1-800-654-2452 (US and Canada). From outside of the US and Canada: 1-314-447-8871. Fax: 1-314-447-8029. For print support, E-mail: JournalsCustomerService-usa@elsevier.com. For online support, E-mail: JournalsOnlineSupport-usa@elsevier.com.**

Reprints. For copies of 100 or more, of articles in this publication, please contact the Commercial Reprints Department, Elsevier Inc., 360 Park Avenue South, New York, NY 10010-1710. Tel.: 212-633-3812; Fax: 212-462-1935; E-mail: reprints@elsevier.com.

The Pediatric Clinics of North America is also published in Spanish by McGraw-Hill Inter-americana Editores S.A., Mexico City, Mexico; in Portuguese by Riechmann and Affonso Editores, Rua Comandante Coelho 1085, CEP 21250, Rio de Janeiro, Brazil; and in Greek by Althayia SA, Athens, Greece.

The Pediatric Clinics of North America is covered in *MEDLINE/PubMed (Index Medicus)*, *Excerpta Medica, Current Contents, Current Contents/Clinical Medicine, Science Citation Index, ASCA, ISI/BIOMED*, and *BIOSIS*.

Printed and bound by CPI Group (UK) Ltd, Croydon, CR0 4YY
Transferred to Digital Print 2012

Contributors

GUEST EDITORS

PASQUALE CASALE, MD
Chief, Division of Urology; Professor, Columbia University, Columbia University Medical Center, Morgan Stanley Children's Hospital, New York, New York

WALID A. FARHAT, MD, FRCSC, FAAP
Associate Professor, Department of Surgery, University of Toronto; Pediatric Urologist, Division of Urology, The Hospital for Sick Children, Toronto, Ontario, Canada

AUTHORS

DARIUS J. BÄGLI, MDCM, FRCSC, FAAP, FACS
Professor of Surgery, Senior Associate Scientist, Divisions of Developmental & Stem Cell Biology and Urology, The Hospital For Sick Children & Research Institute; Institute of Medical Science, and Faculty of Medicine, University of Toronto, Toronto, Ontario, Canada

LINDA A. BAKER, MD
Professor of Urology and Pediatric Urologist, Department of Urology, University of Texas Southwestern Medical Center, Children's Medical Center at Dallas, Dallas, Texas

JOHN W. BROCK III, MD
Monroe Carell Jr. Chair and Professor of Urologic Surgery, Division of Pediatric Urology, Vanderbilt University, Nashville, Tennessee

EARL CHENG, MD
Attending Physician, Division of Urology, Children's Memorial Hospital; Professor of Urology, Northwestern University, Feinberg School of Medicine, Chicago, Illinois

DOUGLASS B. CLAYTON, MD
Assistant Professor of Urologic Surgery, Division of Pediatric Urology, Vanderbilt University, Nashville, Tennessee

LAWRENCE COPELOVITCH, MD
Assistant Professor of Pediatrics, Division of Nephrology, Department of Pediatrics, The Children's Hospital of Philadelphia, Philadelphia, Pennsylvania

FERNANDO F. FONSECA, MD
Department of Urology, Children's Hospital, Boston Harvard Medical School, Boston, Massachusetts

JANELLE A. FOX, MD
Fellow, Division of Pediatric Urology, Children's Hospital of Pittsburgh of UPMC, University of Pittsburgh, Pittsburgh, Pennsylvania

ISRAEL FRANCO, MD, FAAP, FACS
Professor of Urology, Pediatric Urology Associates, New York Medical College, Valhalla,
New York

DOMINIC FRIMBERGER, MD
Associate Professor of Urology, Section of Pediatric Urology, Robotics, University of
Oklahoma Health Sciences Center, Oklahoma City, Oklahoma

CANDACE F. GRANBERG, MD
Pediatric Urology Fellow, Department of Urology, University of Texas Southwestern
Medical Center, Children's Medical Center at Dallas, Dallas, Texas

GWEN M. GRIMSBY, MD
Urology Resident, Mayo Clinic, Arizona

LINDSEY HERREL, MD
Resident in Urology, Department of Urology, Emory University School of Medicine,
Atlanta, Georgia

RON KEREN, MD, MPH
Division of General Pediatrics, Center for Pediatric Clinical Effectiveness, Children's
Hospital of Philadelphia; Center for Clinical Epidemiology and Biostatistics, University
of Pennsylvania School of Medicine, Philadelphia, Pennsylvania

ANDREW J. KIRSCH, MD, FAAP, FACS
Clinical Professor and Chief of Pediatric Urology, Division of Pediatric Urology,
Department of Urology, Emory University School of Medicine, Children's Healthcare
of Atlanta, Atlanta, Georgia

MARTIN A. KOYLE, MD, FAAP, FACS, FRCS (Eng.)
Program Director, Division of Pediatric Urology, Hospital for Sick Children, Professor
of Surgery, University of Toronto, Toronto, Ontario, Canada

BRADLEY P. KROPP, MD
Professor and Interim Chairperson, Chief, Section of Pediatric Urology, University
of Oklahoma Health Sciences Center, Oklahoma City, Oklahoma

SARAH M. LAMBERT, MD
Assistant Professor, Department of Urology, Columbia University, The Morgan Stanley
Children's Hospital of New York, New York, New York

ARMANDO J. LORENZO, MD, MSc, FRCSC, FAAP, FACS
Pediatric Urology, Hospital for Sick Children; Assistant Professor, Department of Surgery,
University of Toronto, Toronto, Ontario, Canada

LAURA STANSELL MERRIMAN, MD
Fellow, Pediatric Urology, Division of Pediatric Urology, Department of Urology, Emory
University School of Medicine, Children's Healthcare of Atlanta, Atlanta, Georgia

HRAIR-GEORGE O. MESROBIAN, MD, MSc
Professor, Division of Pediatric Urology, Department of Urology, Medical College and
Children's Hospital of Wisconsin, Milwaukee, Wisconsin

SHAMA P. MIRZA, PhD
Assistant Professor, Department of Biochemistry, Medical College and Children's
Hospital of Wisconsin, Milwaukee, Wisconsin

THOMAS B. NEWMAN, MD, MPH
Professor of Epidemiology & Biostatistics and Pediatrics, Chief, Department of Epidemiology and Biostatistics, School of Medicine, University of California, San Francisco, California

HIEP T. NGUYEN, MD, FAAP
Department of Urology, Children's Hospital, Boston Harvard Medical School, Boston, Massachusetts

MICHAEL C. OST, MD
Associate Professor, Chief, Division of Pediatric Urology, Children's Hospital of Pittsburgh of UPMC; Vice Chairman, Department of Urology, University of Pittsburgh, Pittsburgh, Pennsylvania

KIRK PINTO, MD, FAAP
Pediatric Urology, Urology Associates of North Texas and Cook Children's Hospital, Fort Worth, Texas

JOAO L. PIPPI SALLE, MD, PhD
Division Head, Professor of Surgery, Division of Urology, Department of Surgery, The Hospital for Sick Children, University of Toronto, Toronto, Ontario, Canada

MICHAEL L. RITCHEY, MD
Professor of Urology, Mayo Clinic Arizona; Chief of Surgery, Phoenix Children's Hospital, Phoenix, Arizona

RODRIGO L.P. ROMAO, MD
Clinical Fellow, Division of Urology, Department of Surgery, The Hospital for Sick Children, University of Toronto, Toronto, Ontario, Canada

DAVID E. SANDBERG, PhD
Professor and Director, Division of Child Behavioral Health, Department of Pediatrics & Communicable Diseases and Program for Disorders of Sex Development, University of Michigan, Ann Arbor, Michigan

DONALD SHIFRIN, MD, FAAP
Clinical Professor of Pediatrics, University of Washington School of Medicine, Seattle, Washington

FABIO Y. TANNO, MD
Department of Urology, Children's Hospital, Boston Harvard Medical School, Boston, Masschusetts

ROBERT M. TURNER II, MD
Resident, Department of Urology, University of Pittsburgh, Pittsburgh, Pennsylvania

DIANE K. WHERRETT, MD
Assistant Professor, Division of Endocrinology, Department of Paediatrics, The Hospital for Sick Children, University of Toronto, Toronto, Ontario, Canada

Contents

Prenatal ultrasound is an integral part of caring for pregnant women in the United States. Although surprisingly few data exist to support the clinical benefit of screening ultrasound during pregnancy, its use continues to rise. Urologic anomalies are among the most commonly identified, with overall detection sensitivity approaching 90%. Prenatal hydronephrosis is the most frequently identified finding and predicting postnatal pathology based on its presence can be difficult. As the degree of fetal hydronephrosis increases so does the risk of true urinary tract pathology. Diagnoses that require more urgent care include causes of lower urinary tract obstruction and bladder and cloacal exstrophy.

The urological care of the neurogenic bladder consists of 2 components: medical management with preservation of renal function and quality-of-life issues with achieving dryness and independence of bladder and bowel management. Both components are equally important for patients to live a healthy and fulfilled life. This report explores the diagnosis of the neurogenic bladder; quality-of-life issues that caregivers and patients should expect; the importance of primary care knowledge of the neurogenic bladder and treatment; surgical options; the transition of pediatric patients to adult care; and the importance of caregiver and patient understanding of their disease, treatment options, and responsibilities.

Problems of the groin and genitalia are a common presenting complaint in both pediatrician's offices and emergency departments. The authors endeavor to provide a comprehensive review of the most common inguinal and genital anomalies encountered by the pediatrician, with a special focus on examination and management.

Functional lower urinary tract problems, bladder and bowel problems, or dysfunctional elimination syndrome are all terms that describe the common array of symptoms that include overactive bladder syndrome, voiding

setting; increase of the knowledge base about genetic mechanisms of normal and abnormal sex development; critical appraisal about the timing and nature of genital surgery in patients with DSD. Herein, the authors present a comprehensive review with up-to-date data about the approach to the newborn with ambiguous genitalia as well as the diagnosis and management of the most common DSD.

In 2005, the Lawson Wilkins Pediatric Endocrine Society and the European Society for Pediatric Endocrinology convened a conference on intersex to review clinical management practices and data from long-term health-related and gender-related outcomes research and to identify key areas for future research. Romao and colleagues provide an overview of the evolving changes after publication of this guidance, informed by experiences in their multidisciplinary clinic. This commentary highlights and expands on several of the topics explored, with a special emphasis on the psychosocial aspects of care for persons affected by disorders of sex development and their families.

Childhood urolithiasis is an evolving condition with an increasing incidence and prevalence over the last 2 decades. Over that time the underlying cause has shifted from predominantly infectious to metabolic in nature. This review describes the pathophysiology, underlying metabolic abnormalities, clinical presentation, evaluation, and management of childhood urolithiasis. A comprehensive metabolic evaluation is essential for all children with renal calculi, given the high rate of recurrence and the importance of excluding inherited progressive conditions.

Over the past 3 decades, minimally invasive stone surgery has completely overtaken open surgical approaches to upper tract pediatric urolithiasis. Progressing from least to most minimally invasive, extracorporeal shock wave lithotripsy, ureteroscopy, and percutaneous nephrolithotomy are the surgical methods of today for kidney and ureteral stones. The choice of treatment modality is individualized in children, considering patient age, stone size, number, location, and anatomic and clinical contributing factors. The purpose of this article is to review these techniques for pediatric upper urinary tract stones and summarize outcomes and complications.

Urinary tract infections are common occurrences in the pediatric age group and are a cause of significant morbidity and expense. The understanding of the consequences and sequelae of febrile urinary tract infections led to revision of standard protocols initiated by the American Academy of Pediatrics (AAP) in 1999. A less invasive protocol of radiologic evaluation has been the major outcome of the revised AAP guidelines. Emphasis on prevention of recurrent febrile urinary tract infections has also led to therapeutic programs that are centered less around the use of prophylactic antibiotics than has previously been the practice.

The past decade has seen a remarkable retreat from previous dogma regarding urinary tract infections (UTIs). Less aggressive imaging is now recommended because although vesicoureteral reflux (VUR) is frequently found in children with a history of febrile UTIs, most VUR resolves spontaneously and we do not have evidence that treatment of the rest improves outcome. Available evidence suggests urine testing for UTI can be less aggressive as well, focusing on those with the most risk factors for UTI, those with the most severe illness, and those at highest risk of complications.

The surgical armamentarium of the pediatric urologist has changed greatly in the past 2 decades on account of new technology and careful adaptation of minimally invasive techniques in children. Conventional laparoscopy, robotic-assisted laparoscopy, laparoendoscopic single-site surgery, and endourologic surgery have, to varying degrees, provided new approaches to urologic surgery in the pediatric population. This article reviews the technology and adaptations behind these recent advances as well as their current applications in management of urologic disease in children.

Functional bladder problems in children are often insidious and are frequently ignored by the child, by parents, and by many caregivers. Consideration of both the urinary and bowel outlets, and more recently, of the corticospinal tracts and brain reveal great complexity in this condition. In this article, the author addresses many of these issues in depth with a familiar personal experience derived from many years of dedicated consideration of these problems. Bladder dysfunction in the child is in many ways the pediatric urologist's hypertension diagnosis. Like antihypertensive therapy, bladder retraining strategies must be adhered to for life.

This article reviews common pediatric urologic cancers involving the genitourinary system. Rhabdomyosarcoma may occur in the bladder, prostate, paratesticular regions, vagina, or uterus. Some of these locations, such as the paratesticular region, have a more favorable outcome. Benign neoplasms account for the majority of pediatric testicular tumors and most are managed with testis-sparing surgery. Most genitourinary malignancies are expected to have a good outcome. One focus of treatment is organ preservation but not at the expense of a good oncologic outcome. Late sequelae of anticancer therapy are a concern and every attempt is made to decrease the intensity of tumor treatment.

The modern management of pediatric genitourinary malignancies has resulted in survival rates that are dramatically better than figures from just a few decades ago. This is largely due to advances in multimodal treatment, collaborative efforts, and multidisciplinary management. Nevertheless, issues related to long-term side effects, treatment-related morbidity, and progression or recurrences remain important and pressing in terms of research directions and areas for improvement. In this Editorial Comment the author attempts to employ the current state of the art, masterfully summarized in the accompanying review by Drs Grimsby and Ritchey, to provide a view of trends that are likely to become increasingly important in the future, highlighting common patterns in treatment philosophy seen in other areas of oncology: more selective or patient-tailored treatment strategies, refined protocols and —whenever possible— tissue sparing and minimally invasive surgical interventions.

Although few children are severely ill when evaluated in the pediatric office, developing the skills to recognize an infant or child who requires hospitalization is critical. Some children will require treatment in an emergency department or direct admission to an inpatient facility, whereas other children can be managed as outpatients. Determining when an infant requires an inpatient admission is particularly important because the metabolic reserve is less abundant in the newborn. Patients with hemodynamic instability must be emergently addressed. This article outlines the most common urgent and emergent pediatric urological conditions with the goal to direct initial evaluation and treatment.

Despite its long history and common practice, circumcision remains a controversial procedure. This article reviews the history of this operation, examines the controversy that surrounds it, and emphasizes the performing practitioner's responsibility to the patient and his family in guiding them through the complicated decision making surrounding newborn circumcision.

PEDIATRIC CLINICS
OF NORTH AMERICA

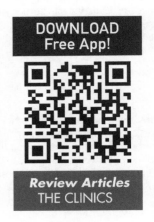

Preface: What Pediatricians Need to Know about Urology

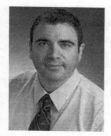 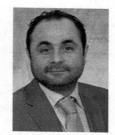

Pasquale Casale, MD   Walid A. Farhat, MD, FRCSC
Guest Editors

Over the past two decades, the pediatric urology subspecialty has been revolutionized with new diagnostic and therapeutics advances. We are honored to be the editors of this particular issue focusing on pediatric urology for the *Pediatrics Clinics of North America*. Although this issue examines some of the important advances that have been made in the field of pediatric urology, we opted to concentrate more on evolving pediatric urology problems. In order to provide additional insight into these topics, we invited some authors to further cover these topics through editorial comments.

Common general pediatric urology pathologies (undescended testicles and hernias with hypospadias) are covered by Kirsch et al, while Dr Pinto from Texas revisits the historical topic of circumcision with more current data and evidence-based recommendations.

The routine use of prenatal ultrasound may have had the most significant impact on pediatric urology practice. Therefore Brock et al from Vanderbilt provides the pediatricians with an insightful run of all the possible diagnoses, approaches, and possible dispositions when urological anomalies are suspected. Since hydronephrosis is one of the most common prenatal ultrasound findings, we dedicated an article by Dr Mesrobian from Wisconsin to providing an update on how to best manage patients with an obstruction, highlighted with the most recent advances on the role of noninvasive diagnostic studies, such as urinary proteomics.

With the newly published AAP guidelines for the management of infants and children with urinary tract infection, it was compulsory to dedicate an article to addressing this topic from a pediatric urologist's point of view, presented by Drs Koyle from Toronto and Shifrin from Seattle, accompanied with an overarching editorial comment by Tom Newman from San Francisco. The treatment of VUR is better standardized today and the role of surgery is better defined. Subsequently, Nguyen et al from Boston provide an evidence-based approach for the management of VUR, while Dr Keren elaborates further by addressing some of the points that general pediatricians need to know, focusing on this evolving subject.

Frimberger et al from Oklahoma and Chicago present an update on the management of children with neurogenic bladder as well as an update on recent advances

Pediatr Clin N Am 59 (2012) xv–xvi
http://dx.doi.org/10.1016/j.pcl.2012.06.001
0031-3955/12/$ – see front matter © 2012 Elsevier Inc. All rights reserved.

in this area. Israel Franco from New York updates us on the pathophysiology of voiding dysfunction, coupled with an interesting commentary by Dr Bagli from Toronto.

Urolithiasis in children is on the rise and Dr Copelovitch from Philadelphia wrote a state-of-the-art article on the medical approach to children with urolithiasis, while Baker et al delineated the surgical approaches to children with stones, hence improving on the pediatrician's knowledge to counsel and tailor treatment options for those children. Dr Ritchey et al from Phoenix provided a review of common and uncommon pediatric urogenital tumors with the current treatment options, while Dr Lorenzo from Toronto added insights into future surgical options that minimize morbidity while maintaining and even enhancing excellent survival.

Finally, a topic of intense controversy and uncertainty is the intersex topic, which was covered by an endocrinologist and a pediatric urologist from Toronto. Romao et al touched on all the necessary information that pediatricians may need to know to adequately manage a patient with ambiguous genitalia with a thorough literature review of advances in the field, while Dr Sandberg from Michigan shed further light on the behavioral issues that surround patients with intersex.

Although pediatric urologists currently spend more time in the office treating nonsurgical conditions such as enuresis, voiding dysfunction, reflux, and prenatally diagnosed hydronephrosis, there have been major leaps in surgical techniques. The incorporation of new technologies, such laparoscopic approaches and robotic surgery, has changed the landscape of this subspecialty, hence markedly improving morbidity while maintaining the excellent outcomes. Ost et al give an overview of all the surgical innovations and advanced technologies used in the field of pediatric urology such as minimally invasive and robotic surgery.

We sincerely thank all of the contributors for their hard work and hope that this issue will help generate interest in this wonderful subspecialty.

Pasquale Casale, MD
Division of Urology
Columbia University
Columbia University Medical Center
Morgan Stanley Children's Hospital
3959 Broadway, 11th Floor
New York, NY 10032, USA

Walid A. Farhat, MD, FRCSC
University of Toronto
Division of Urology
The Hospital for Sick Children
Toronto, Ontario, Canada M5G 1X8

E-mail addresses:
Pc2581@mail.cumc.columbia.edu (P. Casale)
walid.farhat@sickkids.ca (W.A. Farhat)

Prenatal Ultrasound and Urological Anomalies

Douglass B. Clayton, MD*, John W. Brock III, MD

KEYWORDS

- Ultrasonography • Congenital anomalies • Hydronephrosis
- Urinary bladder neck obstruction • Urethral obstruction

KEY POINTS

- Fetal ultrasound is a routine part of prenatal care in the United States despite limited evidence of clinical benefit.
- Prenatal ultrasound use is rising in North America and urologic anomalies are among the most commonly detected findings.
- Hydronephrosis is the most frequently identified fetal urologic abnormality but the severity and clinical implications of prenatal hydronephrosis can vary greatly. As the severity of hydronephrosis increases so does the risk for clinically significant urinary tract pathology.
- The majority of fetuses with a urologic anomaly can be managed expectantly and only a small minority of fetuses will require urgent attention.
- Fetuses with suspected lower urinary tract obstruction comprise the group that may need urgent pediatric urology consultation and may even require fetal intervention.

INTRODUCTION

The performance of ultrasonography during pregnancy in the United States has become commonplace in the obstetric care of women. In reality, the practice of prenatal ultrasound exists largely outside the control of pediatricians or pediatric urologists. Despite the embracement of prenatal screening for organ system anomalies as routine by the medical community as a whole, the long-term clinical impact of identifying congenital anomalies prenatally remains undefined for many diagnoses. For some anomalies, inconsistent correlation between prenatal ultrasound appearance and postnatal clinical outcome leads to uncertainty in the aggressiveness with which postnatal evaluation should be pursued. By contrast, select anomalies may benefit from prenatal

Disclosures: Neither author has any financial or commercial relationships to disclose.
Division of Pediatric Urology, Vanderbilt University, 4102 Doctor's Office Tower, 2200 Children's Way, Nashville, TN 37232, USA
* Corresponding author.
E-mail address: douglass.b.clayton@vanderbilt.edu

Pediatr Clin N Am 59 (2012) 739–756
doi:10.1016/j.pcl.2012.05.003
0031-3955/12/$ – see front matter

diagnosis by allowing for prompt and immediate tertiary care after birth or by providing the opportunity for fetal intervention before delivery.

For practicing pediatricians, a common clinical scenario likely exists. A newborn with a prenatally diagnosed urologic finding is now under the care of a pediatrician in the newborn nursery. Several questions likely come to mind. How much information was obtained about this anomaly before delivery? Should more or less information have been acquired before birth? Did the parents receive counseling from a pediatric urologist during gestation? How should this anomaly classified? Is it mild or is it severe? What are the next steps in the care of the neonate?

The severity of congenital urologic anomalies can be highly variable. In some children, the correct diagnosis and subsequent course of action is clear from the start, yet in other patients, such decisions may be less obvious. This review hopes to provide a clear reference for pediatricians as they see newborn babies with prenatally diagnosed urologic issues in their practice. The complexities of the postnatal evaluation in neonates with a urologic anomaly, specifically PNH, are beyond the scope of this article and are not addressed.

ULTRASOUND USE IN NORTH AMERICA

Few medical technologies have had such rapid incorporation into the care of patients as has prenatal ultrasonography. Although some parents incorrectly view the early second-trimester ultrasound as an opportunity to diagnose fetal gender, its purpose is to screen for organ system anomalies. Prenatal ultrasound in obstetric care has its temporal roots in England, where, in the late 1950s, it was used for detecting abdominal masses in women.[1] In the early 1960s, investigators in Glasgow began measuring fetal cephalic growth in gravid women.[2] A 1970 report describing the prenatal diagnosis of polycystic kidneys was a seminal event in the prenatal identification of organ anomalies.[3] The mainstream incorporation of sonographic fetal anomaly screening in obstetrics occurred as a result of several clinical trials conducted over the past 30 years.[4–7] The ability to prove the clinical benefit of routine screening for organ anomalies remains elusive. A randomized trial from Europe compared prenatal ultrasound screening with expectant management and reported improved fetal survival after prenatal diagnosis of organ anomalies, but this survival improvement was highly influenced by pregnancy terminations that occurred after severe anomalies were detected.[5] To date, the only randomized trial in the United States evaluating routine ultrasound screening during pregnancy failed to conclusively demonstrate that the use of prenatal ultrasound and subsequent prenatal anomaly diagnosis has a positive impact on clinical outcome.[4] Furthermore, 2 separate meta-analyses were also unable to demonstrate that routine use of ultrasound in low-risk or unselected pregnant women leads to a reduction in adverse outcomes or provides clinical benefit.[8,9]

Routine prenatal ultrasound use is on the rise. From 1995 to 2006 in the United States, the mean number of prenatal sonograms performed per pregnancy reportedly increased from 1.5 to 2.7. By the year 2006, women with high-risk pregnancies underwent twice as many studies, having an average of 4.2 ultrasounds per pregnancy.[10] Similar US reports document an approximate doubling of prenatal ultrasounds performed over a 7-year period, from 1998 to 2005.[11] Likewise, in Canada, a 55% increase in prenatal ultrasound use was recognized between 1996 and 2006.[12]

SCREENING SENSITIVITY

The combination of routine prenatal ultrasound and improving ultrasound technology ensures that more organ anomalies are detected before birth. Perhaps the best available data regarding the frequency of organ system anomalies come from 2 separate large-scale ultrasound screening studies, the Eurofetus study and the EuroScan study, performed in obstetric centers throughout Europe in the 1990s.[13,14] In both studies, approximately 2% of all pregnancies were affected by a congenital anomaly. The frequency of detecting anomalies on prenatal ultrasound is heavily contingent on the organ system studied and the experience of the center performing the study.[15] In the Eurofetus study, a second-trimester screening ultrasound detected 61% of post-natally confirmed anomalies before birth, with 44% detected before 24 weeks.[13] By contrast, in the only randomized trial of prenatal ultrasound screening ever performed in the United States, the Routine Antenatal Diagnostic Imaging with Ultrasound trial, the sensitivity for detecting organ system anomalies before 24 weeks of gestation was only 16% and was 35% irrespective of gestational age.[4] The sensitivity for detecting urologic anomalies before birth seems universally high.[16] **Table 1** shows the relative distribution of anomalies by organ system identified at birth in the Eurofetus study.[17] Of the 954 urogenital anomalies detected in Eurofetus, 88.5% were identified prenatally. By contrast, heart and great vessel anomalies were identified only 27% of the time.[17]

NORMAL FETAL URINARY TRACT APPEARANCE

Reviewing the normal appearance of the fetal urinary tract is a prerequisite to discussing congenital anomalies of genitourinary system. **Fig. 1** depicts the normal ultrasound appearance of the fetal kidney and bladder on prenatal ultrasound. The healthy fetal kidney is typically not visualized on a transabdominal ultrasound until at least week 15 of gestation.[18] Fetal renal length varies during development (see **Fig. 1**).[19] The anterior posterior diameter (APD) of the fetal renal pelvis is a measurement that has been increasingly used to categorize fetal renal dilatation as normal or abnormal. Fetal renal APD measurements less than 4 mm in the second trimester and less than 7 mm in the third trimester are considered physiologic levels of fetal renal dilatation.[20] In the normal fetus, the ureters are not visible on prenatal ultrasound whereas normal ureteral diameter in neonates is reported to be 5 mm or less.[21] The fetal bladder is visible on transvaginal ultrasound in 87% of cases by 12 weeks of gestation and care should be taken to ensure the bladder is identified during the second-trimester screening ultrasound.[22] If the bladder is not visualized, repeat imaging later in the study or on a subsequent repeat ultrasound should confirm its presence or absence. Bladder enlargement, also termed megacystis may be noted on prenatal ultrasound and can suggest urinary tract obstruction. Measurements that define a normal fetal bladder size have not been concretely defined. From weeks 10 to 14, suggested normal parameters for bladder size include either a longitudinal

Table 1			
Most common congenital organ anomalies by system			
System	Total Number	Postnatal Frequency (%)	Prenatal Ultrasound Sensitivity (%)
Musculoskeletal anomalies	1043	23	36
Heart and great vessels	953	21	27
Urinary tract abnormalities	954	21	88
Central nervous system	738	16	88

Data from Grandjean H, Larroque D, Levi S. Sensitivity of routine ultrasound screening of pregnancies in the Eurofetus database. The Eurofetus Team. Ann N Y Acad Sci 1998;847:118–24.

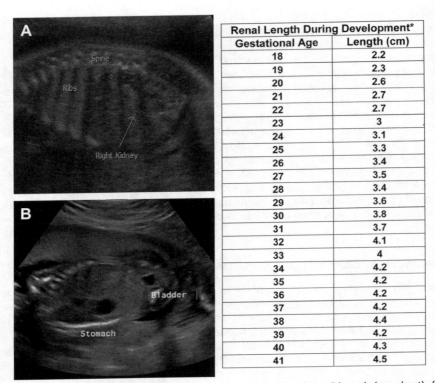

| Renal Length During Development* ||
Gestational Age	Length (cm)
18	2.2
19	2.3
20	2.6
21	2.7
22	2.7
23	3
24	3.1
25	3.3
26	3.4
27	3.5
28	3.4
29	3.6
30	3.8
31	3.7
32	4.1
33	4
34	4.2
35	4.2
36	4.2
37	4.2
38	4.4
39	4.2
40	4.3
41	4.5

Fig. 1. Normal fetal urinary tract appearance and normal fetal renal length (see chart). (*A*) Appearance of healthy right kidney on a 25-week ultrasound. Renal length measures 3.24 cm. (*B*) Appearance of the normal fetal bladder in a healthy 21-week male fetus. (*Data from* Cohen HL, Cooper J, Eisenberg P, et al. Normal length of fetal kidneys: sonographic study in 397 obstetric patients. AJR Am J Roentgenol 1991;157(3):545–8.)

bladder diameter of less than 6 mm or a diameter measuring less than 10% of crown-rump length.[23,24] Normal bladder size in the second and third trimesters remains undefined. A normal bladder in the second trimester has been characterized subjectively as one of small size that empties during a 45-minute time frame.[25] Amniotic fluid levels can be a surrogate marker for fetal urinary tract function. Although fetal urine production begins by 8 to 10 weeks of gestation, it is only beyond 16 weeks of development that the amniotic fluid is primarily composed of fetal urine.[18,26] Thus, abnormalities in the amniotic fluid levels in the second and third trimesters may be harbingers of urinary tract problems.

PRENATAL UROLOGIC ANOMALIES

A variety of urologic diagnoses may be detected before birth. The certainty of prenatal suspicion, however, can only be confirmed with accurate postnatal evaluation and diagnosis. A follow-up report from the EuroScan study detailed the diagnoses in 1130 patients with urologic anomalies diagnosed from a population of 709,030 births.[27] **Table 2** lists the most common diagnoses in the 609 patients with isolated urologic anomalies and the percentage of each diagnosis that were detected prenatally.[27]

Table 2
Most common congenital urologic anomalies (n = 609)

Anomaly	Percentage of Total	Percentage Detected Prenatally
All anomalies (n = 609)	—	82
Hydronephrosis	51	84
Multicystic dysplastic kidney	17	97
Unilateral renal agenesis	10	62
Duplicated kidney	6	95
Renal ectopia	4	56
Posterior urethral valves	4	70
Solitary renal cyst	4	76
Bladder exstrophy	3	53

Data from Wiesel A, Queisser-Luft A, Clementi M, et al. Prenatal detection of congenital renal malformations by fetal ultrasonographic examination: an analysis of 709,030 births in 12 European countries. Eur J Med Genet 2005;48(2):131–44.

The gestational age at which urologic anomalies are first identified is of variable importance. Almost universally, the presence of oligohydramnios in the second trimester is a poor prognostic sign for fetal survival.[28–31] Fetal megacystis may be seen as early as the first trimester, and spontaneous resolution is reported common in fetuses with longitudinal diameters less than 12 mm.[23] In the second and third trimesters, megacystis alone has little predictive value. Rather, the clinical picture of the fetus, from a urologic perspective, should be derived from the ultrasound appearance of the entire urinary tract and the amniotic fluid level, not simply the size of the bladder. The importance of timing in the initial identification of PNH (ie, second-trimester detection vs third-trimester detection) and its correlation with true urinary tract pathology is uncertain. With the majority of screening ultrasounds occurring during the second trimester, women with a normal second-trimester ultrasound are unlikely to undergo a repeat ultrasound in the third trimester. A few studies, however, have shown that PNH severity on a third trimester scan may be more predictive of clinical outcome than the appearance on a second-trimester study.[20,32]

This discussion of specific prenatal urologic diagnoses begins with hydronephrosis. The remainder of the review focuses on those diagnoses that can be managed expectantly and those that require more urgent attention in the fetal and neonatal period.

Hydronephrosis

PNH is the most commonly identified prenatal urinary tract abnormality. Unfortunately, hydronephrosis is not actually a diagnosis but rather a sign of some other underlying problem in the urinary tract. A recent meta-analysis of 17 studies identified 1678 fetuses with PNH of a total screened population of 104, 572 (1.6% prevalence of PNH). Of these 1678, 36% had identifiable urinary tract pathology on postnatal evaluation.[33] Several factors make the interpretation of PNH controversial, including the lack of diagnostic specificity, the variable methods for classifying its severity, and the inconsistent postnatal clinical outcomes with varying degrees of dilatation, particularly in children with mild or moderate PNH.

Hydronephrosis Grading

Accurately classifying the degree of upper urinary tract dilatation in the fetus and neonate can be difficult. Ideally, PNH would be graded using one objective scale that could then accurately predict the risk of true postnatal pathology. Fetuses would be stratified into prognosis groups accordingly, which help guide the postnatal evaluation of the fetus. Unfortunately, no one system to date conclusively allows for such determinations. In general, as the degree of PNH increases so does the risk for persistent postnatal pathology.[33]

As discussed previously, the APD of the renal pelvis is a commonly used method for defining PNH. For proper APD calculations, measurements should be obtained from a transverse axial image of the renal pelvis at approximately the level of the renal hilum.[20] Renal APD measurements can vary depending the gestational age of the fetus, and the thresholds for concern must change as well. An early report from George Washington University used renal APD threshold values of 4 mm before 33 weeks and 7 mm after 33 weeks to define hydronephrosis. The study found both of these gestational age–based APD thresholds nearly 100% sensitive for detecting PNH but poorly specific for predicting both the postnatal persistence of hydronephrosis and the need for postnatal surgery.[20] Repeat analysis of the data in a separate report identified APD measurements greater than 15 mm at any time during gestation as a crucial indicator of severe PNH and correlated with a real risk for postnatal obstructive pathology.[34] The importance of 15 mm of APD has been affirmed by other series and is a measurement that can be used in practice to identify children with severe PNH that should certainly have prompt follow-up with a urologist soon after birth.[35,36] **Fig. 2** depicts the appropriate measurement of fetal renal APD and a subsequent classification scheme proposed in a recent consensus statement on PNH published by the Society for Fetal Urology (SFU). The classification system is based on renal APD measurements in the second and third trimesters.[36]

Both prenatally and postnatally, the severity of hydronephrosis is often characterized using subjective descriptors that include terms, such as *pelviectasis*, *caliectasis*, *pelvocaliectasis*, *mild hydronephrosis*, *moderate hydronephrosis*, and *severe hydronephrosis*. A more objective method for postnatal grading of hydronephrosis was published by the SFU in 1993.[37] The goal of the SFU 5-point classification scheme

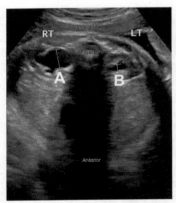

Degree	Second Trimester	Third Trimester
Mild	4 – <7 mm	7 – < 9 mm
Moderate	7 – <10 mm	9 - <15 mm
Severe	>10 mm	>15 mm

Fig. 2. Fetal renal APD and hydronephrosis grading. (*A*) Measurement of the renal APD in the transverse axial plane in a 38-week fetus with bilateral hydronephrosis. Measurement (*A*) in the right kidney demonstrates a renal APD of 15 mm and measurement (*B*) in the left kidney is 9.4 mm. The table represents a classification scheme for grading hydronephrosis. (*Data from* Nguyen HT, Herndon CD, Cooper C, et al. The Society for Fetal Urology consensus statement on the evaluation and management of antenatal hydronephrosis. J Pediatr Urol 2010;6(3):212–31.)

aimed at removing the subjectivity of these commonly used descriptors by replacing them with more concrete definitions. **Fig. 3** depicts the 5-point grading scale and associated images for each classification. When defining hydronephrosis, measurement of the renal pelvis APD is preferable during the fetal period, and the SFU grading scale is appropriate for evaluating postnatal images.

Etiology of Hydronephrosis

The problem with identifying PNH is subsequently determining which patients harbor a substantial risk for true postnatal pathology versus patients with benign or transient hydronephrosis of fetal development that is likely to resolve. A positive correlation exists between increasing hydronephrosis grade and true postnatal pathology. Data from a meta-analysis found that the PNH defined as mild, moderate, or severe hydronephrosis (using trimester-based renal APD measurements for each classification) conferred a 12%, 45%, and 88% risk, respectively, for a subsequent diagnosis of true urinary tract pathology.[33] The most common causes of PNH are illustrated in **Table 3**.

EXPECTANT MANAGEMENT

Urologic anomalies detected prenatally do not always warrant serial evaluation in utero or immediate postnatal care by a urologist. Many fetuses can be managed expectantly with urologic consultation taking place in the first few weeks of life. Particularly in fetuses with moderate to severe PNH, it is reasonable to consider starting prophylactic antibiotics postnatally at least until a urologic consultation can be performed. Additionally, a renal ultrasound should be repeated after birth in any infant diagnosed with PNH. It is recommended the ultrasound be done at least 48 hours after birth to allow for resolution of neonatal dehydration, which can underestimate the degree of hydronephrosis present postnatally.[38]

Ureteropelvic Junction Obstruction

Among the possible pathologic causes of PNH, ureteropelvic junction (UPJ) obstruction is the most common. Most frequently, UPJ obstruction is caused by a narrowed segment of the ureter at the junction between the proximal ureter and the renal pelvis. The segment often has disordered peristalsis and impaired emptying.[39] Other causes of UPJ obstruction include mucosal folds, ureteral polyps, and compression of the ureter from blood vessels as they cross anteriorly over the UPJ. The diagnosis of UPJ obstruction is supported by an ultrasound appearance demonstrating dilatation of the renal pelvis and/or calyces with additional findings of a normal bladder and a lack of ipsilateral ureteral dilatation.[40] **Fig. 4** demonstrates the fetal appearance of hydronephrosis in a kidney ultimately requiring a pyeloplasty during infancy for UPJ obstruction. PNH caused by a UPJ obstruction is notably asymptomatic in newborn patients. Again, renal APD measurements greater than 15 mm are useful to classify PNH as severe. Although fetuses with isolated unilateral hydronephrosis are often monitored by maternal fetal medicine specialists with serial ultrasound in utero, the benefit of this approach is unproved. Fetuses suspected of having a unilateral UPJ obstruction do not require delivery in a tertiary care center presuming all other aspects of the pregnancy are normal and urologic consultation can be obtained within the first few weeks of life. Yet, rare cases of suspected bilateral UPJ obstruction may warrant delivery in a tertiary hospital. In general, few children with PNH suggesting a UPJ obstruction ultimately require surgical repair. Increasing grades of hydronephrosis (SFU grade 3 or grade 4) and increasing renal APD suggests a greater need for

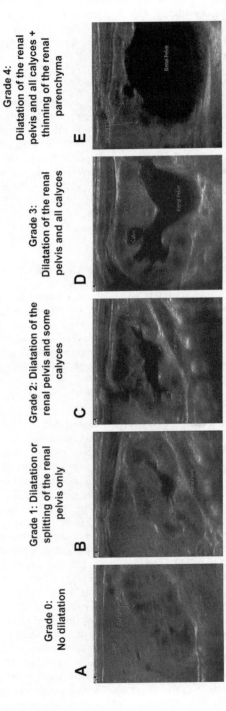

Grade 0:
No dilatation

Grade 1: Dilatation or splitting of the renal pelvis only

Grade 2: Dilatation of the renal pelvis and some calyces

Grade 3: Dilatation of the renal pelvis and all calyces

Grade 4: Dilatation of the renal pelvis and all calyces + thinning of the renal parenchyma

A   B   C   D   E

Fig. 3. (*A–E*) SFU hydronephrosis grading scale. (*Adapted from* Fernbach SK, Maizels M, Conway JJ. Ultrasound grading of hydronephrosis: introduction to the system used by the Society for Fetal Urology. Pediatr Radiol 1993;23(6):478–80; with permission.)

Table 3
Most common causes of prenatal hydronephrosis

Etiology	Percentage
Transient hydronephrosis of fetal development	41–88
Ureteropelvic junction obstruction	10–30
Vesicoureteral reflux	10–20
Ureterovesical junction obstruction	5–10
Duplex collecting system	5–7
Posterior urethral valves	4–6

Data from Nguyen HT, Herndon CD, Cooper C, et al. The Society for Fetal Urology consensus statement on the evaluation and management of antenatal hydronephrosis. J Pediatr Urol 2010;6(3):212–31.

postnatal surgery.[41] In a clinical trial of neonates with PNH demonstrating an APD greater than 15 mm, randomization to either surgery or conservative follow-up revealed that less than 20% of patients followed conservatively required surgical intervention for obstruction.[42]

Vesicoureteral Reflux

Vesicoureteral reflux (VUR) is a common cause of PNH, but definitively diagnosing VUR prenatally is not possible using ultrasound prenatally or postnatally. In the general pediatric population, it is thought that 1% of patients have VUR.[43] Evaluating for all possible causes of PNH requires a postnatal voiding cystourethrogram (VCUG) because the presence of a normal postnatal ultrasound does not eliminate the possibility of VUR. Between 15% and 40% of children with PNH and a subsequently normal postnatal ultrasound may still harbor VUR.[44–46] Furthermore, guidelines for the

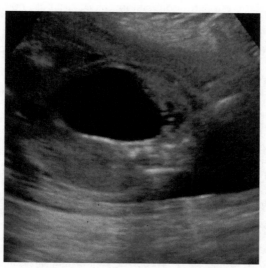

Fig. 4. PNH. Appearance of unilateral left hydronephrosis in a 25-week-old male infant with a right UPJ obstruction. Renal APD measurement was 19 mm. The patient underwent pyeloplasty at 4 months of age.

management of VUR published by the American Urological Association demonstrate that the incidence of VUR in patients with PNH does not differ based on the appearance of the postnatal renal ultrasound. These guidelines demonstrate that the grade of VUR in patients evaluated with a VCUG for PNH either grade 1 or grade 2 in one third, grade 3 in on thrid, and grade 4 or grade 5 in one third.[47]

Multicystic Dysplastic Kidney

As seen in **Table 3**, ultrasound is highly sensitive for detecting multicystic dysplastic kidney (MCDK) before birth. Fetuses with an MCDK may be incorrectly thought to have PNH. Characteristics that define an MCDK and differentiate it from PNH include (1) an ultrasound demonstrating multiple cystic lesions of variable size that do not communicate, (2) the absence of intervening functioning parenchyma between the cysts, and (3) a postnatal nuclear medicine renogram demonstrating a lack of cortical function. Two theories exist to explain the development of MCDK. One theory suggests MCDK form as a result of severe obstruction in the urinary tract early in gestation.[48] Such obstruction may include a UPJ obstruction or obstruction of the ureter as it enters the bladder (ie, ureterovesical junction obstruction). A second theory proposes disordered urinary tract development at the level of the ureteric bud.[49] In any case, it is important to distinguish MCDK from hydronephrosis. Postnatally, the diagnosis must be confirmed using repeat ultrasound with or without a nuclear medicine renal scan. The lack of renal uptake of radiotracer on a renal scan using dimercaptosuccinic acid (DMSA) or technetium 99m mercaptoacetyltriglycine (^{99m}Tc-MAG3) supports the diagnosis. **Fig. 5** demonstrates the prenatal and postnatal ultrasound appearance of an MCDK and a renogram demonstrating the absence of functional renal tissue on the side of the MCDK. The initiation of prophylactic antibiotics is generally recommended for newborns with prenatally diagnosed MCDK, at least until a voiding cystourethrogram has been performed, due to the association of MCDK with contralateral UPJ obstruction and VUR into the solitary functioning renal unit. Yet, data have suggested the need to perform a VCUG is negligible if serial ultrasounds of the contralateral kidney remain normal.[50] No defined follow-up protocol exists for patients with MCDK. The current management of patients with MCDK consists of observation using serial ultrasound. The rate of involution of an MCDK, as documented using ultrasound, is reported to be at least 60% within 10 years.[51]

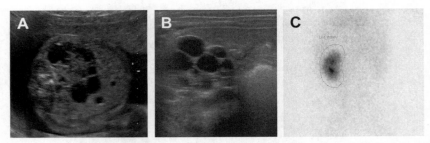

Fig. 5. Prenatal and postnatal imaging of MCDK. (*A*) Appearance of a left MCDK as seen on prenatal ultrasound at 22 weeks' gestation. (*B, C*) Postnatal imaging of an infant with MCDK. (*B*) Postnatal imaging of a right MCDK with multiple cysts that fail to communicate with bright echogenic intervening parenchyma. (*C*) Nuclear medicine renal scan documenting a lack of function in the right kidney.

Megaureter

PNH may present in association with significant ureteral dilatation. The presence of severe ureteral dilatation, assuming the bladder is normal in appearance and other signs of LUTO are absent, suggests a diagnosis of megaureter. Abnormal postnatal ureteral size has been previously defined as a ureteral diameter greater than 7 mm.[21] Megaureters are broadly classified as obstructed, refluxing, obstructed, and refluxing or nonobstructed and nonrefluxing.[39] Megaureters that do not demonstrate VUR on voiding cystourethrogram postnatally are termed, *primary obstructive megaureters*. The cause of primary obstructive megaureter is thought to be disordered development of the distal ureter and its junction with the bladder, a so-called ureterovesical junction obstruction, which is similar to a UPJ obstruction. The need for postnatal surgical intervention in patients with prenatally diagnosed megaureter seems low. Several series demonstrate that 70% of patients with prenatally diagnosed primary megaureter do not require surgical intervention.[52-54] Predictors of the need for surgery for primary megaureter include increasing ureteral diameter, increasing grades of ipsilateral hydronephrosis, and decreased ipsilateral renal function on a nuclear medicine renal scan.[52,54]

Ureterocele

A ureterocele is an abnormal cystic dilatation of the distal ureter that can cause obstruction of the kidney that is associated with it. The vast majority of ureteroceles are identified in association with a kidney that has a duplicated collecting system. Most commonly, the ureter subtending the upper pole of the duplication drains into the ureterocele. On prenatal ultrasound, a ureterocele is suspected when a cystic lesion is seen within the bladder, particularly when hydronephrosis is also visualized. Prior to the permeation of prenatal ultrasound, many infants with an undiagnosed ureterocele presented with febrile urinary tract infections, which led to the discovery of the ureterocele. In almost all cases, a child with a ureterocele diagnosed prenatally can be expectantly managed with urologic consultation taking place after birth. Rarely, a large ureterocele associated with renal collecting system duplication has been reported to cause in utero bladder outlet obstruction that mimics posterior urethral valves (PUV).[55]

Renal Agenesis

Renal agenesis may be bilateral or unilateral and is theorized to occur when the ureteric bud fails to interact appropriately with the metanephric blastema during the first month of fetal development.[56] Bilateral renal agenesis, reported to occur in 1 to 3 of every 10,000 live births, is incompatible with life because the absence of urine production leads to oligohyrdamnios and poor lung development.[11,57] Unilateral renal agenesis is more common, occurring in 1 of every 1000 live births.[58] Gestational development is not expected to be impaired by the congenital absence of one kidney. Beyond general counseling of the implications of having only one kidney, it is important to recognize potential additional urologic associations that are known to occur in patients with unilateral renal agenesis. In approximately half of patients with unilateral agenesis, contralateral kidney abnormalities exist, including VUR in 28% and UPJ obstruction in 7%.[59] Internal genital duct abnormalities may also be identified. Male anomalies affect wolffian duct structures, including ipsilateral abnormalities of the vas deferens, seminal vesicle, and epididymis.[58] Female genital abnormalities include uterine and vaginal duplication anomalies, vaginal agenesis, ovarian anomalies, and fallopian tube anomalies.[60,61]

URGENT MANAGEMENT

Although most fetuses with urologic anomalies identified using ultrasound can be managed conservatively, a small population of patients requires more urgent care and evaluation. Specialty care required in these cases may begin in the fetal period or immediately after birth. Some conditions may require fetal intervention or early induction of delivery.

Lower Urinary Tract Obstruction

The fetus with findings suspicious for lower urinary tract obstruction (LUTO) should raise concerns and should be followed closely during gestation because the child's condition may necessitate specialty care that includes serial ultrasound during gestation, immediate tertiary care after birth, or in utero intervention to relieve obstruction. **Box 1** lists factors that suggest the possibility of LUTO. Almost invariably, male fetuses are affected by in utero LUTO. The 3 most common diagnoses causing LUTO are PUV, urethral atresia, and prune-belly syndrome (PBS) (also known as Eagle-Barrett syndrome).[62] **Table 4** shows the relative distribution of these diagnoses in causing LUTO in a comprehensive meta-analysis of fetal LUTO series. Distinguishing between these diagnoses before birth can be challenging using ultrasound because significant overlap may occur in the clinical presentation of each entity. It is clear that although ultrasonography provides good sensitivity in detecting LUTO, its specificity is low. In one study, the sensitivity and specificity of distinguishing PUV prenatally were 94% and 43%, respectively.[63]

In general, the ultrasound findings most suggestive of fetal LUTO include male gender, hydronephrosis (either unilateral or bilateral), enlargement of the fetal bladder (megacystis), dilated posterior urethra (keyhole sign), and oligohydramnios.[64] **Fig. 6** depicts the appearance of several of these findings. Among these commonly detected ultrasonographic parameters, oligohydramnios has proved the most predictive of both postnatal survival and postnatal renal function.[30,65,66] When signs of obstruction are present in the setting of decreasing amniotic fluid volumes or frank oligohydramnios, referral to a maternal fetal medicine specialist and a pediatric urologist is warranted. In utero intervention in select fetuses is aimed at decompressing the fetal bladder and improving amniotic fluid levels to allow for sufficient pulmonary development. Various methods for decompressing the bladder exist but the most common method is the placement of a vesicoamniotic shunt, which diverts urine from the fetal

---

Box 1
Factors suggestive of LUTO on prenatal ultrasound

- Male fetus
- Hydronephrosis (either unilateral or bilateral)
- Ureteral dilatation
- Enlargement of the bladder
- Bladder wall thickening
- Dilated posterior urethra (keyhole sign)
- Second trimester
- Oligohydramnios
- Previously normal amniotic fluid now decreasing

Table 4
Postnatal diagnoses in patients with suspected fetal LUTO

Diagnosis	Percentage
Posterior urethral valves	43
Urethral atresia	14
Prune belly syndrome	8
Diagnosis unknown or not obstructive	35

Data from Morris RK, Malin GL, Khan KS, et al. Systematic review of the effectiveness of antenatal intervention for the treatment of congenital lower urinary tract obstruction. BJOG 2010;117(4):382–90.

bladder to the amniotic space.[67] Infants with LUTO that survive the fetal period, irrespective of fetal intervention, remain at high risk for compromised renal function.[38] In a systematic review and meta-analysis, fetal intervention for LUTO improved perinatal survival in select fetuses with LUTO but did not demonstrate an ability to improve renal function among postnatal survivors.[51] The common causes of fetal LUTO are described later.

Posterior Urethral Valves

PUV occurs in 1 of every 8000 live male births and is the most common cause of prenatal LUTO.[68] LUTO in boys with PUV is a consequence of a congenital obstructing membrane in the posterior urethra causing complete or partial bladder outlet obstruction.[69]

Progressive obstruction during gestational development can cause megacystis, bladder wall fibrosis, unilateral or bilateral hydronephrosis, renal dysplasia, and pulmonary insufficiency. PUV continues to be a common cause of end-stage renal disease in the pediatric population with the lifetime risk estimated at approximately 30%.[70]

Urethral Atresia

Urethral atresia, although rare in general, is the second most common cause of LUTO in the fetus with oligohydramnios. The exact incidence of UA is difficult to define, likely due to the nearly universal lethal nature of the diagnosis, without some manner of decompressing the bladder either by in utero procedure or the presence of a patent urachus.[71]

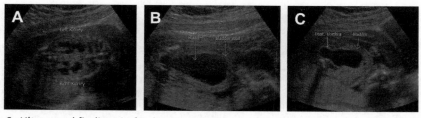

Fig. 6. Ultrasound findings in fetal LUTO. Select prenatal images from a 20-week male fetus with postnatally confirmed PUV. (*A*) Bilateral hydronephrosis. (*B*) Enlarged bladder (megacystis) with bladder wall thickening. (*C*) Dilated posterior urethra (keyhole sign).

Prune-Belly Syndrome

PBS is a triad of urologic findings characterized by deficiency or absence of abdominal wall musculature (causing a prune-like abdominal appearance), urinary tract dilatation of varying severity, and intra-abdominal testicles. The incidence of PBS is estimated at 3.8 per 100,000 live male births.[72] The presence of LUTO is more variable in patients with PBS in comparison with PUV and urethral atresia; thus, the role of fetal intervention for these patients is less defined.[73] Obstruction, when present, is theorized to occur as a result of hypoplasia and redundancy within the prostatic urethra that impairs emptying during voiding.[74] Additionally, urethral atresia has been reported in association with PBS.[75] Irrespective of the presence or absence of LUTO, fetuses with PBS are at high risk for prematurity, fetal death, perinatal mortality, and renal failure.[76]

SEVERE BLADDER ANOMALIES

Severe bladder anomalies include bladder exstrophy and cloacal exstrophy. Both of these rare conditions can be diagnosed prenatally. Bladder exstrophy affects approximately 1 in 50,000 live births whereas cloacal exstrophy is seen in 1 in 200,000 live births.[77] Bladder exstrophy is characterized by malformation of the anterior abdominal wall musculature and bony aspects of the pelvis that result in an anteriorly exposed flat bladder plate, pubic symphysis diastasis, and deficiency of the rectus fascia. Additionally, the external genitalia are malformed. In cloacal exstrophy, the bladder is separated into halves with the hindgut found in-between. A segment of ileum is most often seen in the midportion of this plate.[77] Despite the severe nature of these anomalies, it is estimated that only 10% of patients with bladder or cloacal exstrophy are ultimately diagnosed in utero[78] Select ultrasound criteria have been proposed to aid in the diagnosis of both bladder and cloacal exstrophy.[79,80] The early identification of fetuses with bladder or cloacal exstrophy can have an impact on the initial care of infants. In general, fetuses suspected of having cloacal or bladder exstrophy should be delivered in a tertiary care center to allow for appropriate neonatal intensive care as well as surgical consultation. At the least, these infants require aggressive critical care and resuscitation and many need surgery in the neonatal period.

SUMMARY

Screening ultrasounds are now an inseparable component of prenatal care in the United States. Because ultrasonography is so sensitive for identifying urologic anomalies, prenatal diagnosis of a variety of urologic conditions can be expected to continue. The vast majority of fetuses with urologic anomalies can be managed expectantly. It is important to recognize those findings that suggest a need for urgent care either in utero or immediately after delivery.

REFERENCES

1. Donald I, Macvicar J, Brown TG. Investigation of abdominal masses by pulsed ultrasound. Lancet 1958;1(7032):1188–95.
2. Willocks J. The use of ultrasonic cephalometry. Proc R Soc Med 1962;55:640.
3. Garrett WJ, Grunwald G, Robinson DE. Prenatal diagnosis of fetal polycystic kidney by ultrasound. Aust N Z J Obstet Gynaecol 1970;10(1):7–9.
4. Ewigman BG, Crane JP, Frigoletto FD, et al. Effect of prenatal ultrasound screening on perinatal outcome. RADIUS Study Group. N Engl J Med 1993; 329(12):821–7.

5. Saari-Kemppainen A, Karjalainen O, Ylostalo P, et al. Ultrasound screening and perinatal mortality: controlled trial of systematic one-stage screening in pregnancy. The Helsinki Ultrasound Trial. Lancet 1990;336(8712):387–91.
6. Eik-Nes SH, Salvesen KA, Okland O, et al. Routine ultrasound fetal examination in pregnancy: the 'Alesund' randomized controlled trial. Ultrasound Obstet Gynecol 2000;15(6):473–8.
7. Crowther CA, Kornman L, O'Callaghan S, et al. Is an ultrasound assessment of gestational age at the first antenatal visit of value? A randomised clinical trial. Br J Obstet Gynaecol 1999;106(12):1273–9.
8. Bricker L, Neilson JP, Dowswell T. Routine ultrasound in late pregnancy (after 24 weeks' gestation). Cochrane Database Syst Rev 2008;4:CD001451.
9. Whitworth M, Bricker L, Neilson JP, et al. Ultrasound for fetal assessment in early pregnancy. Cochrane Database Syst Rev 2010;4:CD007058.
10. Siddique J, Lauderdale DS, VanderWeele TJ, et al. Trends in prenatal ultrasound use in the United States: 1995 to 2006. Med Care 2009;47(11):1129–35.
11. Hsieh MH, Lai J, Saigal CS. Trends in prenatal sonography use and subsequent urologic diagnoses and abortions in the United States. J Pediatr Urol 2009;5(6):490–4.
12. You JJ, Alter DA, Stukel TA, et al. Proliferation of prenatal ultrasonography. CMAJ 2010;182(2):143–51.
13. Grandjean H, Larroque D, Levi S. The performance of routine ultrasonographic screening of pregnancies in the Eurofetus Study. Am J Obstet Gynecol 1999; 181(2):446–54.
14. Clementi M, Stoll C. The Euroscan study. Ultrasound Obstet Gynecol 2001;18(4): 297–300.
15. Levi S. Ultrasound in prenatal diagnosis: polemics around routine ultrasound screening for second trimester fetal malformations. Prenat Diagn 2002;22(4): 285–95.
16. Levi S. Mass screening for fetal malformations: the Eurofetus study. Ultrasound Obstet Gynecol 2003;22(6):555–8.
17. Grandjean H, Larroque D, Levi S. Sensitivity of routine ultrasound screening of pregnancies in the Eurofetus database. The Eurofetus Team. Ann N Y Acad Sci 1998;847:118–24.
18. Cohen HL, Kravets F, Zucconi W, et al. Congenital abnormalities of the genitourinary system. Semin Roentgenol 2004;39(2):282–303.
19. Cohen HL, Cooper J, Eisenberg P, et al. Normal length of fetal kidneys: sonographic study in 397 obstetric patients. AJR Am J Roentgenol 1991;157(3): 545–8.
20. Corteville JE, Gray DL, Crane JP. Congenital hydronephrosis: correlation of fetal ultrasonographic findings with infant outcome. Am J Obstet Gynecol 1991; 165(2):384–8.
21. Hellstrom M, Hjalmas K, Jacobsson B, et al. Normal ureteral diameter in infancy and childhood. Acta Radiol Diagn (Stockh) 1985;26(4):433–9.
22. Rosati P, Guariglia L. Transvaginal sonographic assessment of the fetal urinary tract in early pregnancy. Ultrasound Obstet Gynecol 1996;7(2):95–100.
23. Sebire NJ, Von Kaisenberg C, Rubio C, et al. Fetal megacystis at 10-14 weeks of gestation. Ultrasound Obstet Gynecol 1996;8(6):387–90.
24. McHugo J, Whittle M. Enlarged fetal bladders: aetiology, management and outcome. Prenat Diagn 2001;21(11):958–63.
25. Montemarano H, Bulas DI, Rushton HG, et al. Bladder distention and pyelectasis in the male fetus: causes, comparisons, and contrasts. J Ultrasound Med 1998; 17(12):743–9.

26. Yiee J, Wilcox D. Abnormalities of the fetal bladder. Semin Fetal Neonatal Med 2008;13(3):164–70.
27. Wiesel A, Queisser-Luft A, Clementi M, et al. Prenatal detection of congenital renal malformations by fetal ultrasonographic examination: an analysis of 709,030 births in 12 European countries. Eur J Med Genet 2005;48(2):131–44.
28. Barss VA, Benacerraf BR, Frigoletto FD Jr. Second trimester oligohydramnios, a predictor of poor fetal outcome. Obstet Gynecol 1984;64(5):608–10.
29. Hobbins JC, Romero R, Grannum P, et al. Antenatal diagnosis of renal anomalies with ultrasound. I. Obstructive uropathy. Am J Obstet Gynecol 1984;148(7): 868–77.
30. Reuss A, Wladimiroff JW, Stewart PA, et al. Non-invasive management of fetal obstructive uropathy. Lancet 1988;2(8617):949–51.
31. Robyr R, Benachi A, Daikha-Dahmane F, et al. Correlation between ultrasound and anatomical findings in fetuses with lower urinary tract obstruction in the first half of pregnancy. Ultrasound Obstet Gynecol 2005;25(5):478–82.
32. Thornburg LL, Pressman EK, Chelamkuri S, et al. Third trimester ultrasound of fetal pyelectasis: predictor for postnatal surgery. J Pediatr Urol 2008;4(1):51–4.
33. Lee RS, Cendron M, Kinnamon DD, et al. Antenatal hydronephrosis as a predictor of postnatal outcome: a meta-analysis. Pediatrics 2006;118(2):586–93.
34. Coplen DE, Austin PF, Yan Y, et al. The magnitude of fetal renal pelvic dilatation can identify obstructive postnatal hydronephrosis, and direct postnatal evaluation and management. J Urol 2006;176(2):724–7 [discussion: 727].
35. Wollenberg A, Neuhaus TJ, Willi UV, et al. Outcome of fetal renal pelvic dilatation diagnosed during the third trimester. Ultrasound Obstet Gynecol 2005;25(5):483–8.
36. Nguyen HT, Herndon CD, Cooper C, et al. The Society for Fetal Urology consensus statement on the evaluation and management of antenatal hydronephrosis. J Pediatr Urol 2010;6(3):212–31.
37. Fernbach SK, Maizels M, Conway JJ. Ultrasound grading of hydronephrosis: introduction to the system used by the Society for Fetal Urology. Pediatr Radiol 1993;23(6):478–80.
38. Wiener JS, O'Hara SM. Optimal timing of initial postnatal ultrasonography in newborns with prenatal hydronephrosis. J Urol 2002;168(4 Pt 2):1826–9 [discussion: 1829].
39. Carr MC, Casale P. Anomalies and surgery of the ureter in children, vol. 4. Philladelphia: Elsevier; 2011.
40. Roth JA, Diamond DA. Prenatal hydronephrosis. Curr Opin Pediatr 2001;13(2): 138–41.
41. Thomas DF. Prenatal diagnosis: what do we know of long-term outcomes? J Pediatr Urol 2010;6(3):204–11.
42. Dhillon HK. Prenatally diagnosed hydronephrosis: the Great Ormond Street experience. Br J Urol 1998;81(Suppl 2):39–44.
43. Arant BS Jr. Vesicoureteric reflux and renal injury. Am J Kidney Dis 1991;17(5): 491–511.
44. Gloor JM, Ramsey PS, Ogburn PL Jr, et al. The association of isolated mild fetal hydronephrosis with postnatal vesicoureteral reflux. J Matern Fetal Neonatal Med 2002;12(3):196–200.
45. Phan V, Traubici J, Hershenfield B, et al. Vesicoureteral reflux in infants with isolated antenatal hydronephrosis. Pediatr Nephrol 2003;18(12):1224–8.
46. Herndon CD, McKenna PH, Kolon TF, et al. A multicenter outcomes analysis of patients with neonatal reflux presenting with prenatal hydronephrosis. J Urol 1999;162(3 Pt 2):1203–8.

47. Skoog SJ, Peters CA, Arant BS Jr, et al. Pediatric vesicoureteral reflux guidelines panel summary report: clinical practice guidelines for screening siblings of children with vesicoureteral reflux and neonates/infants with prenatal hydronephrosis. J Urol 2010;184(3):1145–51.

48. Johnston JH, Evans JP, Glassberg KI, et al. Pelvic hydronephrosis in children: a review of 219 personal cases. J Urol 1977;117(1):97–101.

49. Mackie GG, Stephens FD. Duplex kidneys: a correlation of renal dysplasia with position of the ureteral orifice. J Urol 1975;114(2):274–80.

50. Ismaili K, Avni FE, Alexander M, et al. Routine voiding cystourethrography is of no value in neonates with unilateral multicystic dysplastic kidney. J Pediatr 2005; 146(6):759–63.

51. Aslam M, Watson AR. Unilateral multicystic dysplastic kidney: long term outcomes. Arch Dis Child 2006;91(10):820–3.

52. Chertin B, Pollack A, Koulikov D, et al. Long-term follow up of antenatally diagnosed megaureters. J Pediatr Urol 2008;4(3):188–91.

53. Shukla AR, Cooper J, Patel RP, et al. Prenatally detected primary megaureter: a role for extended followup. J Urol 2005;173(4):1353–6.

54. McLellan DL, Retik AB, Bauer SB, et al. Rate and predictors of spontaneous resolution of prenatally diagnosed primary nonrefluxing megaureter. J Urol 2002; 168(5):2177–80 [discussion: 2180].

55. Austin PF, Cain MP, Casale AJ, et al. Prenatal bladder outlet obstruction secondary to ureterocele. Urology 1998;52(6):1132–5.

56. Kerecuk L, Schreuder MF, Woolf AS. Renal tract malformations: perspectives for nephrologists. Nat Clin Pract Nephrol 2008;4(6):312–25.

57. Potter EL. Bilateral Absence of ureters and kidneys: a report of 50 cases. Obstet Gynecol 1965;25:3–12.

58. Shapiro E. Anomalies of the upper urinary tract, vol. 4. Philladelphia: Elsevier; 2012.

59. Cascio S, Paran S, Puri P. Associated urological anomalies in children with unilateral renal agenesis. J Urol 1999;162(3 Pt 2):1081–3.

60. Acien P, Acien M. Unilateral renal agenesis and female genital tract pathologies. Acta Obstet Gynecol Scand 2010;89(11):1424–31.

61. Pope JC. Renal dysgenesis and cystic disease of the kidney, vol. 4. Philladelphia: Elsevier; 2012.

62. Biard JM, Johnson MP, Carr MC, et al. Long-term outcomes in children treated by prenatal vesicoamniotic shunting for lower urinary tract obstruction. Obstet Gynecol 2005;106(3):503–8.

63. Bernardes LS, Aksnes G, Saada J, et al. Keyhole sign: how specific is it for the diagnosis of posterior urethral valves? Ultrasound Obstet Gynecol 2009;34(4):419–23.

64. Holmes N, Harrison MR, Baskin LS. Fetal surgery for posterior urethral valves: long-term postnatal outcomes. Pediatrics 2001;108(1):1–7.

65. Oliveira EA, Diniz JS, Cabral AC, et al. Prognostic factors in fetal hydronephrosis: a multivariate analysis. Pediatr Nephrol 1999;13(9):859–64.

66. Sarhan O, Zaccaria I, Macher MA, et al. Long-term outcome of prenatally detected posterior urethral valves: single center study of 65 cases managed by primary valve ablation. J Urol 2008;179(1):307–12 [discussion: 312–3].

67. Morris RK, Malin GL, Khan KS, et al. Systematic review of the effectiveness of antenatal intervention for the treatment of congenital lower urinary tract obstruction. BJOG 2010;117(4):382–90.

68. Hodges SJ, Patel B, McLorie G, et al. Posterior urethral valves. ScientificWorld-Journal 2009;9:1119–26.

69. Krishnan A, de Souza A, Konijeti R, et al. The anatomy and embryology of posterior urethral valves. J Urol 2006;175(4):1214–20.
70. Heikkila J, Holmberg C, Kyllonen L, et al. Long-term risk of end stage renal disease in patients with posterior urethral valves. J Urol 2011;186(6):2392–6.
71. Gonzalez R, De Filippo R, Jednak R, et al. Urethral atresia: long-term outcome in 6 children who survived the neonatal period. J Urol 2001;165(6 Pt 2):2241–4.
72. Routh JC, Huang L, Retik AB, et al. Contemporary epidemiology and characterization of newborn males with prune belly syndrome. Urology 2010;76(1):44–8.
73. Freedman AL, Bukowski TP, Smith CA, et al. Fetal therapy for obstructive uropathy: diagnosis specific outcomes [corrected]. J Urol 1996;156(2 Pt 2):720–4.
74. Caldamone A, Woodard J. Prune belly syndrome. In: Wein AJ, Kavoussi LR, Novick AC, et al, editors. Campbell-Walsh Urology, vol. 4. Philladelphia: Elsevier; 2012. p. 3310–24 [Chapter: 123].
75. Reinberg Y, Chelimsky G, Gonzalez R. Urethral atresia and the prune belly syndrome. Report of 6 cases. Br J Urol 1993;72(1):112–4.
76. Granberg CF, Harrison SM, Dajusta D, et al. Genetic Basis of Prune Belly Syndrome: screening for HNF1beta Gene. J Urol 2012;187(1):272–8.
77. Baker LA, Grady RW. Exstrophy and epispdias. London: Informa; 2007.
78. Jayachandran D, Bythell M, Platt MW, et al. Register based study of bladder exstrophy- epispadias complex: prevalence, associated anomalies, prenatal diagnosis and survival. J Urol 2011;186(5):2056–60.
79. Austin PF, Homsy YL, Gearhart JP, et al. The prenatal diagnosis of cloacal exstrophy. J Urol 1998;160(3 Pt 2):1179–81.
80. Gearhart JP, Ben-Chaim J, Jeffs RD, et al. Criteria for the prenatal diagnosis of classic bladder exstrophy. Obstet Gynecol 1995;85(6):961–4.

The Current Management of the Neurogenic Bladder in Children with Spina Bifida

Dominic Frimberger, MD[a],*, Earl Cheng, MD[b],
Bradley P. Kropp, MD[c]

KEYWORDS

- Neurogenic bladder • Spina bifida • Congenital defects • Spinal cord injury
- Bladder management • Life quality

KEY POINTS

- Before surgery is considered, conservative protocols have to be maximized because two-thirds of patients can become continent by clean intermittent catheterization and medication alone. Fecal continence and bowel management is an integral part of spina bifida treatment.
- Reconstructive lower tract surgery remains the best-studied, most successful, permanent, and long-term satisfactory surgery to deal with urinary and stool incontinence.
- The urological care of patients with spina bifida consists of 2 components: the medical management with preservation of renal function and the quality-of-life issues with achieving dryness and independence of bladder and bowel management. Both components are equally important for patients to live a healthy and fulfilled life.
- Continuous education and care of the families and patients are necessary to motivate them for participation in treatment plans and to avoid frustration and unrealistic expectations.
- Achieving continence is a long road that requires understanding and compliance that is best delivered by a team of specialists.

Neurogenic bladder is a complicated symptom complex that is part of many congenital and acquired disease processes. Common conditions in children include central nervous system diseases and spinal cord lesions as well as functional and structural obstructive uropathology. The neurogenic bladder does not only affect the continence status of patients but, more importantly, it also adversely affects the upper urinary tract potentially causing renal dysfunction. Because of the complexity of the illness and potential grave problems, long-term management is best performed by a specialist.

[a] Section of Pediatric Urology, Robotics, University of Oklahoma Health Sciences Center, 920 Stanton L. Young Boulevard WP3150, Oklahoma City, OK 73104, USA; [b] Children's Memorial Hospital, 2300 Children's Plaza Box 24, Chicago, IL 60614, USA; [c] Section of Pediatric Urology, University of Oklahoma Health Sciences Center, 920 Stanton L. Young Boulevard WP3150, Oklahoma City, OK 73104, USA
* Corresponding author.
E-mail address: Dominic-frimberger@ouhsc.edu

Pediatr Clin N Am 59 (2012) 757–767
doi:10.1016/j.pcl.2012.05.006
0031-3955/12/$ – see front matter © 2012 Elsevier Inc. All rights reserved.

However, because the patients are commonly first encountered in the primary care community, an initial management protocol for primary providers that addresses all patients is useful until the referral takes place. It can be difficult to determine the exact reason for the neurogenic bladder and a detailed patient history and a physical examination often paired with radiographic imaging is necessary. Patients with dysfunctional elimination syndrome rarely require extensive testing and can be, most of the time, separated from patients with neurogenic bladders by careful history and examination. It is very important not to coin every child with voiding issues as a patient with a neurogenic bladder to avoid overtesting and stigmatization. Once the suspicion of a neurogenic bladder is confirmed, video-urodynamic testing is the most accurate method to objectively evaluate the lower urinary tract.

Neurogenic bladder defects are generally classified according to neurologic defects or functional impairment. Neurologic defects can be described by the Loop theory of Bradley[1]; in 1974, he differentiated between 4 different loops of neuronal connection. According to his theory, the disruption of each loop causes specific forms of neurogenic bladder dysfunctions.[1] Other investigators based their classifications and observations on urodynamic findings.[2,3] Also, anatomic and neurologic descriptions help to understand the mechanism of the defect, the functional classification systems have more use for clinical decision making.[4] Especially in children, the most important question remains whether or not the bladder can empty spontaneously while maintaining safe pressures or if drainage has to be provided.

The causes and presentation of a neurogenic bladder in a child is different from adult forms. In most cases, the pediatric neurologic bladder is caused by congenital problems, and many investigators differentiate between a neurologic and a neuropathic bladder. A neurogenic bladder is one from a true neurologic deficit like spina bifida (SB), and a neuropathic bladder is one that acts like a neurogenic bladder but is not caused by an innervation problem. Examples of neuropathic bladders include those caused by a urinary obstruction, like in posterior urethral valves, or lack of bladder tissue, like bladder exstrophy. Acquired forms caused by trauma, infection, or behavioral issues are more comparable with adult clinical pictures. The timing of intervention is important because delay of treatment can cause irreversible damage, especially to the upper tracts. Many congenital defects are obvious, whereas others, like posterior urethral valves, might not be detected until problems occur. Prenatal ultrasounds (US), careful postnatal examination, and the education of primary care providers and parents all help in diagnosing problems early.

Myelodysplasia includes a variety of neural tube defects that differ in their severity depending on site and gravity of the defect. Myelomeningocele (SB) is likely the most common congenital diagnosis for the development of a neurogenic bladder in children. The level of the defect on the spine is strongly associated with survival and the development of cognitive and motor skills, with cervicothoracic levels performing significantly lower in comparison with lumbosacral defects.[5,6] In contrast to the general motor function, the bladder and bowel function do not have a direct correlation with the level of the lesion. Therefore, even patients with SB with the ability to walk often have poorly functioning bladder and bowels that prevents them from achieving spontaneous continence.

The prevalence of SB in Europe is declining because of prenatal management, but the numbers in the United States remain high, with an estimated 1 per 1000 births in 1993.[7] A newer study of 10 regions in the United States demonstrated a prevalence of SB in children aged 0 to 19 years to be 3.07 per 10,000 in 2002. The total number of cases of the same age group living the United States in 2002 was estimated at 24.860.[8] The aggressive promotion of folic acid supplements during all pregnancies, but especially in families with a history of SB, plays a big role in the decline in numbers of newborns with SB. Today, infant survival rates with SB have increased to 92% in 2001 up from 83% in 1983.[9,10] As a result of improved surgical treatments and early medical care, children with SB can expect longer lives today than in the past. This encouraging fact also means that primary care providers have to be more knowledgeable about the medical problems because these children not only grow in numbers but also transition into adulthood.

PRENATAL DIAGNOSIS AND FETAL SURGERY

Routine prenatal US examinations allow for earlier diagnosis of affected fetuses with SB conditions. Lately, Chaoui and colleagues[11] reported that they identified 5 cases of SB at 11 to 13 weeks' gestation by assessing the intracranial translucency and the posterior brain during routine US. A few months earlier, a different group found that at 11 to 13 weeks' gestation most fetuses with SB have measurable abnormalities in the posterior brain.[12] The early detection of SB fueled the desire for intrauterine repair to allow for regular development and improve the prognosis.

To prospectively evaluate the value of intrauterine surgery, a multicenter, randomized controlled trial was established by the National Institutes of Health and limited to 3 centers in the United States. The endpoints of this Management of Myelomeningocele Study (MOMS) included fetal and infant mortality, the need for a ventriculoperitoneal shunt at 1 year of age, and the evaluation of mental and motor development at 30 months of age.

The study began in 2003 and enrolled 183 women who were pregnant with a fetus with SB. In a randomized fashion, half of the affected individuals underwent fetal surgery, whereas the other half had standard postnatal closure of their defect. The results of the study were published in March 2011 in the *New England Journal of Medicine*. There were no maternal deaths and the rates of adverse neonatal outcomes were generally similar between the two groups. Two perinatal deaths occurred in each group. The rates for shunt placement were 40% in the prenatal-surgery group and 82% in the postnatal-surgery group. The prenatal surgery group had better motor function compared with the postnatal surgery group, and parent evaluation confirmed these findings. However, there was no significant differences in cognitive scores. Prenatal surgery was associated with an increased risk of preterm delivery and uterine dehiscence at delivery. The data and safety monitoring committee of the study met on December 7, 2010 and recommended termination of the trial because of the efficacy of prenatal surgery. Of great importance is that all 3 centers of the study have a multidisciplinary team of experts and followed a standard protocol to perform fetal surgery. The investigators caution: "The results of this trial should not be generalized to patients who undergo procedures at less experienced centers or who do not meet the eligibility criteria."[13] No comments were made concerning the effect of the prenatal surgery on the bladder development. Currently, a separate arm of the MOMS trial is looking at bladder function, and results should be available in the next 5 years.

INITIAL BLADDER MANAGEMENT: EXPECTANT VERSUS PROACTIVE

The spinal defect is usually closed in the first 24 hours of life and the bladder drained for that period. Concerning the bladder function, 2 general scenarios are observed. One group of patients with SB will have an overactive sphincter and develop high detrusor leak point pressures greater than 40 cm H_2O and are, therefore, at risk for upper tract damage. The other group will have little sphincter resistance with low detrusor leak point pressures, resulting in free urine flow into the diaper with little risk to the upper tract.

Depending on the policy of the treating institution, 2 different management options are followed. The expectant approach has a more observational and conservative stance, whereas the proactive approach aims to actively influence bladder development. Both options are considered safe for the development of renal function but differ in their perceived benefit for bladder development and later continence. Both approaches require a detailed physical examination, evaluating the presence of a palpable bladder or kidney. Also, a bladder and renal US is obtained to evaluate bladder filling and hydronephrosis. In the case of a negative physical examination and the absence of hydronephrosis, the expectant approach does not initiate clean intermittent catheterization (CIC), video urodynamic studies, or anticholinergic medication. Regular follow-up with examination, creatinine value, and US are initiated, and the parents educated toward the occurrence of urinary tract infections (UTI) and decreased urine output. If hydronephrosis is detected or clinical problems such as infection occur, then urodynamic studies are done to determine if initiation of CIC and pharmacotherapy is needed. The proponents of this approach argue that acting on symptoms is sufficient to protect renal function and it is not justified to have all parents perform CIC.[14,15]

The proactive protocol advocates for early urodynamic testing to identify high-risk patients. Patients with increased leak point pressures, detrusor sphincter dyssynergia, or noncompliant bladder muscles are placed on CIC every 3 to 4 hours during the day, and anticholinergic therapy with oxybutynin is initiated.[16] The rationale is to promote detrusor muscle relaxation and development by bladder cycling and ensure bladder drainage to protect the upper tracts and prevent hydronephrosis.[17–21] However, if the bladder environment is safe on urodynamics, some groups will stop CIC and move patients to the expectant protocol.[22,23] Other groups prefer to continue CIC to keep the child used to catheterization and to ensure proper development. Proponents defend their approach by the fact that most patients will need to perform CIC later to achieve continence and it is easier if the child remains used to the procedure.[24] Prophylactic antibiotics have not been proven to be useful in preventing infections, but no uniform treatment protocols exist.[25]

QUALITY OF LIFE

The initial management is centered on the primary goal of preserving renal function. As the child gets older, life quality and especially continence becomes more important. It is important for the caregiver to make the family understand that most interventions to achieve continence mean a higher level of involvement for everybody. Medical treatment has to be intensified and the child has to be much more involved. Surgical procedures will turn a previously incontinent bladder into a high-volume reservoir that will need to be catheterized. Basically, the family has to understand that surgeries can turn a current, safe incontinent bladder into a continent but very unsafe reservoir if not emptied regularly. Therefore, before initiating changes and continence procedures, patients have to have a high desire to become dry and are willing to accept a new regiment of protocols. Discussions should include the difference between complete and social continence. In the authors' practice, social continence is defined as being continent for several hours without leaking and being continent from stool. Minimal leakage during the day or night is accepted, whereas complete continence is defined as dry for 3 to 4 hours, including nighttime dryness.

Most families have heard about available medications and procedures. The authors inform patients and families in a detailed discussion what tests, surgeries, hospital stays, recovery, postoperative teaching, and changes in their daily protocol will occur.

These consultations can take hours and often require several visits until the family is ready for change. This time is well invested for both caretakers and patients to avoid misunderstandings, frustrations, and to ensure the best possible outcome. Exposing families to social groups like the Spina Bifida Association is equally important to allow discussion and the exchange of information with peers. Often local organizations exist, such as the Greater Oklahoma Disabled Sports Association (Godsa.org), a nonprofit organization that provides sports activities, such as wheelchair basketball. The authors' practice actively supports and promotes these groups and enrolls families into their programs.

Once the decision is made to initiate changes in the management protocol to achieve dryness, a new baseline is established, including video urodynamic testing, US for the urinary tract, and a kidneys, ureter and bladder x-ray for the bowel. CIC, anticholinergics, and bowel management are maximized and their results reevaluated. It is important to include the bowel in the continence program because constipation will adversely affect the bladder and also address the pressing problem of encopresis. Most patients and families will place the importance of continence from stool before urinary dryness. Urine leakage can usually be contained within a diaper and changed at an opportune time. Unlike urine, stool will smell immediately, causing anxiety, and might prevent families from leaving their home environment.[26]

The addition of specialized pediatric nurse practitioners who work with the families extensively is also helpful. This work includes not only explaining the medications and techniques but also providing individualized CIC sessions that address the specific dexterity needs of the child. Catheter type and size is tailored to the specific needs of patients, and bowel management is maximized with oral and rectal options. Regular follow-up in the clinic and on the telephone is provided. This individualized program is time intensive for families and providers, making them understand what it takes to become dry. Investing time and manpower at this stage will deal with anxiety and frustrations early. This investment will not only save time and money later but will also ensure better health and superior postoperative outcomes if surgery does become necessary. This conservative management will be successful in a large number of patients to achieve complete or at least social continence.[27] However, next to continence, independence from caregivers will play a big role as patients become older. Self-catheterization via the urethra can be difficult depending on body shape and genital anatomy. Applying enemas to one self-effectively is almost impossible even for the most mobile patients. The discussion about available surgeries is initiated at this time.

SURGICAL OPTIONS

Generally two-thirds of patients can get socially dry with CIC, whereas the remaining one-third will require surgery. Surgery is divided between well-established traditional surgical reconstruction and the more recent bladder function modulation with medication or neuromodulation.

MINIMAL INVASIVE TREATMENTS AND NEUROMODULATION
Botulinum Toxin

The intravesical injection of botulinum toxin (Botox) is a good temporary measure to enhance bladder capacity and decrease intravesical pressures.[28] Botox is injected into the detrusor muscle endoscopically using a cystoscope under anesthesia. It is performed as an outpatient procedure, is generally well tolerated, and the effects last for several months. Next to its positive effect on the bladder detrusor muscle, many patients report an improvement in bowel function and continence. However, the procedure is not approved by the Food and Drug Administration (FDA). Botox injection can be repeated safely, but because of its temporary effect, it is not a final measure and will require additional procedures later.[29] Neuromodulation therapy aims to treat the abnormal innervation of the bladder, trying to retrain the nerve-muscle interaction to attain more normal bladder function. The available treatments include nonsurgical therapies, such as transurethral electrical bladder stimulation; minimally invasive procedures, such as implantation of a sacral neuromodulation pacemaker device; and operative procedures that reconfigure sacral nerve root anatomy.[30]

Transurethral Electrical Bladder Stimulation

The results of transurethral electrical bladder stimulation have varied. The technique begins with detailed bladder capacity measurements followed by refilling the bladder via an electrocatheter. During the first 90-minute session, various electric parameters, such as intensity of current and frequency, can be adjusted to the individual patient. A series of treatment consists of twenty 90-minute sessions. Follow-up sessions are tailored to the individual patient. In general, bladder stimulation therapy will provide volitional voiding in less than 10% of patients but can be an effective form of treatment for up to 60% of patients. If present, the beneficial effects are generally permanent but the therapy is labor intensive and requires a dedicated family.[30] It is hoped that a better understanding of the mechanism of action will lead to more effective forms of bladder stimulation therapy in the future.

Sacral Neuromodulation

Sacral neuromodulation (InterStim, Medtronic, Minneapolis, MN, USA) is a reversible implantable device that is thought to improve bladder function either by consistent stimulation of the efferent fibers of the sacral nerve roots or by providing rhythmic contractions of the pelvic floor.[31] First, a temporary test system is placed and, if proven successful, replaced by a permanent device. The device consists of a pacemaker, placed in the area of the buttocks, and a neurostimulator lead that is tunneled under the skin to electrically stimulate the S3 nerve root. A prospective randomized study enrolled 42 patients with SB and compared urodynamic outcomes and incontinence. The implanted group demonstrated significantly improved leak point pressure; however, the control group developed significantly improved bladder capacity at 12 months. Some patients in the treatment group also reported improvement in bowel function and a new sensation of a full bladder.[32] Further studies will be necessary to evaluate the true advantage for patients with SB.

Xiao Procedure

Recently, another exciting neurosurgical technique has been developed in which a new neuronal loop is created. This technique was pioneered by Xiao and colleagues[33] in China and has gained international interest. This so-called Xiao procedure describes a limited laminectomy between L4 and S2 and the nerve roots are exposed. The L5 ventral root is identified by electrostimulation producing plantar flexion of the foot and transected at the orifice. The S3 ventral root is transected near the cord. The proximal stump of the ventral root of L5 is then anastomosed to the distal stump of the S3 ventral root. This procedure is performed unilaterally. The originators of this method first reported their successes in adults with spinal cord injuries, showing that via percutaneous electrical stimulation or scratching the skin in the L7 (in animals, humans do not have L7) dermatome, a detrusor contraction could be initiated.[33]

The follow-up data after 3 years showed that 10 of the 15 patients (67%) regained satisfactory bladder control and residual urine decreased from an average of 332 to 31 mL. Overflow incontinence and UTI were no longer clinical issues for these patients.[34] Hence, this same group decided to apply this neurosurgical technique to the SB population. The cohort consisted of 20 children (average age, 11 years); 17 (85%) attained increased bladder storage capacity and emptying functions, including the ability to sense fullness and to initiate bladder emptying with L5 dermatome stimulation, and they were dry 6 months after the procedure. The negative of this trial was that 5 of the 17 children who had success also had signs of partial loss of L5 motor function. In the 3 patients who had no improvement, 2 were noted to have significant scarring in the spinal canal caused by their previous surgeries and, therefore, had inadequate neural rootlet identification. These results are still promising, demonstrating that surgical alteration of the sacral innervation of patients with SB can have significant beneficial effects on bladder function.[35] In 2010, Peters and colleagues[36] published their 1-year results in the first United States trial on 9 patients. Most patients had an improvement in bowel function, but none achieved complete urinary continence. Two patients could stop CIC, and antimuscarinic medication was safely stopped in all. Temporary weakness of lower-extremity muscle groups occurred in 89%, 1 child had persistent foot drop. The investigators concluded that more patients with longer follow-up are needed before the procedure can be universally recommended. To the authors' knowledge, only 2 centers in the United States, 1 in Detroit and 1 in Tampa, are currently offering the procedure.

Reconstructive Bladder and Bowel Surgery

Traditional bladder reconstruction includes enlargement of the bladder with a piece of intestine to increase bladder capacity and lower intravesical pressures permanently. Access of the resulting reservoir can be accomplished either by the native urethra or by a newly created catheterizable channel connecting the bladder with the abdominal skin (cutaneous appendicovesicostomy/Mitrofanoff procedure). At the same time, a cutaneous stoma can be created that allows access to the cecum for the application of antegrade enemas (antegrade continent enema [ACE] procedure). If incontinence persists, additional surgeries might be necessary to achieve long-lasting success.[37]

Bladder Augmentation and Catheterizable Bladder Stoma

Bladder augmentation with a piece of reconfigured intestinal tract will transform a high-pressure low-capacity bladder into a low-pressure reservoir capable of holding 400 to 500 mL of urine. The surgery is a long but standardize procedure offered at most major pediatric urological institutions. Improvements in surgical technique and preoperative and postoperative management have made the procedure safer and reduced the complications. However, short- and long-term complications remain common and include infection, stone formation, intestinal obstruction, electrolyte imbalances, metabolic disturbances, bladder perforation, and possible tumor development.[38] Bladder augmentation will allow patients to store large amounts of urine but also makes it mandatory to empty the reservoir regularly. Because many patients with SB have difficulty accessing their native urethra for CIC, the simultaneous creation of a catheterizable channel is often performed. Several techniques are described depending on patient size and intestine availability. All techniques create a continent channel that connects the bladder with skin via a stoma that can be accessed by patients or caretakers in a sitting position without leaving the wheelchair.

ACE Procedure

This ACE procedure allows patients to empty the bowels on a daily basis via bowel irrigation, therefore, remaining stool continent.[39] Similar to the bladder stomas, a connection between the cecum and the skin is created via a continent channel. These stomas are placed in the umbilicus or lower abdominal wall in a cosmetically hidden position.[40] Patients or caretakers catheterize the cecum via the stoma and infuse normal saline while sitting on the toilet. The amount of fluid and time needed until the bowels are emptied are individually different and need to be tailored to the individual patient's needs.

The surgeries are traditionally accomplished via a long midline incision from below the sternum to the symphysis pubis. With the asset of laparoscopy and robotic assisted laparoscopy, much progress has been made to perform part or the complete surgery with minimal invasive techniques.[41,42]

Bladder Neck Procedures

The bladder neck can either be competent or have little resistance requiring a bladder neck procedure to avoid postoperative urine leakage. Bladder neck procedures either aim to tighten the bladder outlet by creating a muscular channel or by placing a sling to tighten and elevate the bladder neck region. Both procedures create a controlled obstruction to prevent urine flow under low pressures but still allow leakage of urine if the intravesical pressures are high because of excessive bladder filling. Because most patients do not have an adequate native bladder, providing them with a sufficient low-pressure reservoir simultaneous with bladder augmentation is often necessary. However, Snodgrass and colleagues[43] reported the possibility of performing a bladder neck procedure without augmentation. The group observed that in their patients, the bladder usually will eventually gain enough compliance to prevent unsafe intravesical pressures that could harm the upper tracts. As with all major congenital conditions, various management protocols exist and are defended by their proponents passionately. These controversies and educated discussions are highly desirable because they spark more research and advance the field.

Tissue Engineering

Research will continue with the ultimate goal to replace intestinal segments for bladder augmentation. Many groups, including the authors' institutions, pursue possibilities of tissue engineering for bladder regeneration. Bladder augmentation and replacement using laboratory-engineered tissue has been successful in animal models; however, no long-lasting successful human models have been reported. Active laboratory studies creating bladder tissue suitable for transplantation involve biodegradable scaffolds, stem cells, and nanotechnology.[44–47] Intensive collaboration between basic researches and physicians ensures that the balance between basic science and clinical application is assured. This bench-to-bedside approach will keep research focused on the goal to improve the health and long-term life quality of our patients.

TRANSITION OF PEDIATRIC PATIENTS INTO ADULTHOOD

The success in improving the health and life quality of patients with SB has resulted in a new set of problems for patients and their families as well as for the treating physicians. Reconstructive surgery and management protocols require regular and lifelong follow-up. In the past, most patients did not reach adulthood and had been taken care of by pediatric specialties. With improving patient care, patients with SB can expect a normal lifespan but continue to be taken care of by pediatric specialties. Often, tight relationships have been built over the years between the families and the physicians, and surgeons accustomed to the procedures and management have provided care. However, as the patients reach adulthood, transition into adult clinics is necessary. Therefore, models have to be created for pediatric and adult disciplines to work together to streamline care and guarantee high-quality follow-up.[48] Several centers instituted specialized clinics for adult patients cared for by an adult urologist. Exchanges concerning past procedure, new surgeries, management protocols, and research are granted by regular clinics and conferences. However, transition has to occur because adult urologist are more suited to deal with upcoming problems concerning sexuality, benign urological disease, or cancer.

SUMMARY

Much progress and alterations have been made to improve the management, outcome, recovery, and cosmetics of the traditional treatment and continence procedures for patients with SB. Before surgery is considered, conservative protocols have to be maximized because two-thirds of patients can become continent by CIC and medication alone. Fecal continence and bowel management is an integral part of SB treatment. Reconstructive surgery remains the best studied, most successful, permanent, and long-term satisfactory surgery to deal with urinary and stool incontinence. However, complications are common and the families and patients have to understand the need for lifelong management and observation of the created continent reservoir.

The urological care of patients with SB consists of 2 components: the medical management with preservation of renal function and the quality-of-life issues with achieving dryness and independence of bladder and bowel management. Both components are equally important for patients to live a healthy and fulfilled life. Continuous education and care of the families and patients are necessary to motivate them for participation in treatment plans and to avoid frustration and unrealistic expectations. Achieving continence is a long road that requires understanding and compliance best delivered by a team of specialists.

REFERENCES

1. Bradley WE, Timm GW, Scott FB. Innervation of the detrusor muscle and urethra. Urol Clin North Am 1974;1:3–27.
2. Lapides J. Neuromuscular vesical and urethral dysfunction. In: Campbell MF, Harrison JH, editors. Urology. Philadelphia: WB Saunders; 1970. p. 1343–79.
3. Blaivas JG. The neurophysiology of micturition: a clinical study of 550 patients. J Urol 1982;127(5):958–63.
4. Madersbacher H, Wyndaele JJ, Igawa Y, et al. Conservative management in neuropathic urinary incontinence. In: Abrams P, Khoury S, Wein A, editors. Incontinence. 2nd edition. Plymouth (United Kingdom): Health Publication Ltd; 2002. p. 697–754.
5. Lomax-Bream LE, Barnes M, Copeland K, et al. The impact of spina bifida on development across the first 3 years. Dev Neuropsychol 2007;31(1):1–20.
6. Amari F, Junkers W, Hartge D, et al. Prenatal course and outcome in 103 cases of fetal spina bifida: a single center experience. Acta Obstet Gynecol Scand 2010; 89:1276–83.
7. Selzman AA, Elder JS, Mapstone TB. Urologic consequences of myelodysplasia and other congenital abnormalities of the spinal cord. Urol Clin North Am 1993; 20:485–504.

8. Shin M, Besser LM, Siffel C, et al. Prevalence of spina bifida among children and adolescents in 10 regions in the United States. Pediatrics 2010;126:274–9.

9. Wong LY, Paulozzi LJ. Survival of infants with spina bifida: a population study 1979-1994. Paediatr Perinat Epidemiol 2001;15:374–8.

10. Bol KA, Collins JS, Kirby RS. Survival of infants with neural tube defects in the presence of folic acid fortification. Pediatrics 2006;117:803–13.

11. Chaoui R, Benoit B, Heling KS, et al. Prospective detection of open spina bifida at 11-13 weeks by assessing intracranial translucency and posterior brain. Ultrasound Obstet Gynecol 2011;38(6):722–6.

12. Lachmann R, Chaoui R, Moratalla J, et al. Posterior brain in fetuses with open spina bifida at 11 to 13 weeks. Prenat Diagn 2011;31:103–6.

13. Adzick NS, Thom EA, Spong CY, et al. A randomized trial of prenatal versus postnatal repair of myelomeningocele. N Engl J Med 2011;364:993–1004.

14. Hopps CV, Kropp KA. Preservation of renal function in children with myelomeningocele managed with basic newborn evaluation and close followup. J Urol 2003;169: 305–8.

15. Teichman JM, Scherz HC, Kim KD, et al. An alternative approach to myelodysplasia management: aggressive observation and prompt intervention. J Urol 1994; 152:807–11.

16. Dik P, Klijn AJ, van Gool JD, et al. Early start to therapy preserves kidney function in spina bifida patients. Eur Urol 2006;49:908–13.

17. Baskin LS, Kogan BA, Benard F. Treatment of infants with neurogenic bladder dysfunction using anticholinergic drugs and intermittent catheterization. Br J Urol 1990;66:532–4.

18. Kessler TM, Lackner J, Kiss G, et al. Early proactive management improves upper urinary tract function and reduces the need for surgery in patients with myelomeningocele. Neurourol Urodyn 2006;25:758–62.

19. Kasabian NG, Bauer SB, Dyro FM, et al. The prophylactic value of clean intermittent catheterization and anticholinergic medication in newborns and infants with myelodysplasia at risk of developing urinary tract deterioration. Am J Dis Child 1992;146:840–3.

20. Kaefer M, Pabby A, Kelly M, et al. Improved bladder function after prophylactic treatment of the high risk neurogenic bladder in newborns with myelomeningocele. J Urol 1999;162:1068–71.

21. Bauer SB, Hallett M, Khoshbin S, et al. Predictive value of urodynamic evaluation in newborns with myelodysplasia. JAMA 1984;252:650–2.

22. Sidi AA, Dykstra DD, Gonzalez R. The value of urodynamic testing in the management of neonates with myelodysplasia: a prospective study. J Urol 1986;135:90–3.

23. Snodgrass WT, Gargollo PC. Urologic care of the neurogenic bladder in children. Urol Clin North Am 2010;37:207–14.

24. van Gool JD, Dik P, de Jong TP. Bladder-sphincter dysfunction in myelomeningocele. Eur J Pediatr 2001;160:414–20.

25. Zegers BS, Winkler-Seinstra PL, Uiterwaal CS, et al. Urinary tract infections in children with spina bifida: an inventory of 41 European centers. Pediatr Nephrol 2009;24:783–8.

26. Ok JH, Kurzrock EA. Objective measurement of quality of life changes after ACE Malone using the FICQOL survey. J Pediatr Urol 2011;7:389–93.

27. Clayton DB, Brock JW 3rd, Joseph DB. Urologic management of spina bifida. Dev Disabil Res Rev 2010;16:88–95.

28. Kajbafzadeh AM, Moosavi S, Tajik P, et al. Intravesical injection of botulinum toxin type A: management of neuropathic bladder and bowel dysfunction in children with myelomeningocele. Urology 2006;68:1091–6 [discussion: 1096–7].

29. Gamé X, Khan S, Panicker JN, et al. Comparison of the impact on health-related quality of life of repeated detrusor injections of botulinum toxin in patients with idiopathic or neurogenic detrusor overactivity. BJU Int 2011;107:1786–92.

30. Lewis JM, Cheng EY. Non-traditional management of the neurogenic bladder: tissue engineering and neuromodulation. ScientificWorldJournal 2007;7:1230–41.

31. Das AK, White MD, Longhurst PA. Sacral nerve stimulation for the management of voiding dysfunction. Rev Urol 2007;2:43–60.

32. Storrs BB. Selective posterior rhizotomy for treatment of progressive spasticity in patients with myelomeningocele: preliminary report. Pediatr Neurosci 2007;13: 135–7.

33. Xiao CG, de Groat WC, Godec CJ, et al. "Skin-CNS-bladder" reflex pathway for micturition after spinal cord injury and its underlying mechanisms. J Urol 1999; 162:936–42.

34. Xiao CG, Du MX, Dai C, et al. An artificial somatic-central nervous system-autonomic reflex pathway for controllable micturition after spinal cord injury: preliminary results in 15 patients. J Urol 2003;170:1237–41.

35. Xiao CG, Du MX, Li B, et al. An artificial somatic-autonomic reflex pathway procedure for bladder control in children with spina bifida. J Urol 2007;173:2112–6.

36. Peters KM, Girdler B, Turzewski C, et al. Outcomes of lumbar to sacral nerve re-routing for spina bifida. J Urol 2010;184:702–7.

37. Roth CC, Donovan BO, Tonkin JB, et al. Endoscopic injection of submucosal bulking agents for the management of incontinent catheterizable channels. J Pediatr Urol 2009;5:265–8.

38. Frimberger D, Lakshmanan Y, Gearhart JP. Continent urinary diversions in the exstrophy complex: why do they fail? J Urol 2003;170:1338–42.

39. Malone PS, Ransley PG, Kiely EM. Preliminary report: the antegrade continence enema. Lancet 1990;17(336):1217–8.

40. Link BA, Kropp B, Frimberger D. Technical aspects of abdominal stomas. Urol Oncol 2007;25:154–9.

41. Nguyen HT, Passerotti CC, Penna FJ, et al. Robotic assisted laparoscopic Mitro-fanoff appendicovesicostomy: preliminary experience in a pediatric population. J Urol 2009;182:1528–34.

42. Gundeti MS, Acharya SS, Zagaja GP, et al. Paediatric robotic-assisted laparo-scopic augmentation ileocystoplasty and Mitrofanoff appendicovesicostomy (RA-LIMA): feasibility of and initial experience with the University of Chicago technique. BJU Int 2011;107:962–9.

43. Snodgrass W, Barber T. Comparison of bladder outlet procedures without augmen-tation in children with neurogenic incontinence. J Urol 2010;184:1775–80.

44. Roth CC, Mondalek FG, Kibar Y, et al. Bladder regeneration in a canine model using hyaluronic acid-poly(lactic-co-glycolic-acid) nanoparticle modified porcine small intestinal submucosa. BJU Int 2011;108:148–55.

45. Wu S, Wang Z, Bharadwaj S, et al. Implantation of autologous urine derived stem cells expressing vascular endothelial growth factor for potential use in genitouri-nary reconstruction. J Urol 2011;186:640–7.

46. Frimberger D, Morales N, Shamblott M, et al. Human embryoid body-derived stem cells in bladder regeneration using rodent model. Urology 2005;65:827–32.

47. Sharma AK, Bury MI, Fuller NJ, et al. Growth factor release from a chemically modified elastomeric poly(1,8-octanediol-co-citrate) thin film promotes angiogen-esis in vivo. J Biomed Mater Res A 2012;100(3):561–70.

48. Cox A, Breau L, Connor L, et al. Transition of care to an adult spina bifida clinic: patient perspectives and medical outcomes. J Urol 2011;186:1590–4.

Inguinal and Genital Anomalies

Laura Stansell Merriman, MD[a], Lindsey Herrel, MD[b],
Andrew J. Kirsch, MD[a],*

KEYWORDS

- Hernia • Hydrocele • Cryptorchidism • Varicocele • Penile anomalies

KEY POINTS

- Problems of the groin and genitalia are a common presenting complaint in both pediatrician's offices and emergency departments.
- The authors endeavor to provide a comprehensive review of the most common inguinal and genital anomalies encountered by the pediatrician, with a special focus on examination and management. The authors emphasize that the physical examination of the groin and genitalia should compose an important part of every well-child visit.

INTRODUCTION

Problems of the groin and genitalia are a common presenting complaint in both pediatrician's offices and emergency departments. The authors endeavor to provide a comprehensive review of the most common inguinal and genital anomalies encountered by the pediatrician, with a special focus on examination and management.

HERNIA/HYDROCELE

At the regular meeting of the Suffolk District Medical Society on December 26, 1900, Dr E. S. Boland[1] presented his experience in the treatment of infants with hernias. He devised a truss constructed from yarn intended to "assure the natural tendency toward cure in the infantile hernia." This woolen truss was "considered to be a very successful method" in a time when anesthetic risk was formidable.[1]

The evaluation and repair of the pediatric hernia has evolved as efficiencies in surgical technique and advances in pediatric anesthesia have occurred. From the management of infant hernias with yarn trusses to immediate operative repair, we do not often consider hernias with the same urgency as in a previous era.[2] However,

a Division of Pediatric Urology, Department of Urology, Emory University School of Medicine, Children's Healthcare of Atlanta, Atlanta, 5445 Meridian Mark Road, Suite 420, GA 30342, USA; b Department of Urology, Emory University School of Medicine, 1365 Clifton Road, Atlanta, GA 30322, USA
* Corresponding author.
E-mail address: akirschmd@aol.com

Pediatr Clin N Am 59 (2012) 769–781
doi:10.1016/j.pcl.2012.05.005
0031-3955/12/$ – see front matter © 2012 Elsevier Inc. All rights reserved.

it remains that hernias are one of the most common presenting complaints in the pediatrician's clinical practice that will necessitate surgical intervention.

Incidence

The incidence of hernias in the pediatric population ranges from 0.8% to 4.4%.[3] Hernias are more common in boys than girls by a factor of 5, with a predilection to the right side in 60%.[4,5] Approximately 10% to 15% may occur bilaterally, and this is more often observed in premature infants. Hernias are more common overall in premature infants, with an incidence of 2% in girls and up to 30% in boys.[6] It has been reported that the incidence of incarceration within 6 months of birth may approach 30% in premature infants, thus underscoring the necessity of immediate evaluation and planning for possible surgical intervention.

The occurrence of communicating hydrocele is difficult to separate from that of a hernia because they often coexist due to similar pathophysiology. Although simple, noncommunicating hydroceles may be seen in almost 80% of newborn boys, noncommunicating hydroceles are seen in at least 5% of male neonates per a study by Osifo and colleagues[7] when they observed hydroceles in boys presenting for neonatal circumcision.

Pathophysiology

The development of the inguinal canal is contingent on the codevelopment of the coelomic cavity and the descent of the gonad in the case of male gender. As the abdominal wall develops, extensions of each layer contribute to the anatomic structure of the inguinal canal and the spermatic cord.

As the gonad passes through the inguinal canal, a portion of the peritoneum evaginates and follows the path of the testis and gubernaculum. This continuous extension of peritoneum is known as the processus vaginalis. The processus vaginalis ultimately develops into the visceral and parietal layers of the tunica vaginalis. In the case of female gender, the gubernacular equivalent will become the ovarian and round ligaments. Should the processus vaginalis remain patent in girls, it then becomes known as the canal of Nuck. Patency of the processus vaginalis and subsequent formation of hernia or hydrocele has been associated with prematurity, low birth weight, connective tissue anomalies, cystic fibrosis, posterior urethral valves, and other syndromic disorders.[8]

Girls more rarely present with hernias, which is classically represented by the focal enlargement of the labia or groin. The ovary may compose part of the herniated contents. One percent of the time, the gonad will be found to be a testis, which occurs in boys with complete androgen resistance, formerly known as testicular feminization. In this rare disorder, a phenotypic girl, often during an evaluation for amenorrhea, will be found to have a normal XY male karyotype, bilateral intra-abdominal testes, and a foreshortened vagina.

The continuity of the processus vaginalis should obliterate above the level of the gonad, thus eliminating unrestricted access between the potential space within the groin and scrotum and the intraperitoneal contents. It has been reported that complete closure of the processus vaginalis on both sides was observed in only 18% of full-term infants; however, it must be noted that this was an autopsy study of only 19 stillborn infants.[9] A narrowly patent conduit will allow only fluid, thus creating a hydrocele, which is a fluid accumulation within the tunica vaginalis. A widely patent conduit may allow fluid, omentum, bowel, gonads, and so forth, thus creating a hernia.

Hernia

Most children with hernias will present with indirect hernias: the hernia sac traverses through the inguinal canal, lateral to the inferior epigastric vessels as a consequence of a patent processus vaginalis. The diagnosis of direct hernia, a weakness of the abdominal wall protruding through the floor of the inguinal canal, is rare in children.

Associations with the increased risk for a patent processus vaginalis include prematurity, male gender, and increased abdominal pressure as a result of ventriculoperitoneal shunting, peritoneal dialysis, or ascites. In a recent study, Chen and colleagues[10] noted a 13.3% incidence of inguinal hernia repair in 7379 patients with ventriculoperitoneal shunt compared with 4.1% in age-matched controls.

Hydrocele

Hydrocele may be reactive or nonreactive and communicating or noncommunicating. A communicating hydrocele reflects a patent processus vaginalis from the peritoneal cavity to the scrotum or labia. A noncommunicating hydrocele indicates successful postnatal obliteration of the proximal processus vaginalis. This condition is common in infants, and most are reabsorbed before 1 year of age; therefore, observation is clinically appropriate.

A reactive hydrocele, in contrast, is the result of the accumulation of fluid caused by trauma, infection, or other inflammatory conditions. A hydrocele of the spermatic cord results when the neck of the tunica vaginalis obliterates but the processus vaginalis remains patent. Abdominoscrotal hydrocele is the result of retrograde extension of the hydrocele sac into the abdomen. Abdominoscrotal hydroceles have been reported to obstruct the ureters or result in testicular dysmorphism.[11] In some cases, an abdominoscrotal hydrocele may preclude circumcision due to the substantial size.

Metachronous Hernia

The potential occurrence of metachronous hernia is a subject that continues to raise contention in the urologic literature. A review of 918 patients who had undergone contralateral exploration of an asymptomatic side noted a 57% rate of patency of the processus vaginalis.[12] When age is a consideration, infants aged less than 2 months had a 63% patency rate.[13]

However, it is also understood that postnatal obliteration of the processus vaginalis contributes to a decreased prevalence of patency with increasing age. Rowe and colleagues[13] found that the processus vaginalis will spontaneously close in 40% of children within a few months of birth and in 60% of children by 2 years of age. The incidence of a contralateral patent processus vaginalis must be reconciled with the true incidence rate of metachronous symptomatic hernia.

Although some might advocate for immediate surgery to prevent possible incarceration and the need for an operation in the future, others contest that exploration poses an unnecessary risk to the contralateral groin. Ron and colleagues[14] noted that 10 explorations would have to be performed to prevent 1 metachronous patent processus vaginalis. In a review of 904 unilateral hernia repairs, Given and colleagues[15] noted only a 5.6% incidence of contralateral hernia. This finding is supported by a review of the literature performed by Nataraja and colleagues[16] in which they found that the overall risk of a metachronous hernia seems to be 5.76%.

To avoid exploration of the contralateral side, surgeons have used ultrasonography, diagnostic laparoscopy, and insufflation of the abdomen. The Goldstein method exploits the access to the intraperitoneum at the time of ipsilateral hernia repair. Simple insufflation of the intraperitoneal space via the hernia sac allows visual confirmation of patency of the contralateral processus vaginalis.[17] Diagnostic laparoscopy has been hailed as highly accurate and sensitive. A recent meta-analysis noted a 99.4% sensitivity and 99.5% specificity[18]; however, it constitutes a necessary expense related to the surgical equipment. Some have found ultrasound to be useful in the evaluation of the opposite groin. Chen and colleagues[19] found ultrasound to be 97.9% accurate in assessing patency of the processus vaginalis when they used the criteria of a 4-mm widening of the internal ring. However, this practice is not commonly performed.

Clinical Evaluation

An adequate history is imperative to not only establish the diagnosis but to determine the acuity of presentation. Parents may report a bulge in the groin, scrotum, or labia. It may be waxing and waning in nature with crying or straining. The inability to reduce the contents in association with pain, nausea, or vomiting is a significant finding and may require prompt surgical attention. However, typical presentation is that of a boy with painless enlargement of the scrotum or groin.

Thorough physical examination is an essential component of accurate clinical assessment of a child with a hernia. It is important to examine the child in both standing and supine positions. Hernias may be reducible, irreducible, or strangulated. Spontaneous closure will not occur in grossly apparent hernias, which necessitates referral for surgical repair.

Adequate history and physical examination should supplant radiographic evaluation; however, ultrasound may be used in cases of clinical uncertainty. If there is suspicion of a torsion of gonadal structures, evaluation by a urologist or pediatric surgeon should be sought immediately.

Indications for Treatment

The consequences of delayed presentation are incarceration and strangulation. A single surgeon review of more than 6000 cases observed a 12% incidence of incarceration at a mean age of 1.5 years. The risk of incarceration is more pronounced in premature infants, thus requiring definitive surgical planning.[20] A study from Libya evaluated the impact of delayed surgical repair after the reduction of incarcerated inguinal hernias in a pediatric population when circumstances precluded immediate repair. Gahukamble and colleagues[21] reported a similar overall complication rate for those undergoing immediate (within 72 hours) and delayed (within 1 to 3 months) repair. However, the repeat incarceration rate was nearly 16% in those with delayed management. Fortunately, improvements in pediatric anesthesia have rendered operative mortality to nil even in the setting of emergency surgery.

Treatment

The aim of surgery is to obliterate the conduit between the peritoneal cavity and groin. Because the pathophysiology of hydrocele and hernia is similar in the infant and child, they are both generally approached from the groin rather than the scrotum or labia. Ligation of the processus vaginalis at the level of the internal inguinal ring will provide adequate repair in most cases.

Although clinically apparent hernias and many communicating hydroceles necessitate surgical intervention, simple hydroceles are only generally repaired if they have not resolved by 2 years of age or if they are associated with discomfort, secondary inflammation, or parental desire.

The literature reports a 1.2% to 3.8% recurrence rate, with more than half occurring within the first year of initial surgical repair.[4] Risk for recurrence is related to the setting of increased abdominal pressure and the presence of an incarcerated hernia, which may complicate the repair because of tissue edema. Grosfeld and colleagues[22] reported a 12% recurrence rate of hernias in children with ventriculoperitoneal shunts. The population of children with reasons for elevated intra-abdominal pressures, such as shunts, ascites, and peritoneal dialysis, require special attention in the postoperative course.

Recommendations

The ability to differentiate between operative and nonoperative interventions is imperative in the evaluation of the acute and subacute groin/scrotum. Motives for referral include grossly apparent hernia, the history or incident of incarceration of hernia contents, and those in whom diagnosis is in question. Risk of hernia is highest in boys, children who are premature, or in the setting of increased intra-abdominal pressure. Noncommunicating hydrocele will typically resolve before 1 year of age. Referral for hydrocele should occur in the instance of nonresolution after 1 year or in the circumstances of communicating hydrocele or inflammatory features.

CRYPTORCHIDISM

Cryptorchidism is the most common presenting anomaly of the male genitourinary tract. The potential risk of impaired fertility and malignancy is amplified with delayed presentation. The clinical evaluation of the testes is an essential part of the physical examination in boys from infancy to adolescence and should never be overlooked.

Incidence

Cryptorchidism occurs in approximately 3% of full-term boys and 25% to 30% of preterm boys.[23] This incidence decreases to 0.8% to 1.1% within the first year of life because of spontaneous testicular descent.[24,25] Thus, most will descend within the first year of life, with more than 70% reaching the scrotum within the first 3 months postnatally according to a retrospective review by Berkowitz and colleagues.[24] Approximately 1% will remain incompletely descended after the first year of life based on studies of military recruits and observational studies.[24,26] Unilateral undescended testis is 4 times more common than bilaterally undescended testes.

Not all clinical presentations of undescended testes are apparent at birth. There is a 1% to 2% incidence of retractile or ascending testes.[27] This finding highlights the rationale for a thorough physical examination even into adolescence. Vanishing testis may result from an ischemic event or intrauterine testicular torsion. In this circumstance, contralateral orchidopexy remains controversial. Surgical repair or observation is generally at the discretion of the consulting surgeon because no evidence for increased surgical risk to the solitary testis or increased incidence of testicular torsion has been presented.

Cryptorchidism may be associated with prematurity, low birth weight, and exposure to excess estrogen in utero. Ten percent of unilateral maldescent are thought to have a family history of cryptorchidism; however, it is likely that heritability is both polygenic and multifactorial.[28]

Pathophysiology

Androgens are required for the adequate development of the male phenotype, influenced by the SRY gene on the Y chromosome. Because androgens are paracrine hormones, the effects are local and independent of global physiology. The mechanism of testicular descent, which occurs at approximately 28 weeks' gestation, depends on the development and elongation of the gubernaculum. The exact mechanism of testicular descent continues to be debated; however, arrest of descent before traversing the internal ring of the inguinal canal is a rare occurrence, representing less than 10% of cryptorchidisms.

Clinical Evaluation

The evaluation of the testes and scrotum is a vital component of the well-child examination because the risk of a missed diagnosis is not inconsequential. The examination should be performed with anatomic landmarks in mind. The testis may be present intra-abdominally or anywhere along the inguinal canal or upper scrotum. The testis may also have an ectopic gubernacular attachment wherein it may be located in the perineum, femoral canal, subinguinal space, or lateral to the scrotum. The child should be examined in a standing and supine or sitting position. The use of warm water or liquid soap, a cross-legged position, and a warm room may help inhibit the cremasteric reflex and enable the examiner to locate the testis. The examiner should palpate along the inguinal canal while firmly occluding the canal from the possibility of testicular ascent. This can, in effect, trap the testis to aid in the clinical detection. A retractile testis can be positioned reasonably within the scrotum and will remain in place. An ascended testis is a previously descended testis that cannot be manipulated into the scrotum.

A calm distracted child is optimum; however, experience dictates that this will not always be the case. A rapid experienced examiner will be able to detect the position of the testis most of the time. Ultrasonography should not be used as a substitute for physical examination except in cases of ambiguous genitalia when evaluation for Müllerian structures is necessary. Ultrasound cannot distinguish a truly undescended testis from a retractile testis because this requires an astute examiner to palpate and reposition the testis and then assess positional stability or subsequent reascent.[29]

Indications for Treatment

Impaired spermatogenesis

The determination of the optimal timing of surgical repair has centered on the histologic evaluation of the undescended testis. Histopathologic studies observe a significant decrease in intratubular germ cell counts when orchiopexy is performed after 1 year of age.[30] Miliaris and colleagues[31] evaluated 824 boys with cryptorchid testes over a 10-year period. Most of the testes in a suprascrotal position were normal in size or had mild atrophy. Those that were in the intracanalicular, internal ring, or abdominal positions frequently presented with moderate or severe atrophy. The testicular biopsies that were performed noted markedly diminished germ cell counts in children aged older than 4 years. It may be considered most distressing that 80% of their cohort were aged older than 4 years. It has been shown that incompletely descended testes will have impaired spermatogenesis, perhaps caused by the inability to maintain optimum temperatures, alterations in Sertoli cells, and overall delay in maturation.[32,33]

Fertility

Observational studies have found that predicted fertility is approximately 88% if orchiopexy is performed before 2 years of age. However, this decreases to 14% if surgery is delayed until after puberty.[34] The clinical information regarding fertility is difficult to interpret in the literature because most studies are retrospective in nature with heterogeneous data. Certainly the semen parameters of a fertile and infertile man may overlap, thus confounding a direct concrete association between cryptorchidism and infertility. In a series of studies, Lee and colleagues[35] evaluated men with a history of unilateral or bilaterally undescended testes over a 20-year period. They found that 89.7% of the unilateral group and 65.0% of the bilateral group had successfully fathered children. The success rate of the unilateral group mirrored a cohort of age-matched controls. Those with the highest risk of infertility were patients with bilateral cryptorchidism, varicocele, increased age at orchiopexy, and a higher position of the testis in addition to related factors of infertility, such as occurrence of sexually transmitted diseases and prostatic issues.

Cortes and colleagues[36] evaluated 135 men who presented with cryptorchidism in childhood. Testicular biopsy was obtained in 42 bilaterally cryptorchid patients both at the time of orchiopexy and in adulthood. The rates of infertility in the formerly bilateral and unilateral cryptorchid patients were estimated to be 54% and 9%, respectively. The histologic examination confirmed that the mean total number of spermatogonia was less than 30% of the lowest normal value in those with bilateral cryptorchidism. Infertility was suspected in up to one-third of the cohort.

Malignancy

Orchiopexy before puberty has been noted to be protective with a decreased risk of malignancy. A meta-analysis by Walsh and colleagues[37] noted an odds ratio of 5.8 for the occurrence of testicular cancer in men who either underwent postpubertal orchiopexy or never underwent surgical correction.

The risk of malignancy increases with increasing age. In an evaluation of the current literature, Wood and Elder[38] found orchiopexy after 12 years of age or no orchiopexy at all is associated with a 2- to 6-fold likelihood of developing testicular cancer. Testes that remain undescended have a higher risk of malignant transformation into seminoma, whereas those that are surgically repaired are more likely to have nonseminomatous pathologic conditions.

Recommendations

A referral to a pediatric urologist should occur if physical examination is in debate or if a testis remains undescended or impalpable within 1 year of age. An examination should be performed at birth and at 6 months, with a referral to a pediatric urologist should the examination reveal undescended or impalpable testes. Serial examination is most appropriate in those with retractile testes, with a referral when the testis cannot be manipulated to a dependent area of the scrotum. Ultrasound is not generally necessary in the setting of an adequate clinical examination. Thereafter, a confirmatory examination of the testes should be a part of the well-child checkup until puberty.

VARICOCELE

A varicocele is an abnormal dilation of veins within the pampiniform plexus, more particularly the internal spermatic veins of the spermatic cord. Varicoceles contribute to infertility in adulthood; however, 85% of men with varicoceles are fertile.

Incidence

The overall prevalence of varicocele is 15%. This amount varies with age, however, and most are identified during or after the onset of puberty. **Table 1.** shows the incidence of varicocele by age group detailed by Akbay and colleagues.[39]

Patients with primary infertility have a 40% incidence of varicoceles,[40] whereas men with secondary infertility have a rate as high as 81%.[41,42]

Most varicoceles are identified on the left. However, several studies have demonstrated bilateral varicoceles in 7% to 17% of patients.

Table 1 Incidence of varicocele according to age	
Age (y)	Incidence (%)
2–6	0.79
7–10	0.96
11–14	7.8
15–19	14.1

Pathophysiology

Varicoceles arise when reflux is present within the veins of the pampiniform plexus. Incompetence of the valves within these veins allows dilation and increased hydrostatic pressure within the system. The anatomic differences between the left and right spermatic veins are thought to account for the greater incidence of left-sided varicoceles. Additionally, a nutcracker phenomenon has been described whereby the left renal vein is compressed between the superior mesenteric vein and the aorta causing increased pressure within the left spermatic vein.[43,44] Susceptibility to varicoceles has been identified in patients who have a first-degree relative with varicocele, those who are tall and thin, and those with intrinsic venous abnormalities.

The exact pathogenesis behind infertility and impaired spermatogenesis is controversial. Scrotal hyperthermia is postulated to affect both endocrine function of the testis and spermatogenesis. An increase in reactive oxygen species and oxidative stress has also been seen in testes with varicoceles.

Clinical Evaluation

Most adolescents with varicoceles are asymptomatic. Only a small percentage of patients present with pain, characterized by a dragging sensation or dull ache in the scrotum or testis. The diagnosis of a varicocele is made through physical examination. This examination should be performed in a warm room in both standing and supine positions. A varicocele is palpable as tortuosity and fullness of the venous portion of the spermatic cord or, in larger cases, a "bag-of-worms" sensation. Particular attention should be paid to the spermatic cord to confirm decompression of the varicocele when the patient changes from an upright to supine position. Important characteristics to note are the appearance of the overlying skin, grade of varicocele, Tanner stage, the volume of the testes, and testis consistency. The grading system for varicoceles is described in **Table 2**.

Testis volume should be gauged using an objective measuring device, such as ultrasound, calipers, or orchidometers. It is important to accurately and precisely measure the testis volume because testis hypotrophy is one indication for varicocele treatment.

Table 2 Clinical evaluation of varicocele	
Grade	Clinical Findings
Grade 0 (subclinical)	Not palpable on examination, visualized on ultrasound only
Grade 1	Palpable only with Valsalva maneuver
Grade 2	Palpable without Valsalva maneuver
Grade 3	Easily visible

Furthermore, when varicoceles are asymptomatic and observed, testis volume should be recorded over time because testis hypotrophy is an indication for intervention. Identifying testis hypotrophy can be a challenge because testis volume during puberty can vary widely and be asymmetric.

If the examination is equivocal, then scrotal ultrasound may aid in the diagnosis. Identification of a varicocele on ultrasound is suggested by the presence of retrograde flow within the spermatic vein and an enlarged spermatic vein. Both of these measurements should be assessed before and during the Valsalva maneuver. Ultrasonography can also be useful in monitoring testis volume and dimensions over time.

Indications for Treatment

Solid indications for varicocele treatment in adolescents are controversial. However, important factors that should trigger referral to a pediatric urologist should occur in the instance of asymmetric testicular growth or bilateral testis hypotrophy, impairment of spermatogenesis as seen on semen analysis, testicular pain, and the presence of a right-sided varicocele.

Approximately 9% of adolescents with a varicocele present with testis atrophy.[45] Patients who have a solitary testis or otherwise compromised testis function are of particular concern. These patients should be referred to a urologist once a varicocele is identified. Similarly, treatment should be considered if a 10% to 25% or 2- to 3-mL smaller testis is identified on the side with the varicocele.[46,47] Although semen analysis is an excellent tool in adults and more reliable in patients who are Tanner stage 5, spermatogenesis in pubertal or prepubertal patients can be difficult to interpret. A normal semen analysis in this population can be reassuring. Samples should be collected abiding by laboratory recommendations and interpreted according to World Health Organization guidelines. Pain is an infrequent indication for treatment with only 2% to 4% of men with varicoceles present with pain.[48] Importantly, varicoceles that are identified only on the right side should be worked up further. This condition can be an indicator of an abdominal or retroperitoneal process. Patients with a right-sided varicocele only should receive a careful abdominal examination and subsequent abdominal imaging (ultrasound or computed tomography scan).

Treatment

The goal of varicocele treatment is to maximize fertility. Adolescents who are asymptomatic and have an otherwise normal physical examination are candidates for observation. The algorithm for observation should include an annual physical examination with an objective measurement of testis volume. Additionally, annual semen analysis and scrotal ultrasound can be considered as adjuncts to observation. Observation is the treatment option of choice for most patients.

Options for surgical treatment include several different approaches to varicocelectomy. The goal of varicocelectomy is to ligate the veins of the pampiniform plexus. This procedure can be accomplished through several different approaches, including inguinal/subinguinal (open or microscopic) or laparoscopic/retroperitoneal. Complications are uncommon; however, the most common complications that arise after varicocelectomy are the recurrence of the varicocele or hydrocele formation. Rarely testis atrophy or injury to the genitofemoral nerve can result. In the latter, patients experience numbness of the anterior thigh, which usually resolves within 6 months. The risk of these complications varies depending on the approach.

Percutaneous approaches to embolize or sclerose the pampiniform plexus have been used in both antegrade and retrograde fashions. These procedures are generally performed by interventional radiologists, are done using fluoroscopy, and have inherent radiation exposure. Additionally, these techniques are generally less successful than open or laparoscopic procedures.

Recommendations

Varicoceles are a frequently encountered scrotal abnormality in adolescent boys. A careful physical examination, noting the laterality and grade of varicocele with an objective measurement of the testis volume, is important. Annual physical examination along with a scrotal ultrasound is necessary if observation is undertaken. A referral to a pediatric urologist is indicated if there is a solitary testis, testis hypotrophy (>15% volume loss), impaired spermatogenesis, or testis pain.

PENILE ANOMALIES

A range of penile anomalies can be encountered in pediatric patients. Generally, these conditions are noted by the parents or pediatrician during a well-child examination and, although not always emergent, represent conditions under which patients should be referred to a pediatric urologist.

Phimosis

When the opening of the foreskin is too tight to be pulled back over the glans of the penis, so that the meatus is visible, a condition called phimosis is diagnosed. Neonates frequently have a foreskin that is not completely retractable, which is physiologic. Phimosis must be distinguished from paraphimosis, which is an emergency. When paraphimosis is present, the foreskin cannot be reduced; the glans and urethral meatus are visible and frequently edematous and painful at rest. Paraphimosis can compromise blood flow to the glans, and these patients must be seen by a urologist immediately. Phimosis is generally not painful unless the foreskin is being manipulated or balanitis or balanoposthitis is present. Treatment options for patients with phimosis are steroid creams with frequent attempts at retraction to loosen the foreskin, a dorsal slit, or circumcision.

Hypospadias

Hypospadias is a congenital condition of the penis resulting from abnormal development of the urethra, foreskin, and cavernosal bodies. This condition results in a proximally displaced urethral meatus. A wide variance in severity can be seen. Hypospadias is generally seen in association with a prepuce that is not fused ventrally (hooded foreskin) and penile curvature (chordee). Approximately 1 in 250 to 300 boys are born with some degree of hypospadias. All patients with hypospadias should be referred to a pediatric urologist.

A thorough physical examination is the only means for diagnosing hypospadias. This examination should always be completed before circumcision, and circumcision should be aborted if hypospadias is found. Not all cases of hypospadias present with hooded foreskin and chordee, therefore, careful inspection of the urethral meatus is necessary. Megameatus with intact prepuce is a mild form of hypospadias whereby the urethral meatus is enlarged and ventrally displaced but the foreskin is present and normal. Rarely the meatus can be normal and a hooded foreskin or incompletely fused foreskin can be seen. Similarly, chordee can be present as a part of the hypospadias complex or the curvature can be seen as an isolated anomaly. The degree of hypospadias is defined by the location of the urethral meatus, which can be on the glans, penile shaft, scrotum, or even in the perineum. The anomalies that can be seen in conjunction with hypospadias include cryptorchidism, inguinal hernias, and an enlarged prostatic utricle. When hypospadias is seen with an undescended testis or other congenital anomalies, karyotyping should be considered.

The goals of treatment are a urethral meatus positioned at the tip of the glans, a straight penis, a normal glans, and a normal relationship between the penis and the scrotum. There are several surgical repairs that are used to achieve these goals. More severe hypospadias repairs are generally accomplished using staged techniques. Surgical intervention is generally undertaken between 6 and 18 months of age. The complications of repair include urethral stricture, urethrocutaneous fistulae, meatal stenosis, or urethral diverticulum.

Meatal Stenosis

Meatal stenosis is a narrowing in the urethral opening. This condition tends to occur much more frequently in circumcised boys, with an incidence of 1% to 10%. Circumcision allows the glans and the meatus to rub directly on diapers and subsequently inflammation and stenosis can form. The condition is suspected when a report of a strong stream or deviated stream is noticed. Additionally, irritation at the meatus, dysuria, frequent urinary tract infections, and bleeding can be seen. The diagnosis is made by physical examination, which reveals a narrowed meatus. A similar condition, which presents with a deviated stream and an unusual-appearing meatus frequently with an extra flap of skin, is referred to as a meatal baffle. These conditions are treated with a meatotomy or meatoplasty. These procedures are outpatient surgical procedures during which the urethral meatus is enlarged such that urine can flow freely.

SUMMARY

The authors emphasize that the physical examination of the groin and genitalia should compose an important part of every well-child visit.

REFERENCES

1. Boland ES. 'The woolen yarn truss in infantile inguinal hernia.' Boston Medical and Surgical Journal 1901;144:160.
2. Swenson O. Diagnosis and treatment of inguinal hernia. Pediatrics 1964;34: 412–4.
3. Grosfeld JL. Pediatric surgery, vol. 2. 6th edition. Philadelphia: Mosby/Elsevier; 2006.
4. Ein SH, Njere I, Ein A. Six thousand three hundred sixty-one pediatric inguinal hernias: a 35-year review. J Pediatr Surg 2006;41:980–6.
5. Lau ST, Lee YH, Caty MG. Current management of hernias and hydroceles. Semin Pediatr Surg 2007;16:50–7.
6. Rescorla FJ, Grosfeld JL. Inguinal hernia repair in the perinatal period and early infancy: clinical considerations. J Pediatr Surg 1984;19:832–7.
7. Osifo OD, Osaigbovo EO. Congenital hydrocele: prevalence and outcome among male children who underwent neonatal circumcision in Benin City, Nigeria. J Pediatr Urol 2008;4:178–82.
8. Heikkila J, Taskinen S, Toppari J, et al. Posterior urethral valves are often associated with cryptorchidism and inguinal hernias. J Urol 2008;180:715–7.
9. Mitchell GA. The condition of the peritoneal vaginal processes at birth. J Anat 1939;73:658–61.
10. Chen YC, Wu JC, Liu L, et al. Correlation between ventriculoperitoneal shunts and inguinal hernias in children: an 8-year follow-up. Pediatrics 2011;128:e121–6.

11. Cooper CS, Kirsch AJ, Snyder HM 3rd. Early diagnosis and management of neonatal abdominoscrotal hydroceles. Urol Int 1999;62:61–3.
12. Sparkman RS. Bilateral exploration in inguinal hernia in juvenile patients. Review and appraisal. Surgery 1962;51:393–406.
13. Rowe MI, Copelson LW, Clatworthy HW. The patent processus vaginalis and the inguinal hernia. J Pediatr Surg 1969;4:102–7.
14. Ron O, Eaton S, Pierro A. Systematic review of the risk of developing a metachronous contralateral inguinal hernia in children. Br J Surg 2007;94:804–11.
15. Given JP, Rubin SZ. Occurrence of contralateral inguinal hernia following unilateral repair in a pediatric hospital. J Pediatr Surg 1989;24:963–5.
16. Nataraja RM, Mahomed AA. Systematic review for paediatric metachronous contralateral inguinal hernia: a decreasing concern. Pediatr Surg Int 2011;27: 953–61.
17. Powell RW. Intraoperative diagnostic pneumoperitoneum in pediatric patients with unilateral inguinal hernias: the Goldstein test. J Pediatr Surg 1985;20: 418–21.
18. Miltenburg DM, Nuchtern JG, Jaksic T, et al. Laparoscopic evaluation of the pediatric inguinal hernia–a meta-analysis. J Pediatr Surg 1998;33:874–9.
19. Chen KC, Chu CC, Chou TY, et al. Ultrasonography for inguinal hernias in boys. J Pediatr Surg 1998;33:1784–7.
20. Misra D. Inguinal hernias in premature babies: wait or operate? Acta Paediatr 2001;90:370–1.
21. Gahukamble DB, Khamage AS. Early versus delayed repair of reduced incarcerated inguinal hernias in the pediatric population. J Pediatr Surg 1996;31: 1218–20.
22. Grosfeld JL, Cooney DR. Inguinal hernia after ventriculoperitoneal shunt for hydrocephalus. J Pediatr Surg 1974;9:311–5.
23. Kelalis PP, King LR, Belman AB. 2nd edition. Clinical pediatric urology, vol. 2. Philadelphia: Saunders; 1985.
24. Berkowitz GS, Lapinski RH, Dolgin SE, et al. Prevalence and natural history of cryptorchidism. Pediatrics 1993;92:44–9.
25. Scorer CG. The descent of the testis. Arch Dis Child 1964;39:605–9.
26. Baumrucker GO. Incidence of testicular pathology. Bull U S Army Med Dep 1946; 5:312–4.
27. Clarnette TD, Hutson JM. Is the ascending testis actually 'stationary'? Normal elongation of the spermatic cord is prevented by a fibrous remnant of the processus vaginalis. Pediatr Surg Int 1997;12:155–7.
28. Jones IR, Young ID. Familial incidence of cryptorchidism. J Urol 1982;127:508–9.
29. Snodgrass W, Bush N, Holzer M, et al. Current referral patterns and means to improve accuracy in diagnosis of undescended testis. Pediatrics 2011;127: e382–8.
30. Ritzen EM. Undescended testes: a consensus on management. Eur J Endocrinol 2008;159(Suppl 1):S87–90.
31. Miliaras D, Vlahakis-Miliaras E, Anagnostopoulos D, et al. Gross morphologic variations and histologic changes in cryptorchid testes. Pediatr Surg Int 1997; 12:158–62.
32. Lackgren G, Ploen L. The morphology of the human undescended testis with special reference to the Sertoli cell and puberty. Int J Androl 1984;7:23–38.
33. Virtanen HE, Bjerknes R, Cortes D, et al. Cryptorchidism: classification, prevalence and long-term consequences. Acta Paediatr 2007;96:611–6.
34. MacKinnon AE. The undescended testis. Indian J Pediatr 2005;72:429–32.

35. Lee PA. Fertility after cryptorchidism: epidemiology and other outcome studies. Urology 2005;66:427–31.
36. Cortes D, Thorup J, Lindenberg S, et al. Infertility despite surgery for cryptorchidism in childhood can be classified by patients with normal or elevated follicle-stimulating hormone and identified at orchidopexy. BJU Int 2003;91:670–4.
37. Walsh TJ, Dall'Era MA, Croughan MS, et al. Prepubertal orchiopexy for cryptorchidism may be associated with lower risk of testicular cancer. J Urol 2007; 178:1440–6 [discussion: 46].
38. Wood HM, Elder JS. Cryptorchidism and testicular cancer: separating fact from fiction. J Urol 2009;181:452–61.
39. Akbay E, Cayan S, Doruk E, et al. The prevalence of varicocele and varicocele-related testicular atrophy in Turkish children and adolescents. BJU Int 2000;86: 490–3.
40. Madgar I, Weissenberg R, Lunenfeld B, et al. Controlled trial of high spermatic vein ligation for varicocele in infertile men. Fertil Steril 1995;63:120–4.
41. Gorelick JI, Goldstein M. Loss of fertility in men with varicocele. Fertil Steril 1993; 59:613–6.
42. Witt MA, Lipshultz LI. Varicocele: a progressive or static lesion? Urology 1993;42: 541–3.
43. Coolsaet BL. The varicocele syndrome: venography determining the optimal level for surgical management. J Urol 1980;124:833–9.
44. Kim WS, Cheon JE, Kim IO, et al. Hemodynamic investigation of the left renal vein in pediatric varicocele: Doppler US, venography, and pressure measurements. Radiology 2006;241:228–34.
45. Kass EJ, Stork BR, Steinert BW. Varicocele in adolescence induces left and right testicular volume loss. BJU Int 2001;87:499–501.
46. Podesta ML, Gottlieb S, Medel R Jr, et al. Hormonal parameters and testicular volume in children and adolescents with unilateral varicocele: preoperative and postoperative findings. J Urol 1994;152:794–7 [discussion: 98].
47. Sayfan J, Siplovich L, Koltun L, et al. Varicocele treatment in pubertal boys prevents testicular growth arrest. J Urol 1997;157:1456–7.
48. Diamond DA. Adolescent varicocele. Curr Opin Urol 2007;17:263–7.

Functional Bladder Problems in Children

Pathophysiology, Diagnosis, and Treatment

Israel Franco, MD

KEYWORDS

- Functional lower urinary tract problems • Bowel problems
- Dysfunctional elimination syndrome • Overactive bladder syndrome
- Voiding postponement • Stress incontinence
- Giggle incontinence and dysfunctional voiding • Neuropsychiatric disorders

KEY POINTS

- The hallmark of treatment of bladder and bowel problems is the been the use of a bowel program and timed voiding regimen. The use of biofeedback has helped many other children correct their errant voiding patterns.
- The use of drugs to treat OAB shows increased promise and it seems that the sensory limb of the voiding reflex is the primary target for continued pharmacologic treatment.
- Numerous other treatment modalities are available for patients who have failed pharmacologic therapy, therefore no one need go untreated.
- The continued use of stimulation modalities whether peripheral or central needs continued exploration in the future.
- The relationship between neuropsychiatric disorders and OAB is significant, therefore a thorough family history is essential in the initial evaluation to properly treat the patient.

INTRODUCTION

Functional lower urinary tract (LUT) problems, bladder and bowel problems (BBD) or dysfunctional elimination syndrome are all terms that describe the common array of symptoms that include overactive bladder syndrome (OAB), voiding postponement, stress incontinence, giggle incontinence. and dysfunctional voiding. The most common is OAB, which seems to have a peak incidence between 5 and 7 years of age. Ruarte and Quesada[1] and found an incidence of 57.4% in a group of 383 incontinent

An editorial commentary by Dr Darius Bagli, "Is Bladder Dysfunction in Children Science Fiction of Science Fact: Editorial Comment" is based on this article and found in *Pediatric Clinics of North America* (59:4), August 2012.

Pediatric Urology Associates, New York Medical College, 150 White Plains Road, Tarrytown, Valhalla, NY 10591, USA

E-mail address: Franco.PUA@gmail.com

Pediatr Clin N Am 59 (2012) 783–817
doi:10.1016/j.pcl.2012.05.007
0031-3955/12/$ – see front matter

children ranging in age from 3 to 14 years of age. The group consisted of 38.9% boys and 60.1% girls. Daytime wetting is estimated to affect 5 to 7 million children in the United States aged 6 years or older.[1] The impact of daytime wetting in children can be profound. It can affect their life socially, emotionally, and behaviorally and also affects the everyday life of their family.[2] From our understanding of OAB, we know that if it continues over a prolonged period, the bladder wall thickens, which can have an impact in adulthood. As patients become older, its consequences become more profound and require more of an effort to correct.[3,4]

From a pediatric urologist perspective, the child who has OAB has a good chance of becoming an adult who continues to have problems with OAB. This correlation has been reported in 2 published studies. In the first study, Fitzgerald and colleagues[3] revealed that OAB in childhood correlated with adult OAB symptoms. These investigators found that frequent daytime voiding in childhood correlated with adult urgency. A correlation existed between childhood nocturia and adult nocturia. Childhood daytime incontinence and nocturnal enuresis were associated with a more than 2-fold increased association with adult urge incontinence. Also a history of childhood urinary tract infections (UTIs) correlated with a history of adult UTIs. Another study by Minassian and colleagues[4] involving 170 adult women found that there was a higher prevalence of childhood voiding dysfunction in women who had urinary frequency, urgency, stress incontinence, and urge incontinence. These investigators also noted that there was a greater likelihood of their symptomatic patients having a higher body mass index, calculated as weight in kilograms divided by the square of height in meters.

In another study by Stone and colleagues,[5] there was about a one in three chance if patients were wetting by 9 to 10 years of age that they would continue to have OAB-type symptoms by 18 years of age. In this study, all patients were evaluated with urodynamics and magnetic resonance imaging (MRI) of the lumbosacral spine. No lesions were found in the spine to indicate that a spinal problem was the source of the BBD. The implications of these findings underscore the importance of childhood OAB and its potential impact in adulthood. The trend over the years has been to tell parents that these problems are self-limiting and that they will resolve in due time as the child matures. It seems that this theory may not be the case and that some children as they mature are just better at compensating for their problems and eventually drop off the radar screen (our offices) either because of frustration with our inability to treat their problems or because they have developed coping strategies that satisfy their needs for the interim. A better understanding of the potential causes of childhood OAB could prevent undue problems in adulthood and make many children happier, along with their parents and teachers.

This article discusses the updated nomenclature and looks at the pathophysiology of functional bladder disorders from a different perspective than has been the norm in the past. Some standard medical treatments as well as some newer forms of treatment are also outlined. Treatment algorithms for urinary frequency (**Fig. 1**) and urinary incontinence (**Fig. 2**) have been created to help the practitioner manage the patient.

NOMENCLATURE
International Children's Continence Society

The nomenclature in urinary tract function and malfunction has been rife with terms that have been used interchangeably for 1 condition and in other cases to denote specific dysfunctions. This situation has led to confusion when an attempt is made to review the old literature. In 2006, a document was put forth by the International

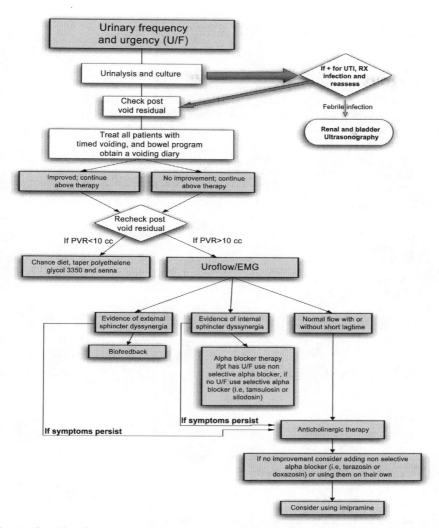

Fig. 1. Algorithm for the management and treatment of urinary frequency and urgency.

Children's Continence Society that standardized the nomenclature and set specific guidelines for the use of certain terms to avoid confusion in future publications.[6]

Frequency

Increased urinary frequency is considered to exist when the patient voids 8 or more times per day and decreased frequency is when the child voids 3 or less times per day. Estimates of voiding frequency are considered to be relevant from age 5 years and older. The estimation of urinary frequency is best made with a voiding diary, which is kept by the parent for younger children.

Incontinence

Incontinence (urinary incontinence) means uncontrollable leakage of urine. It can be continuous or intermittent in nature. Continuous incontinence is usually associated

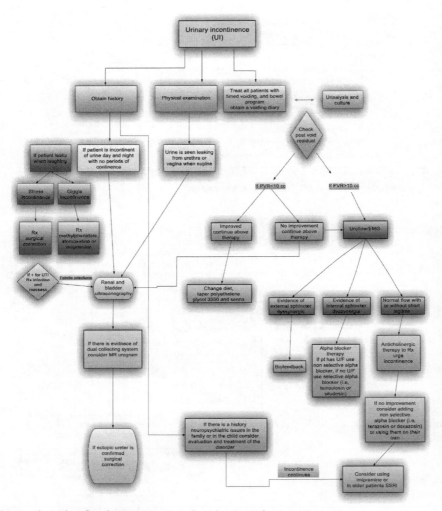

Fig. 2. Algorithm for the treatment and evaluation of urinary incontinence.

with anatomic abnormalities such as ectopic ureters or spina bifida. Intermittent incontinence is urine leakage in discrete amounts. It can occur during the day or at night, and it is applicable to children who are at least 5 years old.

Enuresis
Enuresis means intermittent incontinence while sleeping. In contrast with previous terminology, the terms nocturnal incontinence and enuresis are now synonymous. The term diurnal is no longer used because it can mean daytime or a whole 24-hour period, therefore lending to confusion regarding the time of incontinence. The use of nocturnal has also been discontinued because enuresis now refers only to nocturnal incontinence episodes.

Urgency
Urgency means the sudden and unexpected experience of an immediate need to void. The term is not applicable before the attainment of bladder control or age 5 years,

whichever occurs first. Nocturia means that the child must awaken at night to void. The definition is relevant from the age of 5 years.

Nocturia
Nocturia is common among schoolchildren[7] and it does not necessarily indicate LUT malfunction. The term nocturia does not apply to children who awaken for reasons other than a need to void, for instance children who awaken after an enuretic episode.

Voiding symptoms
The absence of voiding symptoms reported by a child does not mean that there are no such symptoms. They may not reliably have been observed by a caregiver or reported by a child until about age 7 years. The terms splitting or spraying, as used in adult terminology, refer to the appearance of the urine stream and they are of little relevance in childhood, except in instances of meatal stenosis in circumcised boys.

Hesitancy
Hesitancy denotes difficulty in the initiation of voiding or that the child must wait a considerable period before voiding starts. The term is relevant from the attainment of bladder control or age 5 years. Hesitancy may be an indicator of either a delay in the opening of the bladder neck or external sphincter and usually requires further workup with a uroflow/electromyogram (EMG). An extreme form of hesitancy is the shy bladder syndrome, in which the patient is unable to void in public places or with other people present. Hesitancy can be diagnosed with a uroflow/EMG in a noninvasive manner. The measurement of the lag time is considered a means of objectively quantifying hesitancy caused by bladder neck or internal sphincter dyssynergia.

Straining
Straining means that the child applies abdominal pressure to initiate and maintain voiding. If observed, straining is relevant in all age groups.

Weak stream
Weak stream is used for the observed ejection of urine with a weak force and it is relevant from infancy and thereafter.

Intermittency
Intermittency is the term applied when micturition occurs not in a continuous stream, but rather in several discrete spurts. This symptom may be described in all age groups, but it is regarded as physiologic up to age 3 years if not accompanied by straining.

Other Symptoms

Holding maneuvers
Holding maneuvers are observable strategies used to postpone voiding or suppress urgency. The child may or may not be fully aware of the purpose of the maneuvers, but it is usually obvious to caregivers. Common maneuvers are standing on tiptoe, forcefully crossing the legs, or squatting with the heel pressed into the perineum. Grabbing of the penis or even what seems to be masturbation in both males and females may be an attempt at holding maneuvers. Stimulation of the penis or the glans clitoris can cause a reflex suppression of the micturition reflex. The term is relevant from the attainment of bladder control or age 5 years.

Feeling of incomplete emptying
Feeling of incomplete emptying is self-explanatory. It is not relevant before adolescence because younger children usually do not recognize and describe this symptom.

Postmicturition dribble

Postmicturition dribble is the term used when the child describes involuntary urine leakage immediately after voiding has finished. It is applicable after the attainment of bladder control or age 5 years. Vaginal reflux may produce this symptom. It is commonly associated with either external or internal sphincter dyssynergia. It is not uncommon for this symptom to be associated with a spinning top urethra on a voiding cystourethrogram (**Fig. 3**).

Genital and LUT pain

Genital and LUT pain is usually nonspecific and difficult to localize. Pain associated with voiding is commonly seen in patients with some form of dyssynergic voiding. We found that in patients who had bulbar urethritis (dysuria/urethrorrhagia syndrome), the pain at the tip or along the shaft of the penis was most likely caused by dyssynergic voiding and correction of such a voiding pattern eliminated the symptoms.[8] In girls, pain in the vagina or in the urethra can also indicate such an abnormal pattern. Suprapubic pain is more difficult to use as a specific marker. It can be present in the absence of infection and commonly is noted in conjunction with severe urgency. On the other hand, suprapubic pain is not uncommon in the presence of a UTI. Infants may pull their legs up as they void.

Conditions

OAB and urge incontinence

The hallmark of OAB is urgency and, thus, children with this symptom can be said to have an OAB. Incontinence is often also present, as is increased voiding frequency, but these symptoms are not prerequisites for use of the term OAB. Urge incontinence simply means incontinence in the presence of urgency and, thus, it is a term that is applicable to many children with OAB. There is mounting evidence that this is

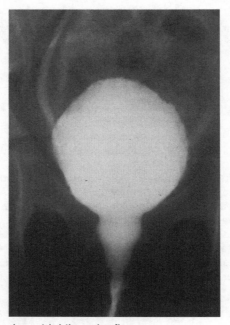

Fig. 3. Spinning top urethra with bilateral reflux.

a sensory problem, and whether it is located in the central nervous system (CNS) or at the bladder level is a matter for debate.

Voiding postponement
Children who are observed by their parents or caregivers to habitually postpone micturition, often in specific situations, using holding maneuvers are said to experience voiding postponement. This symptom is often associated with a low micturition frequency and a feeling of urgency caused by a full bladder. Some children have learned to restrict fluid intake as a method of increasing voiding intervals and at the same time decreasing incontinence. The rationale for the delineation of this entity lies in the observation that these children often experience psychological comorbidity or behavioral disturbances.[9]

Underactive bladder
The old entity lazy bladder is now replaced by the neutral term underactive bladder. This term is reserved for children with low voiding frequency and a need to increase intra-abdominal pressure to initiate, maintain, or complete voiding (ie, straining). The children often produce an interrupted pattern on uroflow measurement and they are usually found to qualify for the term detrusor underactivity if examined with invasive urodynamics.

Dysfunctional voiding
The child with dysfunctional voiding habitually contracts the urethral sphincter during voiding. It is necessary to perform uroflowmetry to confirm the presence of sphincter contraction during voiding. The term describes malfunction during the voiding phase only. It says nothing about the storage phase. It is entirely possible for a child to experience dysfunctional voiding as well as storage symptoms such as incontinence, urgency, or frequency, thereby giving 2 problems that need correction.

Obstruction
Children with an impediment to urine outflow during voiding are said to experience LUT obstruction. It is characterized by increased detrusor pressure and a decreased urine flow rate. In many instances, obstruction is caused by dysfunctional voiding, but anatomic abnormalities such as posterior or anterior urethral valves may be the cause of obstruction.

Stress incontinence
Stress incontinence is the leakage of small amounts of urine at exertion or with increased intra-abdominal pressure, typically associated with Valsalva maneuver. It is rare in neurologically normal children.

Vaginal reflux
Toilet-trained prepubertal girls who wet their underwear within 10 minutes of voiding are said to experience vaginal reflux if no underlying mechanism other than vaginal entrapment of urine is obvious. This symptom is not associated with other LUT symptoms. It is essential to differentiate this symptom from postvoid dribbling, because the treatment is different.

Giggle incontinence
Giggle incontinence is a rare syndrome in which apparently complete voiding occurs specifically during or immediately after laughing. Bladder function is normal when the child is not laughing.

Extraordinary daytime urinary frequency

The term extraordinary daytime urinary frequency applies to children who void often and with small volumes during the daytime only. Daytime voiding frequency is at least once hourly, and average voided volumes are less than 50% of estimated bladder capacity, and usually less. Incontinence is not a usual or necessary component of the condition, and nocturnal bladder behavior is normal for the age of the child. The term is applicable from the age of daytime bladder control or 3 years.

DIAGNOSIS
History and Physical Examination

The evaluation of the child with BBD should start with a history and physical examination. A history is of the utmost in helping to determine what the prevailing symptom is and when the symptoms tend to occur. Generally, it is best to obtain the history from the child if they are cooperative; if not, there may be no choice but to obtain it from the parents. Signs of urgency such as crossing the legs, running to the bathroom, grabbing the penis, rubbing the clitoris, squatting, and sitting on the heels are all signs of urgency. In this case, maintenance of a voiding diary is critical. Urinary frequency is also another manifestation of OAB, and quantifying the number of times that the patient goes to the bathroom and the amount are useful in determining if there is true frequency. Urinary urge incontinence is another classic hallmark of overactive bladder. What typically occurs is that the child has urgency, and some urine leaks out and leaves them with damp underwear, whereas in other cases the urine soaks through their pants. Urge incontinence is commonly seen to occur after lunch. This situation is most likely caused by stimulation of colonic contractions by the gastrocolic reflex. It is understood that there is cross-talk in the spinal cord between the colon and the bladder.[8,10–12] This cross-talk may trigger bladder contractions or at least lead to symptoms of urgency. Patients complain of postvoid dribbling in both sexes; this is a sign of incomplete relaxation of the external sphincter. When the patient is finished urinating, urine typically sits in the posterior urethra until the sphincter completely relaxes and then drips out. This situation typically occurs after the child has pulled up their pants. The physician should also ask about a history of dysuria. Dysuria without evidence of infection is usually caused by dyssynergic voiding.[8] It is commonly associated with microhematuria or in some cases gross terminal hematuria. Many of these children may have a long-standing history (and even a family history) of microhematuria. In some boys, it is not uncommon to find meatal stenosis associated with these 2 findings. Also one should note in the boys if scabbing of the meatus occurs on a regular basis. This symptom is most frequently noted in the morning just before the first void. Many of these boys complain that it feels like the meatus is stuck closed. This feeling is caused by serum that exudes from the irritated bulbar urethra and travels up the urethra, causing the meatus to stick together. In both males and females, there is cystoscopic evidence of denuded urethral mucosa and vascular engorgement of the proximal urethra and the bladder neck that leads to the microhematuria and gross hematuria.

On entering the room, the physician should take close note of the interaction between the child and parent as well as the child and the physician. Excessive anxiety or inappropriate fear should be noted. The parents should be questioned as to whether this type of behavior is commonly present at home or during other stressful situations. A thorough history should be taken with regards to a family history of anxiety, phobias, attention-deficit disorder/attention-deficit/hyperactivity disorder (ADHD), depression, or other neuropsychiatric problems within the first-line family members. In our experience, many parents fail to include these conditions in a typical intake sheet that they are asked to fill out. In some cases, asking which medications the child or parents are taking is an indicator of one of these disease processes.

A thorough history of the bowel habits of the patient should be obtained from the patient directly. Many parents are not cognizant of the true nature of their children's bowel movements and many report that their children's bowel movements are perfectly normal, whereas the children contradict them. Documentation of the size and nature of the bowel movements should be obtained. Use of a diagram is beneficial and facilitates communication with the child (**Fig. 4**). It should be noted if the bowel movements are painful or associated with rectal bleeding. Large massive bowel movements are usually an indicator of infrequent bowel movements. Pain or rectal bleeding can be associated with external sphincter dyssynergia. Patients who have diarrhea or symptoms of colitis can also have issues with an overactive bladder. Chronic periumbilical pain is another sign that there is a problem with constipation or issues with serotonin homeostasis in the gut (commonly seen in Irritable bowel syndrome IBS). Many children may complain of this pain, which disappears as soon as a bowel regimen is instituted. If it does not, then lactose intolerance should be considered as a potential problem, especially if it is associated with gas. We use the Iowa criteria for constipation, as described by Loening-Bauke.[13] Using these criteria, many patients would qualify as being constipated, and it is helpful to explain this to the parents, who typically state that their child is not constipated.

Neuropsychiatric Comorbidity

Children with elimination disorders have an increased rate of comorbid behavioral or psychological disorders. About 20% to 40% of children with daytime urinary incontinence are affected by comorbid behavioral disorders.[14,15] In a large epidemiologic study of a cohort of 8213 children aged 7.5 to 9 years, children with daytime wetting had significantly increased rates of psychological problems, especially separation anxiety (11.4%), attention-deficit (24.8%), oppositional behavior (10.9%), and conduct

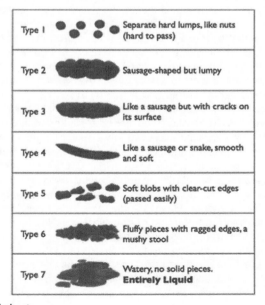

Fig. 4. Bristol stool chart.

problems (11.8%).[16] In the same cohort, 10,000 children aged 4 to 9 years were analyzed. Delayed development, difficult temperament, and maternal depression/anxiety were associated with daytime wetting and soiling.[17] In another population-based study that included 2856 children, the incidence of incontinence was 16.9% within the previous 6 months.[18] In a retrospective study of patients with ADHD, 20.9% wetted at night and 6.5% wetted during the day. The odds ratios were 2.7 and 4.5 times higher, respectively, which means that there is unspecific association of ADHD and both nighttime and daytime wetting.[19] Of possible elimination disorders, children with fecal incontinence (or encopresis) have the highest rates of comorbid behavioral disorders: 30% to 50% of all children have clinically relevant behavioral disturbances.[14,15] In a recent epidemiologic study of more than 8242 7-year-old to 8-year-old children, a wide range of comorbid disorders according to the *Diagnostic and Statistical Manual of Mental Disorders, Fourth Edition* were significantly increased: separation anxiety (4.3%), social phobias (1.7%), specific phobias (4.3%), generalized anxiety (3.4%), depressive disorders (2. 6%), ADHD (9.2%), and oppositional defiant behavior (11.9%). A study by Bael and colleagues[9,20] in 2008 found that, before treatment of nonneurogenic bladder sphincter dysfunction in the European Bladder Dysfunction Group, behavioral problems were present in 19% of the children at a rate of 2:1 compared with a normative population. After treatment of incontinence, the rate decreased to 11%, which was the same as the normative group. The treatment was primarily behavioral therapy and biofeedback. This significant change in score was seen only in the dysfunctional voiders and did not change at all in the patients who had urge syndrome. Conventional wisdom implicates the bladder problem as the source of the behavioral problems in the urge group. The dysfunctional voiders who did respond with resolution of their voiding issues seemed to be put at ease and their behavioral problems resolved. Some patients still persisted with behavioral problems after the dysfunctional issues had been settled. A better explanation based on a neurocentric way of thinking implicates the lack of change in the behavior of these patients to a central defect. The anterior cingulate gyrus (ACG) and the prefrontal cortex (PFC) are the sites most commonly found to have dysfunction in patients with behavioral problems. Regardless of the outcome of their BBD, there should be no expectation that their underlying neuropsychiatric issues will improve with correction of the BBD. On the other hand, the patients with voiding dysfunction could benefit from a bowel program (BP) and biofeedback if their problems are caused by learned aberrant behavior, and correction of such behavior could lead to resolution of their lower urinary tract symptoms (LUTS) as well as some behavioral issues caused by the LUTS. It can also be explained that the behavior of some of the patients with dysfunctional voiding did not improve, and, in this group, voiding dysfunction was most likely linked to the PFC/ACG problem. The association of urinary incontinence and lower psychological well-being in adults has also been noted by Botlero and colleagues.[21] Major depression can predict the onset of urinary incontinence in women in an at-risk population-based sample.[22] One study found increased rates of enuresis in adult bipolar disorder (18%).[12,23] An association with panic disorder and interstitial cystitis has also been described in the literature.[24] In one study,[25] patients who were described as having psychoneuroticism were less likely to respond to treatment of detrusor instability than those who had no form of psychoneuroticism; most good responders and one-third of nonresponders were free of psychiatric issues. Twenty-five percent of the patients in this study had symptoms of irritable bowel syndrome. These findings were no different from our data, which indicate that patients with urge syndrome who are nonresponders have a 50% chance of having some form of neuropsychiatric problem. Daywetting also was found to be a premorbid developmental marker for schizophrenia (SCZ).[26] The investigators found that patients with SCZ had higher rates of childhood enuresis (21%) compared with siblings (11%) or control patients (7%), and the relative risk for enuresis was increased in siblings. Patients with enuresis performed worse on 2 frontal lobe cognitive tests (letter fluency and category fluency) compared with nonenuretic patients. Cerebral defects associated with these disorders tend to cluster around the ACG and PFC, which is where the defects are seen in patients with urgency and urge incontinence.

Physical Examination

The physical examination is helpful in evaluating these children and can be revealing. Examination of the abdomen is critical in determining whether stool is present in the colon. Palpation of the left lower quadrant up to the left upper quadrant typically yields large amounts of stool present in these abdomens. In many cases, the parents deny that their children have any issues with their bowels. Gaseous distention of the colon is just as troublesome and should be noted because it can lead to the same problems as constipation.

Examination of the back typically reveals a normal-appearing back and anocutaneous folds. In rare instances, flattening of the buttocks or abnormal creasing at the sacroiliac joint may be noted, which indicates some type of sacral anomaly (**Figs. 5** and **6**). Observing the child walk can also help identify a potential neurologic problem if the child tends to walk on their toes. High arched feet are also a clue that there may be a neurologic problem. Low-lying sacral dimples are typically not of concern. Only dimples that are associated with tufts of hair or are placed higher up on the back are of concern and should be evaluated with MRI of the lumbar-sacral spine.

Examination of the genitalia should be performed on all children with BBD. One should look at the underwear when it is pulled down to perform the examination. Inspection of the underwear can help gauge the gravity of the problem. Yellow

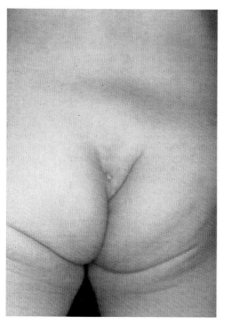

Fig. 5. Abnormal sacral folds.

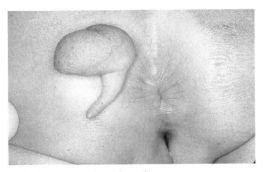

Fig. 6. Fatty tail associated with a tethered cord.

spotting on the front of the undergarment is an indicator of mild urge incontinence and postvoid dribbling, whereas soaked underwear indicates a more profound incontinence problem. In girls, one should look for staining of the underwear with vaginal discharge; the color of the staining is useful in diagnosing vaginitis. Greenish to brownish discoloration indicates chronic bacterial vaginitis, whereas a clear to white discharge is expected in prepubertal girls. The smell of the perineum and underwear are critical clues as well that should not be ignored. The child may have a clean pair of underwear with no discharge, but a foul smell emanating from the perineum is a clue of chronic soiling or discharge.

Stool soiling on the underwear is also important. Mild streaking is an indicator that the patient is hoarding stool. In other cases, stool soiling of the underwear is an indicator of encopresis. Rectal examination is rarely necessary in these children. The only time that a rectal examination is indicated is if there are symptoms of strangury, which could indicate the presence of a rhabdomyosarcoma of the prostate or bladder. Many of these children do not have stool in the rectal vault, but can be loaded with stool higher up in the sigmoid colon or even in the descending colon. Therefore we abstain from rectal examinations on all of our dysfunctional voiders. On the other hand, visual inspection of the anus is a useful tool, which allows us to assess whether the patient has skin tags, fissures, or hemorrhoids; these are indicators of chronic problems with constipation or large bowel movements. Laxity of the anal sphincter is another good sign that the child is passing massive bowel movements. Evidence of an anal wink is a sign of an intact sacral reflex arch (S2–4) and is commonly seen as soon as the buttocks are separated to inspect the anus.

Examination of the penis gives multiple clues that there are problems with the way the child voids. Inspection of the meatus generally reveals meatal stenosis, which is not a true stenosis but rather a urethral membrane that was formed as a result of prolapse of the urethral tissue and eventually becomes keratinized (**Fig. 7**). It is common to see this form of meatal stenosis in all boys who have dysfunctional voiding symptoms as well as urethral syndrome (otherwise known as bulbar urethritis [**Fig. 8**] or urethrorrhagia). We postulate that high-pressure voiding commonly seen in young males allows for prolapse of the urethral tissue like a hemorrhoid prolapses with straining to defecate. Subsequently, over time this tissue becomes keratinized and forms the ventral urethral membrane, similar to the rectal hemorrhoid becoming a skin tag. This ventral urethral membrane is the cause of the deviated urinary stream encountered in most boys with meatal stenosis. It is common to see prolapsed urethral tissue in a neonate and boys circumcised in infancy, which commonly and mistakenly are called meatitis. Meatal prolapse does occur in uncircumcised boys and looks similar

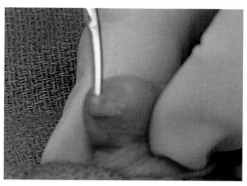

Fig. 7. Ventral urethral membrane (meatal stenosis).

to meatal prolapse in girls but is not so severe. The reason we typically do not see meatal stenosis in uncircumcised boys is that the prepuce prevents chronic irritation of this prolapsed meatal tissue, therefore preventing keratinization of the tissue. Chronic irritation and redness of the penis is usually an indicator that the boy is sitting in wet underwear. In the girls, vaginal irritation is caused by skin irritation from wetting and is rarely if ever caused by fungal infections. Lichen sclerosis is also an indicator that there is chronic irritation of the perineum caused by the patient remaining in wet underwear. Green or foul smelling vaginal discharge with erythema of the vagina is usually an indicator of vaginitis and requires treatment with a cephalosporin. In males, epididymitis is most commonly caused by dyssynergic voiding, which leads to reflux of urine into the ejaculatory ducts. Pain in the groin is also a common sign of dyssynergic voiding, which is usually associated with tenderness along the vas or cord.

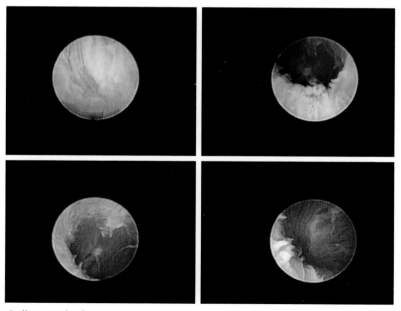

Fig. 8. Bulbar urethral tears in the mucosa associated with urethritis and urethrorraghia.

Urinalysis

The most important clinical test that should be performed in all children who present with BBD is the urinalysis. A simple urinalysis should help determine if the symptoms are caused by infection or BBD. It is not uncommon to see microhematuria in patients who have dyssynergic voiding, which is commonly associated with BBD.

UROFLOW/EMG

The uroflow study is another useful tool in helping to determine if the child is an abnormal voider. Four classic curves are seen: a normal bell curve, the hypervoider curve, the staccato curve, and the plateau curve. The use of the uroflow is further augmented by the concomitant use of an EMG of the perineal muscles. Using this strategy we are able to tell if the child is voiding with external sphincter dyssynergia (increased perineal muscle activity) and even to make the diagnosis of internal sphincter dyssynergia based on lag time and the shape of the flow curve (**Fig. 9**). Children with urgency or urge incontinence show a flow pattern that has an increased external sphincter activity along with a short lag time (**Fig. 10**).

URODYNAMICS

In some instances, urodynamics are performed simultaneously to perform a voiding cystourethrography (VCUG) but in most cases the urodynamic study tells us only what we already know, that is, that there are uninhibited contractions (UICs). Bael and colleagues[27] showed that there was no benefit to performing a urodynamic study

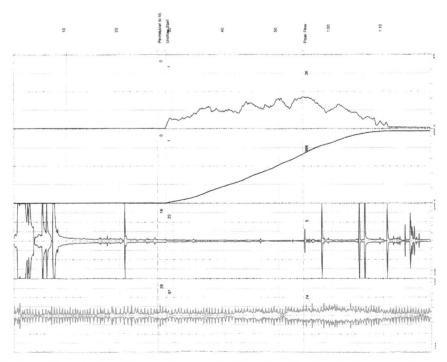

Fig. 9. Uroflow study in 17-year-old male with intermittent testis pain. Presence of internal sphincter dyssynergia is evident because of long lag time before voiding and abdominal straining.

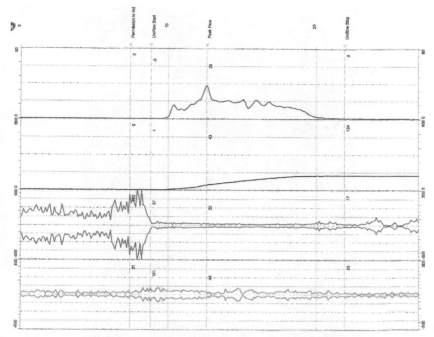

Fig. 10. 5-year-old male with urinary urgency and urge incontinence with characteristic short lag time of the external sphincter before urination.

in children with BBD. The presence of UICs does not rule in or out the presence of a neurologic lesion. The only finding that is of significance is the absence of a detrusor contraction, which would be evident from the uroflow study, which would show a poor flow curve.

IMAGING
VCUG

In many instances, a good VCUG can give information on the dynamics of voiding. The bladder neck can be seen opening and the external sphincter can also be seen as it opens and closes. The presence of the spinning top urethra is a classic example of external sphincter dyssynergia (**Fig. 3**). We find that there is little need to perform urodynamics on children if we use these tests. The presence of an anatomic defect such as valves or an ectopic ureter can be identified on these studies. In refractory patients, it is de rigueur to obtain a VCUG to further help delineate the dynamics of voiding and to make sure no anatomic problem is missed. The VCUG can provide an opportunity to evaluate the amount of stool in the colon. On some occasions, it can also be used to assess the lumbosacral spine.

Lumbosacral Films

Lumbosacral films are useful to help diagnose a sacral anomaly. In patients with severe constipation, the kidney ureter bladder (KUB) may not be adequate to evaluate the spine. We have seen patients have a missed diagnosis of sacral dysraphism because the sacrum is obscured by stool (**Fig. 11**). Once the patient had a lumbosacral film or the KUB had been performed when the bowels had been cleaned out, it was

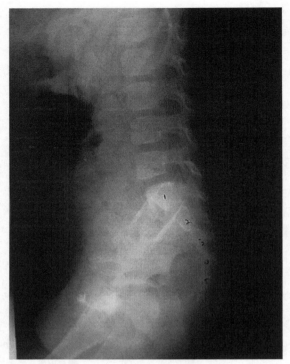

Fig. 11. Sacral anteroposterior film showing the full sacrum; note the large amount of stool present in the abdomen.

clear that a sacral anomaly existed. Spina bifida occulta is rarely associated with incontinence; it is a common finding in the population, and unless the finding is outside the lumbosacral area or the incontinence persists, there is no need to obtain additional studies.

MRI of Spine

Sacral imaging is necessary in a few patients. Patients with obvious lesions of the back should be imaged as described in the physical examination section. On some occasions, patients who lack any outward evidence of abnormalities may need to be imaged if no other source for the BBD is found. In our experience with patients who have BBD, a few have been found to have some cystic lesions in the sacral or lumbar cord, but even in these cases it was believed by the neurosurgeons that these were not causing any neurologic findings requiring surgical intervention. Tethering of the cord without any outward findings is rare and is commonly associated with back pain. In a large follow-up study of patients with intractable BBD symptoms, Stone and colleagues[5] found few patients with any form of tethering. A controversial issue is the finding of a thickened filum terminale, with many of the patients reporting no significant improvement postoperatively.[28]

KUB

The KUB is a plain film of the abdomen, which includes the upper edges of the renal outlines and the area of the bladder and pelvis. This film is useful in helping evaluate the amount of stool present in the abdomen and whether there may be stones in the distal ureter, because such stones can cause frequency and urgency acutely.

Renal and Bladder Ultrasonography

Renal ultrasonography can allow the physician to identify if there is a possibility of a duplication of the kidney, which may be associated with an ectopic ureter. Dilation of a ureter may be another clue that suggests an ectopic ureter. Bladder ultrasonography is helpful in identifying the presence of a ureterocele, which may be useful in ruling out an anatomic source of incontinence. Bladder wall thickening can be discerned from ultrasonography and is a useful indicator that there is detrusor hypertrophy. Another test that is critical in evaluating the child with BBD is the postvoid residual examination. The introduction of this test into the everyday practice of the pediatric urologist has revolutionized the management and treatment of voiding dysfunctions in children. If the child has an increased postvoid residual, then the frequency and urgency are most likely caused by incomplete emptying because of dyssynergic voiding. On the other hand, if an increased residual is not present, then dyssynergia cannot be ruled out, but one has the luxury of treating the patient with the standard protocol without fear of the patient developing a UTI. Measurement of the rectal diameter can also be made on a bladder ultrasonography. Studies indicate that rectal diameter measurements greater than 3-4 cm are commonly seen in patients with BBD.

Pathophysiology

BBD is not completely understood and the feeling is that it most certainly is a multifactorial problem. In some instances, anatomic abnormalities can lead to BBD (these are not discussed in this review), whereas in other cases, functional voiding problems may be the source of the overactive bladder. In other instances, neurologic lesions may lead to the development of overactive bladder.

The prevailing theory in children is that BBD is believed to be caused by a delay in the acquisition of cortical inhibition over uninhibited detrusor contractions in the course of achieving a mature voiding pattern of adulthood. The site of maturational delay is believed to lie in reticulospinal pathways of the spinal cord or in the inhibitory center within the cerebral cortex. Cortical control is normally established between 3 and 5 years of age. Delay in the fine-tuning of bladder sphincter coordination during voiding causes uninhibited detrusor contractions to be met with voluntary external urethral sphincter contractions, the control of which is believed to be acquired at an earlier age.[29] An increase in intravesicle pressure can manifest itself in an array of symptoms that include urgency, urge incontinence, and nocturnal enuresis. OAB triggers bladder overactivity usually in the early filling phase, causing the pelvic floor to respond by voluntary contraction. These voluntary contractions lead to classic holding maneuvers such as leg crossing, penile grabbing, and squatting. It is believed that active external sphincter contraction may possibly cause a temporary reflex relaxation in the detrusor and therefore afford momentary relief from the effects of uninhibited bladder contractions. Persistent isometric contractions of the detrusor against the tightened sphincter or incomplete relaxation of the sphincter lead the bladder muscle to hypertrophy, and this increased hypertrophy gradually decreases functional bladder capacity and increases instability of the bladder, thereby creating a vicious cycle in which the OAB is worsened (**Fig. 12**). The concomitant increased pelvic floor activity may be associated with increased autonomic stimulation of the perineal organs and musculature. This increased activity may be associated with sexual dysfunction in adults.[30–34] We postulate that this increased overactivity may lead to

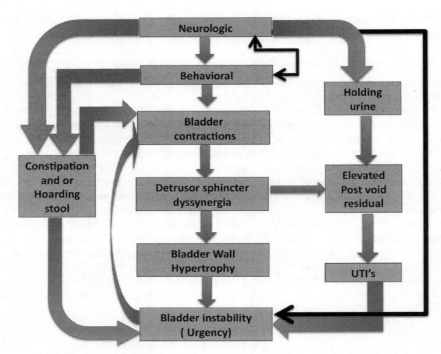

Fig. 12. The interrelationship between bowel, bladder, and CNS and the role they play in bowel and bladder dysfunction.

chronic pelvic pain syndrome (CPPS) and chronic prostatitis in males and interstitial cystitis and other pelvic pain and dysfunction syndromes in females. Urination involves the use of higher cortical centers in the brains, pons, spinal cord, peripheral autonomic somatic and sensory efferent receptors and LUT, and the anatomic components of the LUT itself. Any disorder of these structures may contribute to symptoms of OAB.

Bladder level

OAB may have a myogenic origin; the prevailing theory for many years has been that myogenic abnormalities are a primary cause of overactive bladder. Treatment of these problems is based primarily on the use of acetylcholine (Ach) receptor antagonist (antimuscarinics or anticholinergics) that target muscarinic receptors (**Fig. 13**). However, it seems simplistic to think that there is a primary myogenic problem that affects the bladder without some form of myogenic processes that would affect other smooth muscles. It makes more sense to implicate a process that causes detrusor hyperplasia as a result of neurologic causes or outlet obstruction as the cause of these myogenic problems.

It is also apparent from the recent body of work that urgency and urge incontinence may be caused by sensory issues.[35] More recent data showing that there are sensory receptors in the bladder mucosa are starting to move away from an efferent-based muscular theory to a sensory vesicocentric theory. It seems more reasonable to believe that anticholinergics may work here preferentially, rather than in the muscle. If so, an approach that targets the afferent limb of the micturition process should be the mainstay of treatment. This approach would eventually treat the underlying

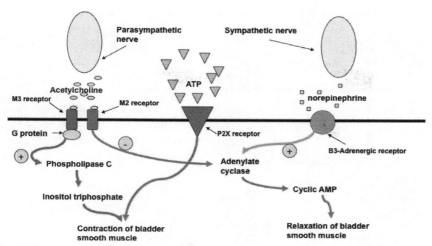

Fig. 13. Current concepts of autonomic efferent innervation contributing to bladder contraction and urine storage.

problem and eradicate the symptoms instead of concentrating only on the symptoms (muscular contractions), as has been the case for many years.

CNS Level

A working model of LUT control by higher brain centers has been pieced together by Griffith and Fowler[36] based on a compilation of functional MRI data in humans (**Fig. 14**). During the storage phase, ascending afferents synapse on the midbrain peri-aqueductal gray (PAG); they are relayed via the hypothalamus and thalamus to the dorsal ACG and to the right insula and to the lateral PFC; in the storage phase, they pass to the medial PFC (MPFC), where the decision to void or not may be made. If the decision is not to void, the situation is maintained by chronic inhibition of the PAG via a long pathway of serotonergic fibers from the MPFC; consequently, the pontine micturition center (PMC) is also suppressed, and voiding does not occur. When the decision to void is made, the MPFC relaxes its inhibition of the PAG and the hyothalamus also provides a safe signal along serotonergic pathways; consequently, the PAG excites the PMC, which in turn sends descending motor output along what seem to be also serotonergic neurons to the sacral spinal cord, which relaxes the urethral sphincter and contracts the detrusor so that voiding occurs. It seems that serotonin is a critical neurotransmitter in the micturition process, and imbalances in this neurotransmitter may lead to issues with micturition.[37]

Right superior frontal damage has been associated with transient urinary incontinence in adulthood.[38] Although bilateral frontal lobe damage is associated with persistent urge incontinence, in patients with SCZ, Hyde and colleagues[26] found that decreased volume of the right superior frontal gyrus was associated with persistent, yet transient, urinary incontinence in childhood (**Fig. 15**). This finding suggests that, at least in patients with SCZ, delayed or abnormal development of the right superior frontal gyrus (BA 9) may mediate childhood enuresis.

Recent work with functional MRI and positron emission tomography scanning indicates that the ACG may play a major role in the modulation of the sensation to void. These studies show that bladder fullness is associated with increased activity in the anterior midbrain.[36,39–44] Disturbances at these sites could explain the refractory

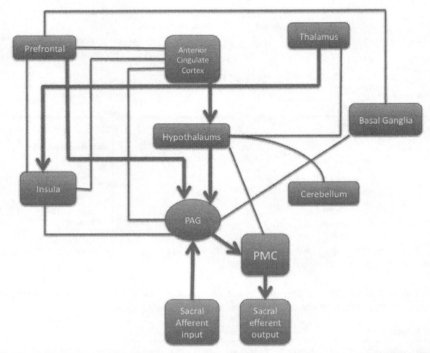

Fig. 14. A working model of LUT control by higher brain centers has been pieced together by Griffith and Fowler. This working model shows probable connections between forebrain and brainstem structures that are involved in the control of the bladder and sphincter in humans. Arrows show probable directions of connectivity but do not preclude connections in the opposite direction. The PMC remains the origin of the final pathway from brain to spinal cord. PAG, periaqueductal gray area; PMC, pontine micturition center.

nature of BBD in these patients. Standard therapy with anticholinergics and bowel regimens would be less likely to correct BBD in these patients. Drugs that would have an effect on the CNS either targeting the ACG or related pathways would be expected to work consistently in this group of patients. The association between cortical thinning and thickening in the ACG and MPFC also helps explain the high incidence of neuropsychiatric comorbidity in these children with functional elimination disorders.

An extensive review of the association of neuropsychiatric disorders and the role that they may play in dysfunctional elimination disorders was published in 2011.[45]

Serotonergic Pathways

A review of the physiology of micturition helps us understand that serotonergic activity emanating from the ACG facilitates urine storage by enhancing the sympathetic reflex pathway and inhibiting the parasympathetic voiding pathway. Sensory input during bladder filling results in an increase in the sympathetic tone. Norepinephrine (NA) release from the hypogastric nerve stimulates β_3 adrenergic receptors in the bladder to cause the smooth muscle to relax, as well as the α adrenoreceptors in the smooth muscle of the bladder neck and proximal urethra to contract. Ach released by the somatic pudendal nerve and the sacral nerve fibers elicits a contraction of the striated urethral sphincter and pelvic floor. Glutamate is believed to be the primary descending neurotransmitter for the storage reflex. Glutamate is released in the ventral horn of the

Gray Matter Volume Decreases in Controls with Enuresis compared with Controls without Enuresis

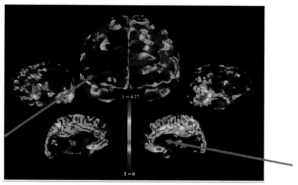

This figure depicts the statistical main effects of regional gray matter volume decreases in healthy controls with a history of childhood enuresis versus those without a history. The central figure is a frontal view, and the other figures, from left to right, are the left lateral, left medial, right medial, and right lateral hemispheric surface views.
The most significant cluster of reduced gray matter volume in healthy controls with enuresis is the left middle temporal gyrus, BA 22. There was also a cluster of decreased gray from the medial frontal gyrus, BA 11 extending into the subgenual cingulate

Fig. 15. Gray matter volume losses seen on functional MRI in controls.

sacral spinal cord (Onuf nucleus). In the Onuf nucleus, serotonergic axons projecting from the CNS synapse with the pudendal nerve. The release of glutamate activates the pudendal nerve and contracts the rhabdosphincter. The Onuf nucleus is densely populated with 5-hydroxytryptamine (5-HT) and NA terminals and contains a high density of 5-HT and NA receptors. There are data that indicate that 5-HT and NA play a modulatory role[46,47] in that they enhance the contraction of the rhabdosphincter but are not able to induce a contraction of the rhabdosphincter on their own.

Neurons expressing 5-HT and NA are concentrated in a few distinct nuclei in the brainstem (ie, medulla and pons). These neurons are involved in the fight-or-flight reflex, facilitating motor activity and inhibiting pain perception. They play a major role in the regulation of mood, pain perception, attention, temperature, gastrointestinal motility, sleep, sexual function, and micturition process.[47] These neurons are seen to connect to cortical centers, primarily in the anterior and posterior cingulate gyrus. Dysfunctions in the ACG and MPFC can lead to improper modulation of autonomic activity and an alteration in pain or sensory perception, which may be a critical component of BBD and LUTS.

BOWEL AND BLADDER INTERACTION
Treatment

Bowel
Children with BBD should be treated as if they are constipated, with initiation of a BP. The BP should include a diet that is high in fiber and high in daily fluid intake. Use of fiber supplements as a primary treatment should be discouraged, because many of the patients do not drink enough fluids during the day to make the supplements of value. In many instances, these children can become more constipated because the extrafiber without fluids, binds the stool even more. If stool is clearly palpable or if a KUB shows large amounts of stool, we instigate a bowel regimen with glycolax every day and a senna laxative once a week in some patients and in those who have significant issues or large

amounts of stool in the colon on KUB, we initiate a regimen that includes polyethylene glycol 3350 and in some cases senna laxatives daily for a 4-6 weeks typically.

In patients who have chronic abdominal pain or persistent constipation problems, we have successfully used tegaserod (a 5-HT$_4$ agonist that is no longer available) in an off-label manner.[48] A marked reduction in postvoid residual was found when the drug was used as well as a diminution in constipation and abdominal pain. These findings seem to confirm the link to a serotonergic mechanism to the BBD.

Once the patients have been on the bowel regimen for 4 to 6 weeks, we make adjustments based on the response to the glycolax as well as the senna. It is imperative to keep the patient on the bowel regimen throughout the treatment course, because it is necessary to keep the bowel emptying well when medications are added. In many instances, the anticholinergics are started as first-line therapy, and they tend to constipate the children. We have seen what appeared to be tachyphylaxis to the anticholinergics when the child had become constipated on the medication, and this had given the impression of recrudescence of the OAB symptoms and failure of the anticholinergics. Many parents argue that their children are not constipated and a KUB may help convince them that they are wrong.

Timed voiding and positive reinforcement

The first step in the treatment of pediatric BBD is to start the patient on a timed voiding regimen. This strategy is critical to help avoid detrusor contractions, which can occur as the bladder starts to reach the critical volume that triggers the contractions. The timed voiding regimen is linked to a positive reinforcement program and a calendar in which the child keeps track of the times that they void. The use of a vibratory watch is also a good option because it does not disturb other children in school and only the patient knows that it has gone off. Some children need to void only 5 times per day, whereas we may recommend that others void every 2 hours during the day. This situation depends on the severity of the symptoms and the functional bladder capacity. Bladder overstretching exercises have been found to be of no use in retraining children with BBD and may even exacerbate the problem by conditioning the child to contract the external sphincter with urination.

BIOFEEDBACK
Biofeedback Therapy

Biofeedback therapy has been used in urology for many years. The use of Kegel exercises was introduced to help patients with stress urinary incontinence. Subsequently, in the mid-1990s, biofeedback was introduced for managing children who had chronic wetting problems as well as an inability to empty the bladder completely. It has become the next line treatment after BPs and timed voiding have been deemed ineffective. We started performing biofeedback therapy in 1997 and our program has been successful.[49] Many children who failed the initial treatment with management of their constipation and showed signs of external sphincter dyssynergia undergo biofeedback therapy. A uroflow study with concomitant abdominal and perineal EMG is performed. This study then indicates the presence of external sphincter dyssynergia by increased activity in the perineal sphincter by EMG probe. If there is no increase in activity in the perineal sphincter probe and there is abdominal straining then the presence of internal sphincter dyssynergia is suggested by the study. If there is internal and external sphincter dyssynergia, treatment consists of the use of α-blockers as well as biofeedback. Each session lasts approximately 45 minutes, with a trained nurse performing the biofeedback therapy. Initial biofeedback therapy included the simple relaxation and contraction exercises while the patient monitored oscilloscopic activity of the perineum. The technology has evolved such that we now use a computerized system with a game-like interactive setting, in which the child attempts to move an icon of their choice (ie, dolphin, car, or bird) within the predetermined ranges that have been set. This system has facilitated the training process and lowered the age at which children can be treated. Preliminary data from our use of this program indicate a reduction in the number of biofeedback sessions required for children to master pelvic floor relaxation. Biofeedback therapy is limited by the ability of the child to cooperate with the health care provider running the session. Children younger than 5 years of age typically are incapable of receiving biofeedback on a regular basis. Occasionally, some children younger than 5 years can be taught to relax their pelvic floor muscles appropriately with biofeedback. Children with significant learning disabilities, behavior problems, and other neurologic problems are not candidates for biofeedback. Biofeedback therapy is useful in the management of BBD primarily by reducing the outlet resistance during voiding that leads to detrusor hypertrophy, thereby leading to detrusor instability. Our data along[23] with more recent work[50,51] reveal that biofeedback therapy is useful in the elimination of reflux in children who show evidence of external sphincter dyssynergia.

STIMULATION
Parasacral Stimulation with Transcutaneous Electrical Nerve Stimulation

Good results have been reported with parasacral transcutaneous electrical nerve stimulation (TENS) for OAB in adults and in children. TENS was first described in 1999 by Walsh and colleagues[52] and Hoebeke and colleagues,[53] respectively. Results with parasacral TENS for OAB have been consistent among the studies. Hoebeke and colleagues tested home parasacral TENS in 15 girls and 26 boys with refractory OAB. The current frequency used was 2 Hz. Parents performed the stimulation for 2 hours every day, for a period of 6 months. Thirteen (32%) children did not respond to the treatment. After 1 year, the rate of complete resolution of daytime incontinence was 51.2%. Bower and colleagues[54] applied home TENS in 17 children, using 1 or 2 sessions daily for 5 months with a frequency of 10 to 150 Hz. Of the children with daytime urinary incontinence, 47% had their symptoms resolved. Barroso and colleagues[55] prospectively randomized 25 girls and 12 boys with an average age of 7.6 years (range, 4–12 years) into the test group (ambulatory parasacral TENS) or sham group (ambulatory TENS on the scapular area).[55] Twenty sessions, 20 minutes each (10 Hz), were performed 3 times per week in each group. After completion of the sessions, the control individuals who were not cured underwent active treatment. A total of 21 patients in the test group and 16 in the sham group underwent treatment. Among the active treatment group, 61.9% of parents reported complete resolution of the symptoms. In the sham group, no parent reported cure ($P<.001$). After sham stimulation, 13 of the 16 patients who underwent parasacral TENS had a full response. Standard urotherapy is time consuming, requires a significant time investment to be effective, and does not work well as the single therapy in children with pronounced OAB. There seems to be efficacy with this modality for patients who are not the most difficult patients to treat.

TIBIAL
Peripheral Nerve Stimulation

Electrical posterior tibial nerve stimulation (PTNS) is based on the traditional Chinese practice of using acupuncture points over the common peroneal posterior tibial nerves to inhibit bladder activity.[56] The posterior tibial nerve is a peripheral mixed sensory motor nerve, originating from the spinal roots L4 to S3, which also contribute to sensory and motor control of the bladder, sphincter, and pelvic floor. PTNS afferent stimulation provides central inhibition of preganglionic bladder motor neurons through a direct route in the sacral cord.[57] This theory has been recently supported by a study on long latency somatosensory-evoked potentials, which reported differences between patients and those in the sham group and hypothesized a plastic reorganization of cortical network triggered by PTNS.[58] Transcutaneous PTNS has been evaluated in clinical trials with variable results. The technique involved using a 34-gauge stainless steel needle, which is inserted approximately 5 cm cephalad to the medial malleolus just posterior to the margin of the tibia. A stick-on electrode is placed on the medial surface of the calcaneus (**Fig. 16**). More substantial data are necessary, but reports in adults indicate that it is beneficial. Limited reports of its use in children have indicated efficacy as well. One study by Hoebeke and colleagues[59] showed that 17 of 28 children who had been refractory to medical treatment had a resolution or improvement in their symptoms. Sixteen of 19 patients who had abnormal frequency showed marked improvement, and overall for the group, mean bladder capacity increased significantly. Degennaro and colleagues[60] Recently, analyzed long-term results of their longitudinal cohort of children, obtaining level 3 evidence evaluating PTNS efficacy and durability of results. Improvement was significantly greater ($P<.002$) in nonneurogenic (78%) than in neurogenic (14%) patients. Among nonneurogenic LUT disease, at 2-year follow-up 5 of 12 (41%) children with OAB and 10 of 14 (71%) with dysfunctional voiding (DV) were completely cured (**Table 1**). By repeating a second PTNS cycle and by maintaining chronic monthly stimulation, 9 additional children (5 with OAB and 4 with DV) resolved LUTS, which relapsed 1 year after the first PTNS cycle. Overall, at long-term follow-up, 10 of 12 children with OAB and 14 of 14 patients with DV were asymptomatic; chronic PTNS was required in 50% and 29% of children, respectively, with OAB or DV, to maintain results.[60] These studies indicate a role for an improvement in BBD in children with peripheral nerve stimulation. On the other hand, our own experience with this modality in a limited number of patients has not been as positive as that of Hoebeke and colleagues or DeGennaro and colleagues. It could be that we selected patients who had failed all other treatment modalities, and difficult patients may not respond so readily.

Cooper and colleagues[61] reported on the use of TENS to treat incontinence and urinary frequency. This treatment does not seem to be highly effective for incontinence and the results were no better than anticholinergics for urinary frequency.

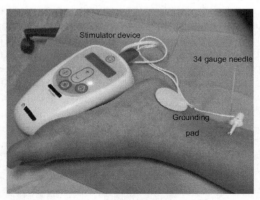

Fig. 16. Percutaneous PTNS using a 34-gauge needle.

Table 1
Studies that have used electrical stimulation

Author/Year	LUTD	Number of Patients[a]	Stimulation	Frequency/Intensity	Treatment Period	Follow-up	LUTS Improvement Rate (%)
Bower et al,[54] 2001	OAB	14	2 h/daily	10 Hz —[a]	1 mo	1 mo	73
Hoebeke et al,[53] 2001	OAB	41	2 h/daily	2 Hz —[a]	6 mo	1 y	51
Barroso et al,[86] 2006	OAB	19	20 min/session 3 sessions/wk	10 Hz 6–42 mA[a]	1–6 wk	1 y	63
Malm Buatsi et al,[61] 2007	OAB	18	20 min/session twice daily	— 0–60 mA[a]	8 ± 7 mo	1 y	73
Lordelo et al,[55] 2010	OAB	21	20 min/session 3 sessions/wk	10 Hz —[a]	7 wk	7 wk	61.9
Hoebeke et al,[59] 2002	OAB	31	30 min/session 1 session/wk	20 Hz 1–10 mA[a]	12 wk	3 mo	Urge: 60 Increase: 17 Frequency: 84
De Gennaro et al,[87] 2004	OAB DV	10 7	30 min/session 1 session/wk	20 Hz 1–10 mA[a]	12 wk	3 mo	OAB: 80 DV: 71
Capitanucci et al,[60] 2009	OAB DV	14 14	30 min/session 1 session/wk	20 Hz 1–10 mA[a]	12 wk + maintenance (1 session/mo)	2 y DV: 100	OAB: 83

[a] Sensory threshold.

SPINAL

Spinal cord stimulation has been used with increasing regularity in adult patients. In 20 prospectively followed patients described by Roth and colleagues,[58] resolution or greater than 50% improvement occurred in 88% of children with urinary incontinence, 63% with nocturnal enuresis, 89% with daytime frequency, and 59% with constipation. Complications commonly cited with Sacral Nerve Stimulation (SNS) are device or wound infection, electrode migration, loss of effect, and lead fracture. Revision rates range between 7% and 18% because of lead migration, faulty connection, and wound infection. Revisions have also been necessary because of uncomfortable buzzing or painful sensations and battery replacement. The role of spinal stimulation in children is yet to be well defined and more studies are needed to find out if it is worthwhile in children.

MEDICATIONS
Anticholinergics

Many classes of drugs have been studied or proposed for the treatment of symptoms of OAB in adults. Five antimuscarinics are currently approved in the United States for the treatment of OAB: darifenacin, oxybutynin, solifenacin, tolterodine, and trospium. (A sixth, propiverine, is available in Europe.) Studies of these agents have shown similar efficacy (70%–75%) for decreasing urge incontinence episodes. Only 2 antimuscarinics have formally achieved approval for use in children (oxybutynin and tolterodine) and 2 are in the process of obtaining approval. Several pitfalls limit the quality of clinical studies: heterogeneity of the patients and their symptoms and the fact that many patients can have more than 1 confounding problem. The clinical trials performed in children have generally used patients with neurogenic voiding problems and have not concentrated on the nonneurogenic patients.

Recent data suggest that antimuscarinics are functioning on the sensory limb of the reflex arc in neurologically intact patients more so than on the motor side.[62] Antimuscarinics are active during the filling/storage phase of micturition when there is no activity in the cholinergic nerves. Ach can be generated and released from the urothelium and also may leak from the cholinergic nerves during bladder filling,[35] binding to M_2 and M_3 receptors. Five subtypes of muscarinic receptors are recognized and the bladder smooth muscle has 2 known subtypes (M_2 [70%–80%] and M_3 [20%–30%]) that predominate. M_3 receptors have been shown to evoke smooth muscle contraction, which is the primary stimulus for bladder contraction. It has been postulated that M_2 and M_3 receptors are involved not only in motor (efferent) activation but also in sensory (afferent) activation. The activation of M_2 receptors may reverse sympathetically mediated smooth muscle relaxation during the filling/storage phase of micturition; there are additional mechanisms by which M_2 receptors may cause smooth muscle contraction. M_1 receptors are found in the brain, glands (eg, salivary), and sympathetic ganglia, which account for most of the side effects noted with antimuscarinic drugs. Although dry mouth is the most common symptom, constipation, gastroesophageal reflux, blurry vision, urinary retention, and cognitive side effects can also occur; these symptoms are generally less bothersome in children. Adverse cognitive effects and delirium caused by antimuscarinic drugs can occur in children, but are generally limited to overdosing situations. In adult trials, quantitative electroencephalographic data suggest that oxybutynin has more CNS effects than trospium or tolterodine.[63,64] Long-acting anticholinergic agents and newer, more selective antimuscarinic agents should be tested for clinically important cognitive side effects.

Oxybutynin is a nonselective antimuscarinic agent that relaxes bladder muscles and has local anesthetic activity. It is available in immediate and extended-release forms, as well as in a transdermal patch. Immediate-release oxybutynin seems to be efficacious for the treatment of neurogenic and nonneurogenic overactivity of the detrusor muscle with urge incontinence. The efficacy of immediate-release oxybutynin has been limited by antimuscarinic side effects (dry mouth) of the parent drug and its active metabolite (N-desethyloxybutynin). Generic immediate-release oxybutynin is inexpensive and may be useful for patients whose symptoms are best managed by a short-acting drug (eg, symptoms that are bothersome only when the patient is away from home or at night). A once daily controlled-release formulation of oxybutynin seems to have the same beneficial effects as immediate-release oxybutynin, with fewer side effects, a benefit ascribed to the more constant levels of the parent drug and, possibly, a lower rate of conversion to the active metabolite in the stomach and small intestine.[64] A transdermal oxybutynin patch is also available that is as efficacious as immediate-release oxybutynin but with half the incidence of dry mouth.[65,66] In 1 placebo-controlled trial, the patch caused local skin erythema in more than half the subjects (3% of cases were severe) and was associated with pruritus in up to 17%.[49] Oxybutynin has been instilled intravesicularly through a catheter to treat severe overactivity of the detrusor muscle in patients with neurogenic bladders, with minimal side effects, but its use is of limited value in children with nonneurogenic problems.

Tolterodine is a muscarinic antagonist that is available in short-acting (twice daily) and long-acting (once daily) preparations. Side effects are similar to those of short-acting oxybutynin, with dry mouth in 20% to 25% of patients, and the rates of discontinuation because of side effects are similar to those for placebo (5%–6%). Randomized controlled trials indicate that propiverine and trospium are effective for the treatment of urge incontinence and have fewer side effects than short-acting oxybutynin.[67–70] Trospium is currently available in the United States; propiverine is not available. Hyoscyamine, like short-acting oxybutynin, may be useful for some patients with intermittent symptoms or under specific circumstances; it can be associated with prominent side effects. Propantheline has proven efficacy for the treatment of urge incontinence, but the need for multiple daily doses and the high incidence of side effects are drawbacks. At least 2 new antimuscarinic drugs (darifenacin and solifenacin) with selective M3-receptor antagonist actions and, theoretically, fewer systemic anticholinergic side effects than currently available agents are yet to be studied in children, with limited anecdotal data available for these drugs in children.

α-Blockers

α-Blockers are playing a larger role in the management of OAB in our practice. Aside from the role that they play in the management of bladder neck dysfunction and urinary retention, we have found them to be useful in ameliorating the symptoms of urgency and urge incontinence in some children.[71] Early work on the benefits of α-blockers on nonneuropathic voiding dysfunction by Austin and Homsy[72] pioneered the introduction of α-blockers into the armamentarium of drugs that are used to treat voiding problems in children. In many cases, terazosin is our first-line drug for urgency and frequency because of its nonselective properties and the potential to cross the blood-brain barrier. More selective α-blockers such as tamusolin and alfuzosin are better suited for management of bladder neck dysfunction, which can lead to detrusor hypertrophy and instability. Because nonselective α-blockers can cause postural hypotension, they require a gradual titration of the dose and must be used carefully. In patients with a family history of easy fainting or postural hypotension, dose titration is essential even with the selective α-blockers. For the most part, children tolerate α-blockade well and we have used terazosin in children as young as 1 year old for bladder neck dysfunction associated with high-grade vesicoureteral reflux or spina bifida. Further research is needed to determine the optimal use of α-blockers and anti-cholinergic drugs alone, together, or combined with behavioral therapy as a treatment of overactive bladder.

Tricyclics

We have found imipramine, a tricyclic antidepressant with both anticholinergic and α-adrenergic effects and, possibly, a central effect on voiding reflexes, to be effective in controlling urge incontinence in some children who were refractory to antimuscarinic therapy.[73] Imipramine can cause postural hypotension and cardiac-conduction abnormalities and thus must be used carefully. Amitriptyline (another tricyclic) has been used more frequently for the management of interstitial cystitis and OAB in adults, and its use in children is limited.

Selective Serotonin Reuptake Inhibitors

Selective serotonin reuptake inhibitors and selective norepinephrine reuptake inhibitors have been useful in older patients with BBD, especially when there is evidence of anxiety disorders of clinical significance. We have found that management of the underlying neuropsychiatric at the central level can resolve the problem in many cases. In other cases, the addition of an antimuscarinic may help the patient achieve continence.

OTHER DRUGS

Although currently available β-agonists have not been shown to be useful for overactive bladder, more selective β$_3$-agonists may have therapeutic value.

Drugs that act by means of adenosine triphosphate-sensitive potassium-channel transporters to hyperpolarize smooth muscle and decrease spontaneous bladder contractions may be useful for suppressing involuntary bladder contractions without interfering with normal voiding.[74] However, first-generation agents in this class have had effects on vascular smooth muscle and can cause hypotension.

Drugs that act on sensory afferent pathways are also being developed and hold promise when used either alone or in combination with other drugs. Vanilloids such as capsaicin and resiniferatoxin activate nociceptive sensory nerve fibers through an ion channel, known as vanilloid receptor subtype. This receptor is a nonselective cation channel that is activated by heat and protons, suggesting that it functions as a transducer of painful thermal stimuli and acidity in vivo. Vanilloid receptors are located predominantly on C-fiber bladder afferents, and activating the receptors initially excites and subsequently desensitizes C-fibers. Resiniferatoxin seems to be more potent and less irritating than capsaicin, but is no longer available for clinical use. Other drugs that block receptors on sensory afferents, such as neurokinin receptor antagonists, might not cause urinary retention, which can occur with antimuscarinic agents.

The role of phosphodiesterase inhibitors in BBD needs further exploration and only time will tell if it may also play a useful role.[75–78]

INJECTABLE THERAPY
Botulinum A Toxin for the Sphincter

Botulinum A toxin is the most potent biologic toxin known. The toxin acts at the neuromuscular junction at the external sphincter to block vesicle transport of Ach, in essence producing chemical denervation. Clinical effects begin within 5 to 7 days and are reversible, because terminal resprouting occurs within 6 months. The clinical success of botulinum A toxin is supported by laboratory research showing marked decreases in the release of labeled NA and Ach in rat bladders and urethras injected with botulinum A toxin. Although the therapeutic effects of inhibiting Ach release are obvious, blocking NA release may provide clinical benefit by inhibiting sympathetic transmission in smooth muscle dyssynergia. For this reason, some of the patients who we have treated who have combined internal and external dyssynergia have responded well to botulinum A toxin injections.[79]

Botulinum A toxin has also been used to inject the bladder to reduce detrusor hyperactivity. Studies in adult patients with spinal cord injury and children with myelodysplasia and spinal cord lesions have indicated success with multiple injections occurring throughout the floor of the bladder. There seems to be no evidence of tachyphylaxis even with multiple repeat injections.[80] Botulinum A toxin injections of the detrusor have been performed for nonneurogenic OAB in symptomatic adults with some success. One of the drawbacks of this treatment is the need for retreatment, because the probable underlying cause is not in the bladder but elsewhere. Hoebeke and colleagues[81] published their experience in 15 children indicating that durable (>12 months) relief of symptoms could be achieved in more than 50% of the patients with a single injection. These findings are encouraging and could help further the treatment of OAB in children in whom the cause is not sphincter dyssynergia.

On the other hand, the use of botulinum A toxin injections for sphincter dyssynergia seems to be beneficial. With the elimination of the dyssynergic voiding pattern, there is elimination of detrusor hypertrophy, which is commonly associated with detrusor overactivity. Botulinum A toxin injection produces a reversible chemical sphincterotomy, which avoids a major surgical procedure with its attendant risks. Botulinum A toxin has been used to treat patients with spinal cord injury with detrusor sphincter dyssynergia (DSD) in adults and children with spina bifida. Its use to treat nonneurogenic DSD was described by Steinhardt[82] in a neurologically normal child in 1997. More recently, a larger series of 20 patients presented by Radojicic and colleagues[83] indicates that the treatment of DSD is clearly helped by the use of botulinum A toxin injections in neurologically normal children. We have had exceptionally good results in children in whom we used botulinum A toxin to treat external sphincter dyssynergia of nonneurogenic origin.[84] We injected 12 patients with botulinum A toxin with 300 units in and around the external sphincter, all 12 patients responded well to the injections, with no adverse effects. Only 1 patient had to be reinjected more then once. One patient on intermittent catheterization was unable to empty her bladder, leaving a postvoid residual of 250 mL at a time. This child is completely dry, has no accidents, and voids to completion 5 years after injection. Another child had been offered augmentation cystoplasty to manage his intractable wetting and severe DSD, leading to chronic epididymitis (**Fig. 17**). In the limited studies that we have available, botulinum A toxin represents a viable option for treating DSD. Correction of the DSD has led to resolution of the associated OAB symptoms.

URETHRAL OVERDISTENTION

Management of OAB and bladder instability by the use of urethral dilation has been going on for many years. Many young girls had their urethras dilated and continue to have their urethras dilated as adults. Many of these women have classic symptoms of overactive bladder, pelvic discomfort, dysuria, and recurrent UTIs. This mechanism of overdilation probably works in a similar fashion to the use of botulinum A toxin at the level of the external sphincter. This temporary sphincterotomy occurs either by overdistention or by tearing of the sphincter muscles. Central neural processes may lead to resetting of receptors in the spinal cord and possibly in the brain, which may lead to decreased activity of the sphincter. This decrease in sphincter activity leads to

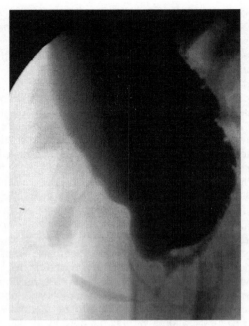

Fig. 17. 10-year-old male with history of recurrent epididymitis and urinary infection, before treatment with botulinum toxin A and ritalin.

improved bladder emptying because of reduced outlet resistance, thereby allowing the detrusor muscle in the bladder to not work so hard. This decrease in detrusor activity in turn is translated to possible reduction in overactivity at the bladder level.[85]

SUMMARY

Pediatric BBD is a common problem that needs to be addressed aggressively in childhood to help prevent potentially irreversible adult complications of the disease. As we gain greater understanding of the disease process, it is clear that, except for a few patients who develop BBD because of some transient bout of constipation or viral illness, it is a problem that tends to linger throughout life and manifests itself in many different ways, ranging from frequency and urgency to the more profoundly affected who go on to develop interstitial cystitis or CPPS.

The hallmark of treatment has been the use of a BP and timed voiding regimen. The use of biofeedback has helped many other children correct their errant voiding patterns and therefore correct their OAB and prevent it from being carried into adulthood. The use of drugs to treat OAB shows increased promise as we understand the disease process more. It seems that the sensory limb of the voiding reflex is the primary target for continued pharmacologic treatment. Numerous other treatment modalities are available for patients who have failed pharmacologic therapy, but in most of these therapies, the problems seem to go back to the sensory limb of the voiding reflex. The continued use of stimulation modalities (whether peripheral or central) needs continued exploration in the future. The complexity and difficulties that are encountered in clinical studies in children need to be overcome to allow greater advancement in this field.

REFERENCES

1. Ruarte AC, Quesada EM. Urodynamic evaluation in children. In: Retik A, Cukier J, editors. International Perspectives in Urology: Pediatric Urology, vol. 14. Baltimore (MD): Williams and wilkins; 1987. p. 114–24.
2. Landgraf JM, Abidari J, Cilento BG Jr, et al. Coping, commitment, and attitude: quantifying the everyday burden of enuresis on children and their families. Pediatrics 2004;113:334–44.
3. Fitzgerald MP, Thom DH, Wassel-Fyr C, et al. Childhood urinary symptoms predict adult overactive bladder symptoms. J Urol 2006;175:989–93.
4. Minassian VA, Lovatsis D, Pascali D, et al. Effect of childhood dysfunctional voiding on urinary incontinence in adult women. Obstet Gynecol 2006;107:1247–51.
5. Stone JJ, Rozzelle CJ, Greenfield SP. Intractable voiding dysfunction in children with normal spinal imaging: predictors of failed conservative management. Urology 2010;75:161–5.
6. Neveus T, von Gontard A, Hoebeke P, et al. The standardization of terminology of lower urinary tract function in children and adolescents: report from the Standardisation Committee of the International Children's Continence Society. J Urol 2006; 176:314–24.
7. Mattsson SH. Voiding frequency, volumes and intervals in healthy schoolchildren. Scand J Urol Nephrol 1994;28:1–11.
8. Herz D, Weiser A, Collette T, et al. Dysfunctional elimination syndrome as an etiology of idiopathic urethritis in childhood. J Urol 2005;173:2132–7.
9. Lettgen B, von Gontard A, Olbing H, et al. Urge incontinence and voiding postponement in children: somatic and psychosocial factors. Acta Paediatr 2002;91: 978–84 [discussion: 895–6].
10. Warne SA, Godley ML, Wilcox DT. Surgical reconstruction of cloacal malformation can alter bladder function: a comparative study with anorectal anomalies. J Urol 2004;172:2377–81 [discussion: 81].
11. Pezzone MA, Liang R, Fraser MO. A model of neural cross-talk and irritation in the pelvis: implications for the overlap of chronic pelvic pain disorders. Gastroenterology 2005;128:1953–64.
12. Ustinova EE, Fraser MO, Pezzone MA. Colonic irritation in the rat sensitizes urinary bladder afferents to mechanical and chemical stimuli: an afferent origin of pelvic organ cross-sensitization. Am J Physiol Renal Physiol 2006;290: F1478–87.
13. Loening-Baucke V. Prevalence rates for constipation and faecal and urinary incontinence. Arch Dis Child 2007;92:486–9.
14. Tekgul S, Nijman RJ, Hoebeke P, et al. Diagnosis and management of urinary incontinence in children. In: Cardozo L, Abrams P, Khoury S, et al, editors. Incontinence. 4th edition. Paris: Health Publications Ltd; 2009. p. 701–92.
15. Gontard AV, Nevéus T. Management of disorders of bladder and bowel control in childhood. London: Mac Keith Press; 2006. p. xi, 355.
16. Joinson C, Heron J, Butler U, et al. Psychological differences between children with and without soiling problems. Pediatrics 2006;117:1575–84.
17. Joinson C, Heron J, von Gontard A, et al. Early childhood risk factors associated with daytime wetting and soiling in school-age children. J Pediatr Psychol 2008; 33:739–50.
18. Sureshkumar P, Jones M, Cumming R, et al. A population based study of 2,856 school-age children with urinary incontinence. J Urol 2009;181:808–15 [discussion: 15–6].

19. Robson WL, Jackson HP, Blackhurst D, et al. Enuresis in children with attention-deficit hyperactivity disorder. South Med J 1997;90:503–5.
20. Bael A, Winkler P, Lax H, et al. Behavior profiles in children with functional urinary incontinence before and after incontinence treatment. Pediatrics 2008;121: e1196–200.
21. Botlero R, Bell RJ, Urquhart DM, et al. Urinary incontinence is associated with lower psychological general well-being in community-dwelling women. Menopause 2010;17:332–7.
22. Melville JL, Fan MY, Rau H, et al. Major depression and urinary incontinence in women: temporal associations in an epidemiologic sample. Am J Obstet Gynecol 2009;201:490 e1–7.
23. Henin A, Biederman J, Mick E, et al. Childhood antecedent disorders to bipolar disorder in adults: a controlled study. J Affect Disord 2007;99:51–7.
24. Weissman MM, Gross R, Fyer A, et al. Interstitial cystitis and panic disorder: a potential genetic syndrome. Arch Gen Psychiatry 2004;61:273–9.
25. Moore KH, Sutherst JR. Response to treatment of detrusor instability in relation to psychoneurotic status. Br J Urol 1990;66:486–90.
26. Hyde TM, Deep-Soboslay A, Iglesias B, et al. Enuresis as a premorbid developmental marker of schizophrenia. Brain 2008;131:2489–98.
27. Bael A, Lax H, de Jong, et al. The relevance of urodynamic studies for urge syndrome and dysfunctional voiding: a multicenter controlled trial in children. J Urol 2008;180:1486–93 [discussion: 94–5].
28. Nogueira M, Greenfield SP, Wan J, et al. Tethered cord in children: a clinical classification with urodynamic correlation. J Urol 2004;172:1677–80 [discussion: 80].
29. Homsy Y, Austin P, editors. Dysfunctional voiding disorders and nocturnal enuresis. London: Martin Dunitz; 2002. p. 345–70.
30. McVary KT, Rademaker A, Lloyd GL, et al. Autonomic nervous system overactivity in men with lower urinary tract symptoms secondary to benign prostatic hyperplasia. J Urol 2005;174:1327–433.
31. Gonen M, Kalkan M, Cenker A, et al. Prevalence of premature ejaculation in Turkish men with chronic pelvic pain syndrome. J Androl 2005;26:601–3.
32. Seftel A. Correlation between LUTS (AUA-SS) and erectile dysfunction (SHIM) in an age-matched racially diverse male population: data from the prostate cancer awareness week (PCAW). J Urol 2005;174:1940.
33. Muller A, Mulhall JP. Sexual dysfunction in the patient with prostatitis. Curr Opin Urol 2005;15:404–9.
34. Rosen H, Swigar ME. Depression and normal pressure hydrocephalus. A dilemma in neuropsychiatric differential diagnosis. J Nerv Ment Dis 1976;163:35–40.
35. Wein AJ, Rackley RR. Overactive bladder: a better understanding of pathophysiology, diagnosis and management. J Urol 2006;175:S5–10.
36. Fowler CJ, Griffiths DJ. A decade of functional brain imaging applied to bladder control. Neurourol Urodyn 2010;29:49–55.
37. Cheng CL, de Groat WC. Role of 5-HT1A receptors in control of lower urinary tract function in anesthetized rats. Am J Physiol Renal Physiol 2010;298: F771–8.
38. Mochizuki H, Saito H. Mesial frontal lobe syndromes: correlations between neurological deficits and radiological localizations. Tohoku J Exp Med 1990; 161(Suppl):231–9.
39. Griffiths D, Tadic SD. Bladder control, urgency, and urge incontinence: evidence from functional brain imaging. Neurourol Urodyn 2008;27:466–74.

40. Kuhtz-Buschbeck JP, van der Horst C, Pott C, et al. Cortical representation of the urge to void: a functional magnetic resonance imaging study. J Urol 2005;174: 1477–81.
41. Matsuura S, Kakizaki H, Mitsui T, et al. Human brain region response to distention or cold stimulation of the bladder: a positron emission tomography study. J Urol 2002;168:2035–9.
42. Griffiths D, Derbyshire S, Stenger A, et al. Brain control of normal and overactive bladder. J Urol 2005;174:1862–7.
43. DasGupta R. Different brain effects during chronic and acute sacral neuromodulation in urge incontinent patients with implanted neurostimulators. BJU Int 2007; 99:700.
44. Kavia R, Dasgupta R, Critchley H, et al. A functional magnetic resonance imaging study of the effect of sacral neuromodulation on brain responses in women with Fowler's syndrome. BJU Int 2010;105:366–72.
45. Franco I. Neuropsychiatric disorders and voiding problems in children. Curr Urol Rep 2011;12:158–65.
46. Oelke M, Roovers JP, Michel MC. Safety and tolerability of duloxetine in women with stress urinary incontinence. BJOG 2006;113(Suppl 1):22–6.
47. Schuessler B. What do we know about duloxetine's mode of action? Evidence from animals to humans. BJOG 2006;113(Suppl 1):5–9.
48. Franco I, Cagliostro S, Collett-Gardere T, et al. Treatment of lower urinary tract symptoms in children with constipation using tegaserod therapy. Urotoday Int J 2010;3:5784–92.
49. Palmer LS, Franco I, Rotario P, et al. Biofeedback therapy expedites the resolution of reflux in older children. J Urol 2002;168:1699–702 [discussion: 702–3].
50. Kibar Y, Demir E, Irkilata C, et al. Effect of biofeedback treatment on spinning top urethra in children with voiding dysfunction. Urology 2007;70:781–4 [discussion: 84–5].
51. Kibar Y, Ors O, Demir E, et al. Results of biofeedback treatment on reflux resolution rates in children with dysfunctional voiding and vesicoureteral reflux. Urology 2007;70:563–6 [discussion: 66–7].
52. Walsh IK, Johnston RS, Keane PF. Transcutaneous sacral neurostimulation for irritative voiding dysfunction. Eur Urol 1999;35:192–6.
53. Hoebeke P, Van Laecke E, Everaert K, et al. Transcutaneous neuromodulation for the urge syndrome in children: a pilot study. J Urol 2001;166:2416–9.
54. Bower WF, Moore KH, Adams RD. A pilot study of the home application of transcutaneous neuromodulation in children with urgency or urge incontinence. J Urol 2001;166:2420–2.
55. Lordelo P, Teles A, Veiga ML, et al. Transcutaneous electrical nerve stimulation in children with overactive bladder: a randomized clinical trial. J Urol 2010;184: 683–9.
56. van Balken MR, Vergunst H, Bemelmans BL, et al. The use of electrical devices for the treatment of bladder dysfunction: a review of methods. J Urol 2004;172: 846–51.
57. Amarenco G, Ismael SS, Even-Schneider A, et al. Urodynamic effect of acute transcutaneous posterior tibial nerve stimulation in overactive bladder. J Urol 2003;169:2210–5.
58. Roth TJ, Vandersteen DR, Hollatz P, et al. Sacral neuromodulation for the dysfunctional elimination syndrome: a single center experience with 20 children. J urol 2008;180:306–11.

59. Hoebeke P, Renson C, Petillon L, et al. Percutaneous electrical nerve stimulation in children with therapy resistant nonneuropathic bladder sphincter dysfunction: a pilot study. J Urol 2002;168:2605–7 [discussion: 7–8].

60. Capitanucci ML, Camanni D, Demelas F, et al. Long-term efficacy of percutaneous tibial nerve stimulation for different types of lower urinary tract dysfunction in children. J Urol 2009;182:2056–61.

61. Malm-Buatsi E, Nepple KG, Boyt MA, et al. Efficacy of transcutaneous electrical nerve stimulation in children with overactive bladder refractory to pharmacotherapy. Urology 2007;70:980–3.

62. Finney SM, Andersson KE, Gillespie JI, et al. Antimuscarinic drugs in detrusor overactivity and the overactive bladder syndrome: motor or sensory actions? BJU Int 2006;98:503–7.

63. Todorova A, Vonderheid-Guth B, Dimpfel W. Effects of tolterodine, trospium chloride, and oxybutynin on the central nervous system. J Clin Pharmacol 2001;41:636–44.

64. Gupta SK, Sathyan G, Lindemulder EA, et al. Quantitative characterization of therapeutic index: application of mixed-effects modeling to evaluate oxybutynin dose-efficacy and dose-side effect relationships. Clin Pharmacol Ther 1999;65: 672–84.

65. Davila GW, Daugherty CA, Sanders SW. A short-term, multicenter, randomized double-blind dose titration study of the efficacy and anticholinergic side effects of transdermal compared to immediate release oral oxybutynin treatment of patients with urge urinary incontinence. J Urol 2001;166:140–5.

66. Dmochowski RR, Davila GW, Zinner NR, et al. Efficacy and safety of transdermal oxybutynin in patients with urge and mixed urinary incontinence. J Urol 2002;168: 580–6.

67. Madersbacher H, Halaska M, Voigt R, et al. A placebo-controlled, multicentre study comparing the tolerability and efficacy of propiverine and oxybutynin in patients with urgency and urge incontinence. BJU Int 1999;84:646–51.

68. Madersbacher H, Murtz G. Efficacy, tolerability and safety profile of propiverine in the treatment of the overactive bladder (non-neurogenic and neurogenic). World J Urol 2001;19:324–35.

69. Mazur D, Wehnert J, Dorschner W, et al. Clinical and urodynamic effects of propiverine in patients suffering from urgency and urge incontinence. A multicentre dose-optimizing study. Scand J Urol Nephrol 1995;29:289–94.

70. Madersbacher H, Stohrer M, Richter R, et al. Trospium chloride versus oxybutynin: a randomized, double-blind, multicentre trial in the treatment of detrusor hyper-reflexia. Br J Urol 1995;75:452–6.

71. Franco I, Cagliostro S, Collett T, et al. The use of alpha blockers to treat urgency/frequency syndrome in children presented at the American Academy of Pediatrics Meeting. San Francisco (CA): October 2007.

72. Austin PF, Homsy YL, Masel JL, et al. alpha-Adrenergic blockade in children with neuropathic and nonneuropathic voiding dysfunction. J Urol 1999;162:1064–7.

73. Young R, Kwon EO, Collett T, et al. Imipramine for refractory pediatric overactive bladder syndrome. Boston: American Academy of Pediatrics; 2008.

74. Martin SW, Radley SC, Chess-Williams R, et al. Relaxant effects of potassium-channel openers on normal and hyper-reflexic detrusor muscle. Br J Urol 1997; 80:405–13.

75. Oger S, Behr-Roussel D, Gorny D, et al. Relaxation of phasic contractile activity of human detrusor strips by cyclic nucleotide phosphodiesterase type 4 inhibition. Eur Urol 2007;51:772–80 [discussion: 80–1].

76. Werkstrom V, Svensson A, Andersson KE, et al. Phosphodiesterase 5 in the female pig and human urethra: morphological and functional aspects. BJU Int 2006;98:414–23.
77. Tadalafil (Cialis) for signs and symptoms of benign prostatic hyperplasia. Med Lett Drugs Ther 2011;53:89–90.
78. Donatucci CF, Brock GB, Goldfischer ER, et al. Tadalafil administered once daily for lower urinary tract symptoms secondary to benign prostatic hyperplasia: a 1-year, open-label extension study. BJU Int 2011;107:1110–6.
79. Smith CP, Chancellor MB. Emerging role of botulinum toxin in the management of voiding dysfunction. J Urol 2004;171:2128–37.
80. Akbar M, Abel R, Seyler TM, et al. Repeated botulinum-A toxin injections in the treatment of myelodysplastic children and patients with spinal cord injuries with neurogenic bladder dysfunction. BJU Int 2007;100:639–45.
81. Hoebeke P, De Caestecker K, Vande Walle J, et al. The effect of botulinum-A toxin in incontinent children with therapy resistant overactive detrusor. J Urol 2006;176: 328–30 [discussion: 30–1].
82. Steinhardt GF, Naseer S, Cruz OA. Botulinum toxin: novel treatment for dramatic urethral dilatation associated with dysfunctional voiding. J Urol 1997;158:190–1.
83. Radojicic ZI, Perovic SV, Milic NM. Is it reasonable to treat refractory voiding dysfunction in children with botulinum-A toxin? J Urol 2006;176:332–6 [discussion: 36].
84. Franco I, Landau-Dyer L, Isom-Batz G, et al. The use of botulinum toxin A injection for the management of external sphincter dyssynergia in neurologically normal children. J Urol 2007;178:1775–9 [discussion: 79–80].
85. Bloom DA, Knechtel JM, McGuire EJ. Urethral dilation improves bladder compliance in children with myelomeningocele and high leak point pressures. J Urol 1990;144:430–3 [discussion: 43–4].
86. Barroso U Jr, Lordêlo P, Lopes AA, et al. Nonpharmacological treatment of lower urinary tract dysfunction using biofeedback and transcutaneous electrical stimulation: a pilot study. BJU Int 2006;98(1):166–71.
87. De Gennaro M, Capitanucci ML, Mastracci P, et al. Percutaneous tibial nerve neuromodulation is well tolerated in children and effective for treating refractory vesical dysfunction. J Urol 2004;171(5):1911–3.

Current Options in the Management of Primary Vesicoureteral Reflux in Children

Fernando F. Fonseca, MD, Fabio Y. Tanno, MD, Hiep T. Nguyen, MD*

KEYWORDS

- Vesicoureteral reflux • Children • Management • Ureteral reimplant • Antibiotics
- Urinary tract infection

KEY POINTS

- Children with VUR have different risks for urinary tract infection and renal injury.
- The majority of children with VUR have low grade reflux and do not have associated renal abnormalities such as dysplasia or scarring.
- Dysfunctional elimination disorders can significantly impact the resolution of reflux.
- Surgical treatment of VUR is indicated in approximately 5-15% of children with reflux.
- In the future, genetic evaluation may help to identify which children with VUR are at the greatest risk for UTI and renal injury.

INTRODUCTION

Urinary tract infection (UTI) is common in children, affecting 2% of boys and 8% of girls.[1] The presentation of UTIs varies from a simple symptomatic cystitis to pyelonephritis and sepsis. In general, children who present with a UTI have a 30% to 50% incidence of anatomic abnormalities and a 30% to 40% rate of UTI recurrence.[2] The risk of renal injury (ie, scarring) is directly related to the number of UTIs, increasing logarithmically after 2 episodes.[3] UTIs are associated with long-term morbidity and with renal scarring in about 5% of affected children.[4] Consequently, the management of children with UTIs

An editorial commentary by Dr Ron Keren, "Editorial Commentary: Management of Primary Vesicoureteral Reflux in Children," is based on this article and found in *Pediatric Clinics of North America* 59:4, August 2012.

Department of Urology, Children's Hospital, Boston Harvard Medical School, Boston, MA 02115, USA

* Corresponding author. Department of Urology, Hunnewell-353, Children's Hospital Boston, 300 Longwood Avenue, Boston, MA 02115.
E-mail address: Hiep.Nguyen@childrens.harvard.edu

Pediatr Clin N Am 59 (2012) 819–834
doi:10.1016/j.pcl.2012.05.012
0031-3955/12/$ – see front matter © 2012 Elsevier Inc. All rights reserved.

has traditionally been focused on identifying and treating the associated anatomic abnormalities, such as vesicoureteral reflux (VUR), in hopes of preventing renal injury.

More recently, however, it has been recognized that the anatomic abnormalities are but one factor that predisposes children to UTIs and put them at risk for renal injury; others, such as bacterial virulence and host biologic susceptibility, may equally play an important role.[5] The interaction between these factors will determine which children with VUR will be at risk for UTIs and renal injury. As a result, there are divergent options in the management of VUR, from surveillance/observation with or without antibiotics prophylaxis to surgical intervention using open endoscopic or laparoscopic approaches.

NONSURGICAL MANAGEMENT OF PRIMARY VUR
Surveillance/Observation

This management option is based on observations derived from animal and large clinical studies over the last 40 years: (1) VUR without associated infection does not induce renal injury or interfere with renal function and (2) VUR may resolve spontaneously with time. Experiment and clinical studies have demonstrated that the renal injury associated with VUR results from the acute inflammatory reaction induced by bacterial infection of the renal parenchyma (reviewed by Peters and Rushton, 2010[6]). Bacterial virulence and host susceptibility factors determine the extent and reversibility of the renal injury. In the absence of high-pressure voiding,[7,8] sterile VUR in itself does not seem to result in renal scarring or impair renal growth[9,10] or glomerular function.[11]

Early clinical studies[12,13] observed that VUR resolved spontaneous in most children, occurring at any age. Consequently, it was difficult to predict when VUR would cease. More recent studies[14,15] demonstrated that specific patient demographic factors, such as age at presentation, gender, grade of the reflux, laterality, mode of clinical presentation, and ureteral anatomy, could help delineate the rate of resolution. Repeat radiological evaluation with a voiding cystourethrogram (VCUG) or radionuclide cystogram should be repeated approximately 12 to 18 months.

Continuous Antibiotic Prophylaxis

During the 1960s and 1970s, several studies observed that renal scarring developed in 21% to 66% of children with VUR who were observed and only treated with antibiotics after an infection was diagnosed.[12,16] Because it was not possible to predict which children were going to develop renal scarring, it was generally recommended that continuous antibiotic prophylaxis (CAP) should be instituted for preventing recurrent UTI. Subsequent studies demonstrated that treatment with CAP significantly reduced the incidence of renal scarring to less than 1% to 3% with low emergence of bacterial resistance.[17,18] CAP was comparable with surgical intervention in preventing UTIs and renal scarring.[19,20]

The most common antibiotics recommended for this purpose include trimethoprim-sulfamethoxazole, nitrofurantoin, and amoxicillin, the later primarily in infants less than 3 months of age. At prophylactic doses, these antibiotics have good urinary levels, are effective against urinary pathogens, have minimal effects on the bowel flora, and overall have minimal side effects (reviewed by Smellie, 1991[21]). Children with VUR on CAP may be screened periodically (1–4 times per year) with follow-up urine cultures.[21,22] Compliance rates with CAP range from 12% to 90%[18,23] and is a common reason for pursuing alternative management options.[24]

While on CAP, infection with an organism resistant to prophylaxis may occur, with rates ranging from 10% to 25%.[25,26] These breakthrough infections are more frequent in girls, in children with bladder/bowel dysfunction,[25,27] and those with existing renal abnormalities on dimercaptosuccinic acid (DMSA) imaging.[28] These infections may be febrile, with lower tract symptoms only, or be completely asymptomatic (detected on surveillance urine culture). After 1 to 2 breakthrough infections, it is generally recommended to seek alternative methods of VUR treatment.

Discontinuation of CAP may be recommended after a certain age, with the rationale that new renal scarring occurs primarily in younger children. It is assumed that the mature kidneys are more resistant to injury from infection than immature ones. The exact age at which it is safe to stop CAP is not known but is assumed to be around 5 to 9 years of age.[29,30] In addition, it has been observed that children with high-grade VUR and bladder/bowel dysfunction[30,31] remain at risk for renal scarring and, thus, should be kept on CAP. Currently, there are no prospective studies that establish safe guidelines for stopping CAP. Consequently, it is important that children with VUR who stopped CAP be monitored for UTI and renal scarring because some patients will remain at risk despite their age.

No Antibiotic Prophylaxis

Recently, the use of CAP in children with VUR, which seemed rational for many decades, has come under increasing scrutiny. Theoretical concerns include the development of antibiotic resistance in the individual and in the community, the carcinogenic potential, and the financial cost. Parental pressure to not use CAP in children with VUR increases as access to unsupervised and general medical information becomes more readily available. Recent studies comparing the nonsurgical management of VUR with and without CAP suggested that in patients with low-grade VUR (grades 1–3), there was no significant difference in the incidence of UTI, acute pyelonephritis, and late renal scarring between the two groups.[32–36] Similarly, a 2011 meta-analysis of the literature demonstrated that long-term low-dose antibiotic prophylaxis compared with no treatment/placebo did not significantly reduce repeat symptomatic or febrile UTI.[37] However, CAP did reduce the risk of new or progressive renal damage as assessed by DMSA imaging.

It is should be noted that many of the studies currently in the literature have significant limitations that prevent the generalization of their conclusions to all children with VUR. Most studies primarily evaluated children with low-grade (grade 1–3) VUR; excluded patients that are at risk for renal damage, such as those with bladder/bowel dysfunction, recurrent UTIs, and preexisting renal scarring on DMSA imaging; and had short follow-up times. Studies recently demonstrated that CAP reduced the risk of febrile UTI and renal scarring in girls and in children with reflux grade 3 to 5 or with bladder/bowel dysfunction.[38,39]

Management of Bladder and Bowel Dysfunction

Dysfunctional elimination disorders (ie, bladder and bowel dysfunction) seem to play a part in the cause and natural history of VUR. In infants, high-grade VUR is observed in association with high voiding pressures and detrusor hypercontractility.[40,41] The resolution of VUR seems to correlate with the improvement in urodynamic parameters. In toilet-trained children, various forms of abnormal bladder function (ie, detrusor over-activity and dyssynergia of the detrusor and urinary sphincter) were similarly observed in association with VUR.[42] Moreover, abnormal bowel function, such as constipation and encopresis, has been correlated with VUR and the risk of UTI (reviewed by Halachmi and Farhat, 2008[43]). Given these findings, the treatment of dysfunctional elimination disorders is generally recommended for children with VUR to decrease the risk of UTI and improve the chance of VUR resolution. Treatment options include behavioral therapy; biofeedback; dietary/fluid modification; and medications, anticho-linergic or alpha-blockers for the bladder and fiber or laxatives for the bowel (reviewed by Peters and colleagues,[44] 2010).

SURGICAL MANAGEMENT OF PRIMARY VUR
Circumcision

Uncircumcised boys aged younger than 1 year are at a greater risk of febrile UTIs.[45] Consequently, circumcision is a treatment option in the management of male infants with VUR. This statement is supported by observations in the International Reflux Study in which there were more boys with breakthrough infections and new scarring in the European arm as opposed to the American arm[20,46]; most of the boys in the American arm were circumcised, whereas those in the European arm were not. Although it may be of benefit, there currently are no prospective studies evaluating the benefit of circumcision in reducing the risk of UTIs in boys with VUR.

Indications for Surgical Intervention

Although the techniques for the surgical correction of VUR were first described in the 1950s, the indications for surgical intervention to this date remain in flux. Although there are ongoing debates, it is generally agreed that the absolute indication for surgical correction is the failure of nonsurgical management as evident by break-through UTIs or patient noncompliance. Relative indications include the following: (1) high-grade (4–5) reflux that failed to spontaneously resolve; (2) VUR associated with other anatomic problems, such as large para-ureteral diverticulum or ureteral duplication; or (3) reflux associated with impaired renal growth or function on serial evaluation. More controversial indications include persistent reflux in girls after puberty and parental/physician preference to avoid the need for follow-up VUR eval-uation or CAP.

Currently, it remains unclear whether surgical intervention is better than CAP in pre-venting UTIs and renal scarring. A 2011 meta-analysis of the literature indicated surgical correction of VUR (open or endoscopic approaches) did not reduce the risk of symptomatic UTIs compared with CAP. Surgical correction was associated with a 57% reduction in febrile UTI by 5 years but did not decrease the risk of new or progressive renal damage.[37] Consequently, the added benefits of surgical correction over CAP remain to be determined. However, as with CAP, it is likely that a limited subgroup of children with VUR with specific characteristics would most benefit from surgical intervention.

Open Ureteral Reimplantation

Traditional open ureteral reimplantation remains the gold standard for surgical treat-ment when VUR must be corrected, with reported success rates of 95% to 98% and low complication rates.[47,48] Several techniques for surgically correcting reflux have been described. Although different methods have specific advantages and complications, they all share the basic principle of creating a passive flap valve mech-anism that allows the ureter to occlude temporarily when intravesical pressure increases. The procedure must also allow for normal ureteral peristalsis and unob-structed drainage into the bladder.

The most popular and reliable intravesical open procedure is the cross-trigonal reimplantation described by Cohen.[49] This technique is a simple and reliable method for surgically correcting all grades of reflux. It is easy to learn and perform and is, therefore, probably safer for less-experienced surgeons. Intravesical mobilization of the ureter is performed, but the ureter is reimplanted across the trigone toward the contralateral ureter (**Fig. 1**). The main issue with this procedure is the difficulty of endoscopically accessing the ureters if they are subsequently required for treating urolithiasis. The other reliable intravesical open procedures are suprahiatal reimplantation (Politano Leadbetter) and infrahiatal reimplantation (Glenn Anderson).

Extravesical ureteral reimplantation was developed simultaneously by Lich and Gregoir.[50] The ureter is completely detached circumferentially from the detrusor muscle fibers, leaving only mucosal attachments to connect the ureter to the bladder, and the detrusor incision is extended down toward the bladder neck to create space for advancing the ureter (**Fig. 2**). After anchoring the ureter to the apex of the detrusorotomy, the detrusor muscle is approximated over the ureter, creating a muscular backing for the submucosal tunnel.[51] The most notorious complication of this procedure is an increased risk of temporary postoperative urinary retention if a simultaneous bilateral extravesical reflux repair is performed[52]; the risk is increased because dissecting the detrusor near the ureterovesical junction may injure the nerve fibers leading to the bladder. In a study comparing 220 patients undergoing bilateral extravesical reimplantation, a modified inverted-Y dissection of the ureter was compared with circumferential mobilization of the ureter. The urinary retention rate was 8.4% for the inverted-Y incision and 15.2% for the standard ureteral mobilization. In this study, the risk factors for urinary retention included male sex, younger age (younger than 2–3 years), and higher grades of reflux.[53]

The success rates for extravesicular and intravesicular ureteral reimplantation are similar and are highest for grades I to III, with most series reporting success rates greater than 95%.[54,55] Most recent studies have discussed methods of reducing the duration of the hospital stay and of Foley catheter placement.[56,57]

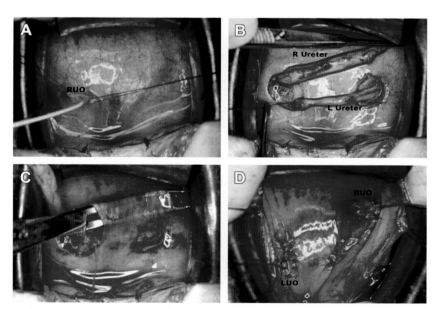

Fig. 1. Cohen cross-trigonal ureteral reimplantation. The ureters are mobilized from an intravesical approach (A) and placed in a cross-trigonal fashion (B). Submucosal tunnels are developed to provide an antireflux mechanism (C). The ureters are secured in their new location (D). LUO, left ureteral orifice; RUO, right ureteral orifice. (*Courtesy of* Dr Joseph G. Borer.)

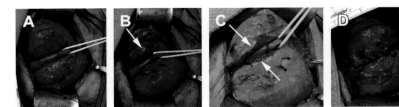

Fig. 2. Extravesical ureteral reimplantation. The ureter is mobilized outside of the bladder (*A*). A submucosal tunnel (*arrow*) is created by incising the detrusor muscle (*B*). The ureter is then placed in the submucosal tunnel (*arrows*) (*C*). The detrusor muscle is then re-approximated over the ureter (*D*).

Endoscopic Treatment of Primary VUR

Endoscopic correction of VUR is a minimally invasive treatment of patients with reflux and UTI or renal damage. Endoscopic subureteric transurethral injection was first described in 1981, with Teflon as the bulking agent.[58] Subsequently, several bulking agents have been used for endoscopic VUR correction, such as polytetra-fluoroethylene (Teflon), polydimethylsiloxane, bovine collagen, calcium hydroxyapatite, polyacrylate-polyalcohol copolymer (Vantris, Promedon, Cordoba, Argentina), and dextranomer/hyaluronic acid (Dx/HA) (Deflux, Oceana Therapeutics, Inc, Edison, NJ, USA). Currently, Deflux is the only material that is currently approved by the Food and Drug Administration (FDA) for treating VUR. Since its FDA-approval, the use of this treatment modality has rapidly increased.[59,60] Some investigators have suggested it as a first-line alternative to antibiotic prophylaxis or surgical treatment despite an absence of methodologically appropriate trials comparing these modalities.[61–63]

The description of the original subureteric Teflon injection (STING) procedure suggests an injection site that is 2 to 3 mm distal to the ureterovesical junction, immediately below the ureteral orifice (**Fig. 3**); the needle enters the bladder mucosa and advances 4 to 5 mm in the submucosal plane, creating a bulge that elongates the intramural ureter.[64] This technique has been shown to be a safe minimally invasive procedure for treating VUR.[62,65,66]

Kirsch and colleagues[67] have modified this procedure by inserting the needle into the floor of the distal ureter with the aid of hydrodistention. This modification was followed by a STING procedure if coaptation of the ureteral orifice was not achieved. The goal of this technique is to completely coapt the ureteral tunnel. The investigators described a ureteral success rate of 92% using the hydrodistention-implantation technique (HIT) compared with 79% with the standard STING procedure, with superior results even in patients with higher-grade reflux. Recently, the HIT technique has been modified to include both proximal and distal intraureteric injections (termed double HIT), which achieves better coaptation of the intramural tunnel. The first injection (the proximal HIT) reaches the floor of the midureteral tunnel, and the distal HIT is performed just within the ureteral orifice. If coaptation does not occur, a complementary STING injection is performed. Kallisvaart and Kirsch[68] recently evaluated 54 patients who underwent double HIT and described 96% clinical and 92% radiographic success rates after 1 year of follow-up.

In a meta-analysis that examined all types of injections (including Dx/HA) in 5527 patients and 8101 renal units, primary success rates of 78.5% for grades I and II, 72.0% for grade III, 63.0% for grade IV, and 51.0% for grade V reflux were reported. In cases when the first treatment was unsuccessful, the second injection had a success rate of 68% and the third had a success rate of 34%. The success rate was lower for

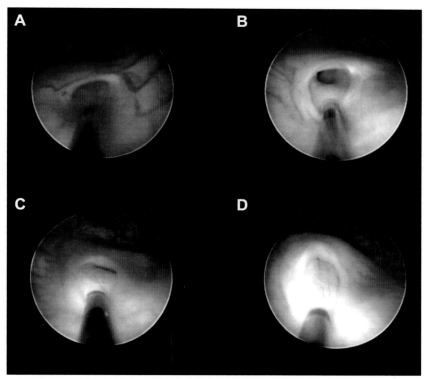

Fig. 3. Endoscopic injection for the treatment of vesicoureteral reflux. The needle is placed 2 to 3 mm distal to the ureteral orifice (*A*) and is advanced an additional 4 to 5 mm into the ureteral wall (*B*). Deflux is then injected to create coaptation of the ureteral wall (*C, D*).

duplicated than for single systems (50% vs 73%) and lower for neuropathic (62%) than for normal bladders (74%).[69]

Independent of the technique used, there has been a learning curve associated with endoscopic VUR correction. Kirsch has reported a 60% success rate in his first 20 patients compared with an 80% success rate in his most recent 20 patients.[70] Herz and colleagues[71] achieved a success rate of 46% in 28 refluxing ureters during the first 6 months of their study. In the subsequent 18 months, the overall correction rate was 93% in 84 ureters. Using multivariate analysis, Lorenzo and colleagues[72] have demonstrated that physician experience was an independent predictor of VUR correction rates.

The complications that follow endoscopic treatment are mainly related to a new contralateral reflux developing after unilateral VUR treatment and to the obstruction of the ureterovesical junction, which is an uncommon event.[73] In long-term follow-up, potential complications include the development of calcification at the site of the Deflux injection and recurrent VUR. In histologic studies, it has been demonstrated that Deflux injection results the formation of a pseudocapsule with granulomatous inflammation and calcification after a mean period of 22 months.[74] Although calcification at the site of the Deflux injection is an expected finding, clinicians inexperienced with Deflux may mistake it for distal ureteral calculi or tumor.[75,76] Finally, several recent studies have put to into question the durability of Deflux treatment. Approximately

20% to 30% of children who were treated with Deflux and had a negative VCUG at 3 months re-presented with UTI and most were found to have recurrent VUR.[77,78]

Laparoscopic/Robotic Ureteral Reimplantation

The initial laparoscopic ureteral reimplantation method used the extravesical Lich-Gregoir technique through a transperitoneal approach.[79,80] The refined technical aspects of this approach were documented in 2000 by Lakshmanan and Fung,[81] who emphasized limiting the tissue dissection and downsizing the ports and instruments. They reported on reimplanting 71 ureters in 47 children using this technique; none of the children had postoperative reflux or obstruction. They emphasized patient selection, advising that this technique may be challenging in the narrow pelvises of children younger than 4 years and that ureters requiring tapering are probably unsuitable. Riquelme and colleagues[82] reported on a series of 15 children treated with extravesical reimplantation; they achieved a 94.7% success rate in their series, even in cases of bilateral reflux or duplex ureters.

Difficulties with port placement and the limitations of the intravesical working space have delayed the development of a minimally invasive cross-trigonal Cohen technique. Gill and colleagues[83] reported on their experiences with this technique using 2 suprapubic ports and a transurethral resectoscope; they achieved VUR resolution in 2 out of 3 patients, demonstrating that this procedure was effective and technically feasible. Gatti and colleagues[84] evaluated 29 children (with 46 refluxing ureters) and performed percutaneous endoscopic trigonoplasty using the Gil-Vernet technique in the first 23 patients and the Cohen technique in the last 6 patients. The long-term follow-up of the patients treated using the Gil-Vernet technique found that the reflux resolution rate decreased from 63% to 47%. They reported an 83% success rate with the Cohen technique, but the operative time was nearly twice as long as for the Gil-Vernet method. Canon and colleagues[85] retrospectively compared 52 children undergoing vesicoscopic ureteral reimplantation through cross-trigonal repair, with 40 children undergoing open reimplantation. The postoperative VUR resolution rate was 91% in the vesicoscopic group versus 97% in the open group. The investigators also described significantly decreased postoperative analgesic requirements and longer mean operative times in the vesicoscopic group (199 vs 92 minutes). The mean hospital stay was similar between the two groups (approximately 2 days).

Using robotic assistance to treat vesicoureteral reflux aims to add the benefits of laparoscopy, such as reduced pain and morbidity, to the advantages of robotics, such as enhanced instrument maneuverability and shorter learning curves for a skill-intensive procedure. The evolution of robotic-assisted laparoscopic ureteral reimplantation (RALUR) has closely mirrored the development of conventional laparoscopy, starting with the extravesical approach. Because of the concerns of an increased risk for urinary retention when using bilateral extravesical reimplantation, an intravesical RALUR technique has also been investigated.

In 2004, Peters was the first to describe RALUR (17 unilateral extravesical and 3 bilateral intravesical procedures) in a pediatric population, reporting reflux correction in 89% of the refluxing units and a postoperative complication rate of 12% (bladder leaks in 2 cases and a transient obstruction in 1 case).[86] In 2008, Casale and colleagues[87] reported on their experiences with bilateral extravesical RALUR in 41 patients. They emphasized identifying and preserving the pelvic plexus, which is located lateral to the ureteral hiatus. A surgical success rate of 97.6% was achieved. No complications occurred, including urinary retention. The mean operative time was 2.33 hours. This study decreased concerns about potential voiding dysfunction after bilateral extravesical reimplantation.

Recently, the authors' group retrospectively evaluated 39 children who had undergone RALUR (19 intravesically and 20) and compared these children with 22 patients undergoing open intravesical and 17 undergoing open extravesical ureteral reimplantation.[88] The operative times for the intravesical and extravesical RALUR patients were significantly longer than those of the open-reimplantation group. The children who underwent intravesical RALUR had fewer or less-intense bladder spasms and less hematuria than did the intravesical open reimplantation group, but there was no statistically significant difference in pain. The intravesical RALUR children also required shorter periods of Foley catheter drainage and had shorter hospital stays. There were no significant differences in these parameters between those who received extravesical RALUR and those who were treated using the open extravesical technique. The overall clinical and radiological success rates for intravesical and extravesical RALUR and open reimplantation were similar.

DECIDING TREATMENT OPTIONS FOR CHILDREN WITH PRIMARY VUR

Interaction between the existence of anatomic abnormalities, such as VUR, bacterial virulence, and host biologic susceptibility, will determine an individual's susceptibility to UTIs and renal injury. A child with a history of UTI, VUR, and bladder/bowel dysfunction has a greater risk of renal scarring than one with UTI or VUR alone.[15,89] Consequently, VUR management must be individualized based on gender, age, grade of reflux, susceptibility to UTI and renal scarring, and bladder/bowel dysfunction to prevent undertreatment of those at high risk and overtreatment of those at low risk (**Table 1**).

THE FUTURE

Over the past 30 years, clinical observations have suggested a genetic basis for VUR.[90] There is a 30% to 50% incidence of VUR in the first-degree relatives of the probands[91,92] and a 100% and 50% concordance rate among monozygotic and dizygotic twins respectively.[93] Over the last decades, many investigators have attempted to elucidate genes implicated in VUR development (reviewed by Carvas and colleagues,[94] 2010). Genes and candidate loci on almost every chromosome have been implicated, which is likely because these previous studies evaluated the many different forms of VUR as one disease. Clinical observations suggest that there are distinct natural history and clinical outcomes in different patient populations with VUR (such as male vs female, those who present with UTI vs prenatal hydronephrosis, and probands vs siblings with reflux). Consequently, it is likely that there are different forms of VUR with different genetic determinates.

In evaluating 98 nuclear families with 1 or more affected sibling pairs with VUR, Briggs and colleagues[95] identified 3 candidate loci on chromosome 5, 13, and 18. In a subanalysis based on gender, boys with VUR were associated with candidate loci on chromosome 1 and 5.[96] In contrast, girls with VUR were associated with candidate loci on chromosome 3, 13, and 15. When analyzing the study population based on the mode of presentation, patients who presented with UTI were associated with a candidate locus on chromosome 18. Finally, when analyzing the study population based on DMSA findings (renal scarring), candidate locus on chromosome 11 for those without renal abnormalities and on chromosome 17 for those with renal abnormalities were identified.[97] Together, these findings suggest that different forms of VUR have distinct genetic susceptibility. Identifying these genetic differences will help to determine an individual's risk for recurrent UTIs and renal injury and allow for more individualized management of VUR.

Table 1
Management and follow-up of children with VUR based on risk-factor assessment

Risk Groups	Presentation	Initial Treatment	Comments	Follow-Up
High	Symptomatic male or female patients after toilet training with high-grade reflux (IV–V), abnormal kidneys and LUTD	Initial treatment is always for LUTD with CAP; intervention may be considered in case of BT infections or persistent reflux	There is a greater possibility of earlier intervention	More aggressive follow-up for UTI and LUTD; full reevaluation after 6 mo
High	Symptomatic male or female patients after toilet training with high-grade reflux, abnormal kidneys and no LUTD	Intervention should be considered	Open surgery has better results than endoscopic surgery	Postoperative VCUG on indication only, follow-up of kidney status until after puberty
Mod	Symptomatic male or female patients before toilet training with high-grade reflux and abnormal kidneys	CAP is the initial treatment; intervention may be considered in case of BT infections or persistence of reflux	Spontaneous resolution is higher in boys	Follow-up for UTI/hydronephrosis and full reevaluation after 12–24 mo
Mod	Asymptomatic patients (PNH or sibling) with high-grade reflux and abnormal kidneys	CAP is the initial treatment; intervention may be considered in cases of BT infections or persistent reflux		Follow-up for UTI/ hydronephrosis and full reevaluation after 12–24 mo
Mod	Symptomatic male or female patients after toilet training with high-grade reflux and normal kidneys with LUTD	Initial treatment is always for LUTD with CAP; intervention may be considered in case of BT; infections, or persistence of reflux	In cases of persistent LUTD despite urotherapy, intervention should be considered. The choice of intervention is controversial	Follow-up for UTI and LUTD, kidney status, full reevaluation after successful urotherapy
Mod	Symptomatic male or female patients after toilet training with low-grade reflux, abnormal kidneys with or without LUTD	The choice of treatment is controversial; endoscopic treatment may be an option; LUTD treatment if needed		Follow-up for UTI LUTD, and kidney status until after puberty
Mod	All symptomatic normal kidneys with low-grade reflux with LUTD	The initial treatment is always for LUTD with or without CAP		Follow-up for UTI and LUTD
Low	All symptomatic patients with normal kidneys, with low-grade reflux, with no LUTD	No treatment or CAP	If no treatment is given, parents should be informed about the risk of infection	Follow-up for UTI
Low	All asymptomatic normal kidneys with low-grade reflux	No treatment or CAP in infants	If no treatment is given, parents should be informed about the risk of infection	Follow-up for UTI

Abbreviations: BT, breakthrough; LUTD, lower urinary tract dysfunction; Mod, moderate; PNH, prenatal diagnosed hydronephrosis.

Data from Tekgul S, Riedmiller H, Gerharz E, et al. Guidelines on paediatric urology. European Association of Urology Web site. Available at: http://www.uroweb.org/gls/pdf/19_Paediatric_Urology.pdf.

SUMMARY

There are many options in the management of primary VUR in children. In view of the few randomized controlled studies available in the literature and the limitations in current studies, more research is needed to determine the benefit of one over another. However, careful analysis of individual characteristics, such as age, gender, grade of VUR, prior history of UTI, preexistence of renal scarring, and bladder/bowel dysfunction, is likely to be helpful in selecting the appropriate management. Independent of the treatment chosen, the main objectives in VUR management remains the same: the prevention of ascending UTIs and pyelonephritis; the improvement of voiding; and most importantly, the prevention of renal scarring and dysfunction.

REFERENCES

1. Hellstrom A, Hanson E, Hansson S, et al. Association between urinary symptoms at 7 years old and previous urinary tract infection. Arch Dis Child 1991; 66:232–4.
2. Winberg J, Andersen HJ, Bergstrom T, et al. Epidemiology of symptomatic urinary tract infection in childhood. Acta Paediatr Scand Suppl 1974;(252): 1–20.
3. Jodal U, Lindberg U. Guidelines for management of children with urinary tract infection and vesico-ureteric reflux. Recommendations from a Swedish state-of-the-art conference. Swedish Medical Research Council. Acta Paediatr Suppl 1999;88:87–9.
4. Normand IC, Smellie JM. Prolonged maintenance chemotherapy in the management of urinary infection in childhood. Br Med J 1965;1:1023–6.
5. Nielubowicz GR, Mobley HL. Host-pathogen interactions in urinary tract infection. Nat Rev Urol 2010;7:430–41.
6. Peters C, Rushton HG. Vesicoureteral reflux associated renal damage: congenital reflux nephropathy and acquired renal scarring. J Urol 2010;184:265–73.
7. Heptinstall RH, Hodson CJ. Pathology of sterile reflux in the pig. Contrib Nephrol 1984;39:344–57.
8. Ransley PG, Risdon RA, Godley ML. High pressure sterile vesicoureteral reflux and renal scarring: an experimental study in the pig and minipig. Contrib Nephrol 1984;39:320–43.
9. Aggarwal VK, Verrier Jones K, Asscher AW, et al. Covert bacteriuria: long term follow up. Arch Dis Child 1991;66:1284–6.
10. Smellie JM, Edwards D, Normand IC, et al. Effect of vesicoureteric reflux on renal growth in children with urinary tract infection. Arch Dis Child 1981;56:593–600.
11. Verrier Jones K, Asscher AW, Verrier Jones ER, et al. Glomerular filtration rate in schoolgirls with covert bacteriuria. Br Med J (Clin Res Ed) 1982;285:1307–10.
12. Lenaghan D. Proceedings: natural history of reflux and long-term effects of reflux on the kidney. Br J Urol 1974;46:115.
13. Mulcahy JJ, Kelalis PP. Non-operative treatment of vesicoureteral reflux. J Urol 1978;120:336–7.
14. Estrada CR Jr, Passerotti CC, Graham DA, et al. Nomograms for predicting annual resolution rate of primary vesicoureteral reflux: results from 2,462 children. J Urol 2009;182:1535–41.
15. Skoog SJ, Peters CA, Arant BS Jr, et al. Pediatric vesicoureteral reflux guidelines panel summary report: clinical practice guidelines for screening siblings of children with vesicoureteral reflux and neonates/infants with prenatal hydronephrosis. J Urol 2010;184:1145–51.

16. O'Donnell B, Moloney MA, Lynch V. Vesico-ureteric reflux in infants and children: results of "supervision", chemotherapy and surgery. Br J Urol 1969;41: 6–13.

17. Goldraich NP, Goldraich IH. Follow-up of conservatively treated children with high and low grade vesicoureteral reflux: a prospective study. J Urol 1992;148: 1688–92.

18. Skoog SJ, Belman AB, Majd M. A nonsurgical approach to the management of primary vesicoureteral reflux. J Urol 1987;138:941–6.

19. Prospective trial of operative versus non-operative treatment of severe vesicoureteric reflux in children: five years' observation. Birmingham Reflux Study Group. Br Med J (Clin Res Ed) 1987;295:237–41.

20. Weiss R, Duckett J, Spitzer A. Results of a randomized clinical trial of medical versus surgical management of infants and children with grades III and IV primary vesicoureteral reflux (United States). The International Reflux Study in Children. J Urol 1992;148:1667–73.

21. Smellie JM. Reflections on 30 years of treating children with urinary tract infections. J Urol 1991;146:665–8.

22. Bloom DA, Bennett CJ. Nonoperative management of vesicoureteral reflux. Semin Urol 1986;4:74–81.

23. Wan J, Greenfield SP, Talley M, et al. An analysis of social and economic factors associated with follow-up of patients with vesicoureteral reflux. J Urol 1996;156: 668–72.

24. Szymanski KM, Oliveira LM, Silva A, et al. Analysis of indications for ureteral reimplantation in 3738 children with vesicoureteral reflux: a single institutional cohort. J Pediatr Urol 2011;7:601–10.

25. Greenfield SP, Ng M, Wan J. Experience with vesicoureteral reflux in children: clinical characteristics. J Urol 1997;158:574–7.

26. Huang FY, Tsai TC. Resolution of vesicoureteral reflux during medical management in children. Pediatr Nephrol 1995;9:715–7.

27. Hanson E, Hansson S, Jodal U. Trimethoprim-sulphadiazine prophylaxis in children with vesico-ureteric reflux. Scand J Infect Dis 1989;21:201–4.

28. Mingin GC, Nguyen HT, Baskin LS, et al. Abnormal dimercapto-succinic acid scans predict an increased risk of breakthrough infection in children with vesicoureteral reflux. J Urol 2004;172:1075–7 [discussion: 7].

29. Belman AB, Skoog SJ. Nonsurgical approach to the management of vesicoureteral reflux in children. Pediatr Infect Dis J 1989;8:556–9.

30. Leslie B, Moore K, Salle JL, et al. Outcome of antibiotic prophylaxis discontinuation in patients with persistent vesicoureteral reflux initially presenting with febrile urinary tract infection: time to event analysis. J Urol 2010;184:1093–8.

31. Alconcher LF, Meneguzzi MB, Buschiazzo R, et al. Could prophylactic antibiotics be stopped in patients with history of vesicoureteral reflux? J Pediatr Urol 2009;5: 383–8.

32. Conway PH, Cnaan A, Zaoutis T, et al. Recurrent urinary tract infections in children: risk factors and association with prophylactic antimicrobials. JAMA 2007; 298:179–86.

33. Garin EH, Olavarria F, Garcia Nieto V, et al. Clinical significance of primary vesicoureteral reflux and urinary antibiotic prophylaxis after acute pyelonephritis: a multicenter, randomized, controlled study. Pediatrics 2006;117:626–32.

34. Montini G, Rigon L, Zucchetta P, et al. Prophylaxis after first febrile urinary tract infection in children? A multicenter, randomized, controlled, noninferiority trial. Pediatrics 2008;122:1064–71.

35. Pennesi M, Travan L, Peratoner L, et al. Is antibiotic prophylaxis in children with vesicoureteral reflux effective in preventing pyelonephritis and renal scars? A randomized, controlled trial. Pediatrics 2008;121:e1489–94.

36. Roussey-Kesler G, Gadjos V, Idres N, et al. Antibiotic prophylaxis for the prevention of recurrent urinary tract infection in children with low grade vesicoureteral reflux: results from a prospective randomized study. J Urol 2008;179:674–9 [discussion 9].

37. Nagler EV, Williams G, Hodson EM, et al. Interventions for primary vesicoureteric reflux. Cochrane Database Syst Rev 2011;6:CD001532.

38. Brandstrom P, Jodal U, Sillen U, et al. The Swedish reflux trial: review of a randomized, controlled trial in children with dilating vesicoureteral reflux. J Pediatr Urol 2011;7:594–600.

39. Craig JC, Simpson JM, Williams GJ, et al. Antibiotic prophylaxis and recurrent urinary tract infection in children. N Engl J Med 2009;361:1748–59.

40. Chandra M, Maddix H, McVicar M. Transient urodynamic dysfunction of infancy: relationship to urinary tract infections and vesicoureteral reflux. J Urol 1996;155: 673–7.

41. Sillen U, Hjalmas K, Aili M, et al. Pronounced detrusor hypercontractility in infants with gross bilateral reflux. J Urol 1992;148:598–9.

42. Hong YK, Altobelli E, Borer JG, et al. Urodynamic abnormalities in toilet trained children with primary vesicoureteral reflux. J Urol 2011;185:1863–8.

43. Halachmi S, Farhat WA. Interactions of constipation, dysfunctional elimination syndrome, and vesicoureteral reflux. Adv Urol 2008;2008:1–3.

44. Peters CA, Skoog SJ, Arant BS Jr, et al. Summary of the AUA guideline on management of primary vesicoureteral reflux in children. J Urol 2010;184: 1134–44.

45. Wiswell TE, Roscelli JD. Corroborative evidence for the decreased incidence of urinary tract infections in circumcised male infants. Pediatrics 1986;78: 96–9.

46. Jodal U, Koskimies O, Hanson E, et al. Infection pattern in children with vesicoureteral reflux randomly allocated to operation or long-term antibacterial prophylaxis. The International Reflux Study in Children. J Urol 1992;148: 1650–2.

47. Elder JS. Guidelines for consideration for surgical repair of vesicoureteral reflux. Curr Opin Urol 2000;10:579–85.

48. Jodal U, Smellie JM, Lax H, et al. Ten-year results of randomized treatment of children with severe vesicoureteral reflux. Final report of the International Reflux Study in Children. Pediatr Nephrol 2006;21:785–92.

49. Cohen SJ. The Cohen reimplantation technique. Birth Defects Orig Artic Ser 1977;13:391–5.

50. Lich R Jr, Howerton LW, Davis LA. Childhood urosepsis. J Ky Med Assoc 1961; 59:1177–9.

51. Zaontz MR, Maizels M, Sugar EC, et al. Detrusorrhaphy: extravesical ureteral advancement to correct vesicoureteral reflux in children. J Urol 1987;138:947–9.

52. Lipski BA, Mitchell ME, Burns MW. Voiding dysfunction after bilateral extravesical ureteral reimplantation. J Urol 1998;159:1019–21.

53. Barrieras D, Lapointe S, Reddy PP, et al. Urinary retention after bilateral extravesical ureteral reimplantation: does dissection distal to the ureteral orifice have a role? J Urol 1999;162:1197–200.

54. Kennelly MJ, Bloom DA, Ritchey ML, et al. Outcome analysis of bilateral Cohen cross-trigonal ureteroneocystostomy. Urology 1995;46:393–5.

55. Minevich E, Tackett L, Wacksman J, et al. Extravesical common sheath detrusor-rhaphy (ureteroneocystostomy) and reflux in duplicated collecting systems. J Urol 2002;167:288–90.
56. Chamie K, Chi A, Hu B, et al. Contemporary open ureteral reimplantation without morphine: assessment of pain and outcomes. J Urol 2009;182:1147–51.
57. Wicher C, Hadley D, Ludlow D, et al. 250 consecutive unilateral extravesical ureteral reimplantations in an outpatient setting. J Urol 2010;184:311–4.
58. Matouschek E. New concept for the treatment of vesico-ureteral reflux. Endoscopic application of Teflon. Arch Esp Urol 1981;34:385–8.
59. Lendvay TS, Sorensen M, Cowan CA, et al. The evolution of vesicoureteral reflux management in the era of dextranomer/hyaluronic acid copolymer: a pediatric health information system database study. J Urol 2006;176:1864–7.
60. Nelson CP, Copp HL, Lai J, et al. Is availability of endoscopy changing initial management of vesicoureteral reflux? J Urol 2009;182:1152–7.
61. Chertin B, Colhoun E, Velayudham M, et al. Endoscopic treatment of vesicoureteral reflux: 11 to 17 years of follow-up. J Urol 2002;167:1443–5 [discussion: 5–6].
62. Puri P, Chertin B, Velayudham M, et al. Treatment of vesicoureteral reflux by endoscopic injection of dextranomer/hyaluronic acid copolymer: preliminary results. J Urol 2003;170:1541–4 [discussion: 4].
63. Stenberg A, Hensle TW, Lackgren G. Vesicoureteral reflux: a new treatment algorithm. Curr Urol Rep 2002;3:107–14.
64. O'Donnell B, Puri P. Treatment of vesicoureteric reflux by endoscopic injection of Teflon. Br Med J 1984;289:7–9.
65. Lackgren G, Wahlin N, Skoldenberg E, et al. Endoscopic treatment of vesicoureteral reflux with dextranomer/hyaluronic acid copolymer is effective in either double ureters or a small kidney. J Urol 2003;170:1551–5 [discussion: 5].
66. Lackgren G, Wahlin N, Skoldenberg E, et al. Long-term follow-up of children treated with dextranomer/hyaluronic acid copolymer for vesicoureteral reflux. J Urol 2001;166:1887–92.
67. Kirsch AJ, Perez-Brayfield M, Smith EA, et al. The modified sting procedure to correct vesicoureteral reflux: improved results with submucosal implantation within the intramural ureter. J Urol 2004;171:2413–6.
68. Kalisvaart JF, Scherz HC, Cuda S, et al. Intermediate to long-term follow-up indicates low risk of recurrence after double HIT endoscopic treatment for primary vesico-ureteral reflux. J Pediatr Urol 2011. [Epub ahead of print].
69. Elder JS, Diaz M, Caldamone AA, et al. Endoscopic therapy for vesicoureteral reflux: a meta-analysis. I. Reflux resolution and urinary tract infection. J Urol 2006;175:716–22.
70. Kirsch AJ, Perez-Brayfield MR, Scherz HC. Minimally invasive treatment of vesicoureteral reflux with endoscopic injection of dextranomer/hyaluronic acid copolymer: the Children's Hospitals of Atlanta experience. J Urol 2003;170:211–5.
71. Herz D, Hafez A, Bagli D, et al. Efficacy of endoscopic subureteral polydimethylsiloxane injection for treatment of vesicoureteral reflux in children: a North American clinical report. J Urol 2001;166:1880–6.
72. Lorenzo AJ, Pippi Salle JL, Barroso U, et al. What are the most powerful determinants of endoscopic vesicoureteral reflux correction? Multivariate analysis of a single institution experience during 6 years. J Urol 2006;176:1851–5.

73. Elmore JM, Kirsch AJ, Lyles RH, et al. New contralateral vesicoureteral reflux following dextranomer/hyaluronic acid implantation: incidence and identification of a high risk group. J Urol 2006;175:1097–100 [discussion: 100–1].

74. Stenberg A, Larsson E, Lackgren G. Endoscopic treatment with dextranomer-hyaluronic acid for vesicoureteral reflux: histological findings. J Urol 2003;169: 1109–13.

75. Nelson CP, Chow JS. Dextranomer/hyaluronic acid copolymer (Deflux) implants mimicking distal ureteral calculi on CT. Pediatr Radiol 2008;38:104–6.

76. Palagiri AV, Dangle PP. Distal ureteral calcification secondary to deflux injection: a reality or myth? Urology 2011;77:1217–9.

77. Chi A, Gupta A, Snodgrass W. Urinary tract infection following successful dextranomer/hyaluronic acid injection for vesicoureteral reflux. J Urol 2008;179: 1966–9.

78. Sedberry-Ross S, Rice DC, Pohl HG, et al. Febrile urinary tract infections in children with an early negative voiding cystourethrogram after treatment of vesicoureteral reflux with dextranomer/hyaluronic acid. J Urol 2008;180:1605–9 [discussion: 10].

79. Ehrlich RM, Gershman A, Fuchs G. Laparoscopic vesicoureteroplasty in children: initial case reports. Urology 1994;43:255–61.

80. Schimberg W, Wacksman J, Rudd R, et al. Laparoscopic correction of vesicoureteral reflux in the pig. J Urol 1994;151:1664–7.

81. Lakshmanan Y, Fung LC. Laparoscopic extravesicular ureteral reimplantation for vesicoureteral reflux: recent technical advances. J Endourol 2000;14:589–93 [discussion: 93–4].

82. Riquelme M, Aranda A, Rodriguez C. Laparoscopic extravesical transperitoneal approach for vesicoureteral reflux. J Laparoendosc Adv Surg Tech A 2006;16: 312–6.

83. Gill IS, Ponsky LE, Desai M, et al. Laparoscopic cross-trigonal Cohen ureteroneocystostomy: novel technique. J Urol 2001;166:1811–4.

84. Gatti JM, Cartwright PC, Hamilton BD, et al. Percutaneous endoscopic trigonoplasty in children: long-term outcomes and modifications in technique. J Endourol 1999;13:581–4.

85. Canon SJ, Jayanthi VR, Patel AS. Vesicoscopic cross-trigonal ureteral reimplantation: a minimally invasive option for repair of vesicoureteral reflux. J Urol 2007; 178:269–73 [discussion: 73].

86. Peters CA. Robotically assisted surgery in pediatric urology. Urol Clin North Am 2004;31:743–52.

87. Casale P, Patel RP, Kolon TF. Nerve sparing robotic extravesical ureteral reimplantation. J Urol 2008;179:1987–9 [discussion: 90].

88. Marchini GS, Hong YK, Minnillo BJ, et al. Robotic assisted laparoscopic ureteral reimplantation in children: case matched comparative study with open surgical approach. J Urol 2011;185:1870–5.

89. Riedmiller H, Androulakakis P, Beurton D, et al. EAU guidelines on paediatric urology. Eur Urol 2001;40:589–99.

90. Zel G, Retik AB. Familial vesicoureteral reflux. Urology 1973;2:249–51.

91. Noe HN. The long-term results of prospective sibling reflux screening. J Urol 1992;148:1739–42.

92. Noe HN, Wyatt RJ, Peeden JN Jr, et al. The transmission of vesicoureteral reflux from parent to child. J Urol 1992;148:1869–71.

93. Kaefer M, Curran M, Treves ST, et al. Sibling vesicoureteral reflux in multiple gestation births. Pediatrics 2000;105:800–4.

94. Carvas F, Silva A, Nguyen HT. The genetics of primary, nonsyndromic vesicoureteral reflux. Curr Opin Urol 2010;20:336–42.
95. Briggs CE, Guo CY, Schoettler C, et al. A genome scan in affected sib-pairs with familial vesicoureteral reflux identifies a locus on chromosome 5. Eur J Hum Genet 2010;18:245–50.
96. Marchini GS, Onal B, Guo CY, et al. Genome gender diversity in affected sib-pairs with familial vesico-ureteric reflux identified by single nucleotide polymorphism linkage analysis. BJU Int 2011;109(11):1709–14.
97. Onal B, Miao X, Ozonoff A, et al. Protective locus against renal scarring on chromosome 11 in affected sib-pairs with familial vesicoureteral reflux identified by single nucleotide polymorphism linkage analysis. Br J Urol, in press.

Management of Primary Vesicoureteral Reflux in Children
Editorial Commentary

Ron Keren, MD, MPH[a,b],*

KEYWORDS

- Vesicoureteral reflux • Febrile urinary tract infection • Recurrent UTI • Renal injury

KEY POINTS

- Decisions must be made about the clinical management of children with vesicoureteral reflux (VUR) and a standardized risk-specific treatment approach is needed that can provide clinicians with an opportunity to standardize care and measure and continuously improve outcomes for these children.
- Clinicians and researchers must begin to think outside of the proverbial VUR box. Clinicians are beginning to understand that there are a variety of abnormalities in host defenses that might predispose some children to recurrent urinary tract infection.
- Knowledge of these deficiencies in specific host defenses may lead to therapies designed to compensate for them.
- There is also much to be learned about host inflammatory response to kidney infection, to explain why some children suffer extensive kidney injury with pyelonephritis, whereas others with the same amount of acute inflammation avoid scarring altogether.

The current paradigm for the management of children diagnosed with vesicoureteral reflux (VUR) after a febrile urinary tract infection (UTI) rests on the assumption that long-term renal insufficiency can be avoided by preventing recurrent UTIs with continuous antimicrobial prophylaxis (CAP) or surgically correcting VUR.[1] The International Reflux Study found that surgical correction of VUR offered no additional benefit compared with CAP alone,[2] although it did not test whether CAP was better than

This editorial commentary was written in response to the article written by Drs Fernando F. Fonseca, Fabio Y. Tanno, and Hiep T. Nguyen, entitled, "Current Options in the Management of Primary Vesicoureteral Reflux in Children" in *Pediatric Clinics of North America* (59:4), August 2012.

^a Division of General Pediatrics, Center for Pediatric Clinical Effectiveness, Children's Hospital of Philadelphia, 3535 Market Street, Room 1524, Philadelphia, PA 19104, USA; ^b Center for Clinical Epidemiology and Biostatistics, University of Pennsylvania School of Medicine, Philadelphia, PA, USA
* Children's Hospital of Philadelphia, 3535 Market Street, Room 1524, Philadelphia, PA 19104.
E-mail address: keren@email.chop.edu

no intervention at all. The best evidence regarding the effectiveness of CAP is from the meta-analysis of randomized controlled trials conducted for the 2011 American Academy of Pediatrics[5] (AAP) "Clinical Practice Guideline for the Diagnosis and Management of the Initial UTI in Febrile Infants and Children 2 to 24 Months," which did not detect a statistically significant benefit of prophylaxis in preventing recurrence of febrile UTI/pyelonephritis in infants without reflux or those with grades I, II, III, or IV VUR. Among the studies included in that meta-analysis, the trial by Craig and colleagues[3] had the strongest design (placebo controlled, adequate power, and stringent UTI definition), and it showed only a modest protective effect of CAP for children with VUR (6% 1-year absolute risk reduction in recurrent UTIs, from 17% down to 11%) that lasted for only the first 6 months of therapy. In 2013, the results of the Randomized Intervention for Children with Vesicoureteral Reflux (RIVUR) trial will be published.[4] If this multicenter placebo-controlled trial of prophylactic trimethoprim/sulfamethoxazole for children aged 2 months to 6 years with grades I to IV VUR shows the same marginal benefit of CAP, pediatricians, urologists, and nephrologists will need to reconsider the assumptions that informed the dominant paradigm for managing VUR in the last few decades.

More specifically, they will have to acknowledge that children who develop a UTI can be divided into 2 groups. The first, which comprises most children and the subjects of recent clinical trials, are those with low-grade VUR (grades I–III) and no or minimal kidney scarring at the time of UTI diagnosis. The evidence suggests that only 5% to 30% of these children go on to develop a second UTI,[5] a vanishingly small percentage of them develop renal scarring of any clinical significance,[6,7] and CAP has little, if any, effect on their clinical outcomes. For this reason, the recently revised AAP guideline recommended that (1) the initial work-up of children with first febrile UTI should consist of a renal ultrasound only, which should detect most high-grade VUR and significant renal scarring or anatomic abnormalities of the genitourinary tract; and (2) CAP can be deferred in children with normal renal ultrasound. With this change in recommendations around imaging of young children with first febrile UTI, the large proportion of children who are likely to have a benign clinical course will be spared an invasive voiding cystourethrogram (VCUG), years of CAP, and possibly surgery to correct VUR.

The second group of children, which represents the minority with first UTI, consists of those with high-grade VUR (grades IV–V), more extensive kidney scarring at baseline, and a predisposition to multiple breakthrough UTIs. These children are at the highest risk of suffering clinically significant renal injury, but, because there are so few of them, they are not well represented in recent clinical trials and thus there is considerable uncertainty about what, if any, therapy can effectively protect them from long-term renal insufficiency. They are also the ones most likely to find their way to the offices of pediatric urologists, and so they feature prominently in the pediatric urologic literature, including the review article by Fonseca and colleagues elsewhere in this issue. Given the problem of small numbers, and the reluctance of most physicians and parents to agree to randomization of these high-risk children, it will be difficult to conduct clinical trials to define best practices for them. Some of these children have genetically determined developmental abnormalities of the kidneys and urinary tract, which manifest after birth as VUR and renal dysplasia/hypoplasia.[8] In these children, the UTIs are an epiphenomenon rather than the cause of the renal abnormalities,[9] and there may be little that can be done to prevent the development of renal insufficiency. For others, surgical correction of VUR may remove an important risk factor for recurrent UTI and prevent subsequent kidney injury.

The greatest contribution of the review by Fonseca and colleagues is that it articulates the idea that the risk of recurrent UTI and subsequent renal insufficiency varies considerably among children with first UTI, and that the intensity (and potential harms) of any intervention must be matched to that risk. However, their review omits 2 important considerations: first, that most children with first UTI (and nearly all the children that a primary care pediatrician encounters) are in the low-risk group; and, second, that there is little to no high-quality evidence to support their recommendations for the small number of children in the moderate-risk and high-risk groups. Nonetheless, decisions must be made about the clinical management of these children and a standardized risk-specific treatment approach such as the one the authors outline, can provide clinicians with an opportunity to standardize care and measure and continuously improve outcomes for these children. Given the lack of feasibility to conduct randomized controlled trials in this patient population, the best hope for progress in understanding how to manage them is for pediatric urologists to establish a national registry of high-risk children, documenting their clinical characteristics, treatments, and outcomes in a thorough and consistent manner. Such registries have been successful in facilitating discussion, evaluating practices, and improving outcomes for other uncommon conditions, such as cystic fibrosis,[10] inflammatory bowel disease,[11] and congenital heart disease.[12]

Although comparisons of treatments for high-risk children are difficult outside of national registries, there is still much to be learned about the factors that contribute to renal injury in these children. Clinicians and researchers must begin to think outside of the proverbial VUR box. It is beginning to be understood that there are a variety of abnormalities in host defenses that might predispose some children to recurrent UTI.[13] Knowledge of these deficiencies in specific host defenses may lead to therapies designed to compensate for them. There is also much left to be learned about host inflammatory response to kidney infection to explain why some children suffer extensive kidney injury with pyelonephritis, whereas others with the same amount of acute inflammation avoid scarring altogether.[14] The National Institute of Diabetes and Digestive and Kidney Diseases recently funded a trial to determine whether steroids can modify the inflammatory and scarring response to acute pyelonephritis (clintrials.gov identifier NCT01391793). If steroids are found to be effective, future research should explore the ability of more targeted and powerful biologic agents to control the inflammation and scarring associated with kidney infection. In addition, there is still hope that advances in genetics may help to accurately stratify children according to their risk of recurrent UTI and kidney injury, even before they have their first UTI, thus allowing earlier tailoring of their therapy to their risk status.

REFERENCES

1. Keren R. Imaging and treatment strategies for children after first urinary tract infection. Curr Opin Pediatr 2007;19(6):705–10.
2. Olbing H, Claesson I, Ebel KD, et al. Renal scars and parenchymal thinning in children with vesicoureteral reflux: a 5-year report of the International Reflux Study in Children (European branch). J Urol 1992;148(5 Pt 2):1653–6.
3. Craig JC, Simpson JM, Williams GJ, et al. Antibiotic prophylaxis and recurrent urinary tract infection in children. N Engl J Med 2009;361(18):1748–59.
4. Keren R, Carpenter MA, Hoberman A, et al. Rationale and design issues of the Randomized Intervention for Children with Vesicoureteral Reflux (RIVUR) study. Pediatrics 2008;122(Suppl 5):S240–50.
5. Urinary tract infection: clinical practice guideline for the diagnosis and management of the initial UTI in febrile infants and children 2 to 24 months. Pediatrics 2011;128(3):595–610.

6. Salo J, Ikaheimo R, Tapiainen T, et al. Childhood urinary tract infections as a cause of chronic kidney disease. Pediatrics 2011;128(5):840–7.
7. Wennerstrom M, Hansson S, Jodal U, et al. Renal function 16 to 26 years after the first urinary tract infection in childhood. Arch Pediatr Adolesc Med 2000;154(4): 339–45.
8. Woolf AS. Clinical impact and biological basis of renal malformations. Semin Nephrol 1995;15(4):361–71.
9. Craig JC, Williams GJ. Denominators do matter: it's a myth–urinary tract infection does not cause chronic kidney disease. Pediatrics 2011;128(5):984–5.
10. Cystic Fibrosis Foundation Patient Registry. 2010 annual data report. Bethesda (MD): Cystic Fibrosis Foundation; 2011. Available at: http://www.cff.org/research/ClinicalResearch/PatientRegistryReport. Accessed May 23, 2012.
11. Crandall W, Kappelman MD, Colletti RB, et al. ImproveCareNow: the development of a pediatric inflammatory bowel disease improvement network. Inflamm Bowel Dis 2011;17(1):450–7.
12. Caceres M, Braud RL, Garrett HE Jr. A short history of the Society of Thoracic Surgeons national cardiac database: perceptions of a practicing surgeon. Ann Thorac Surg 2010;89(1):332–9.
13. Zasloff M. Antimicrobial peptides, innate immunity, and the normally sterile urinary tract. J Am Soc Nephrol 2007;18(11):2810–6.
14. Ragnarsdottir B, Lutay N, Gronberg-Hernandez J, et al. Genetics of innate immunity and UTI susceptibility. Nat Rev Urol 2011;8(8):449–68.

Hydronephrosis: A View from the Inside

Hrair-George O. Mesrobian, MD, MSc[a],*, Shama P. Mirza, PhD[b]

KEYWORDS

- Hydronephrosis • Prenatal • Kidney • Evaluation and management
- Urinary proteome

KEY POINTS

- Obstructive diseases of the urinary tract in the newborn can lead to infant death, kidney failure, and in those who survive, chronic kidney disease and early heart disease in adolescence and adulthood.
- In the Western Hemisphere, despite the availability of prenatal maternal sonography and advanced imaging, obstructive diseases of the urinary tract account for most cases of end-stage kidney disease and consume a large chunk of health care expenditure in this segment of the population.
- Early diagnosis by virtue of maternal sonography (secondary to hydronephrosis) affords opportunities to arrest or slow down the progression of renal functional deterioration. However, renal function can deteriorate by as much as 50% before it can be detected.
- Despite the magnitude of the problem, the renal response to human obstructive uropathy and subsequent disease progression remain poorly understood. This obscurity is compounded by the fact that current methods of diagnosis of renal impairment are insensitive (serum creatinine level) or invasive (tissue biopsy).
- Early detection and prevention of progressive renal damage are feasible and important strategies with long-term benefits to the individual and society.[1] Urinary tract obstruction leading to hydronephrosis consists of a spectrum of conditions resulting in a range of renal functional impairment.

INTRODUCTION

Obstructive diseases of the urinary tract in the newborn can lead to infant death, kidney failure, and in those who survive, chronic kidney disease and early heart disease in adolescence and adulthood.[2] In the Western Hemisphere, despite the availability of prenatal maternal sonography and advanced imaging, obstructive diseases of the urinary tract account for most cases of end-stage kidney disease and consume a large chunk of health care expenditure in this segment of the population.[3] Early diagnosis by virtue of maternal sonography (secondary to hydronephrosis) affords

[a] Division of Pediatric Urology, Department of Urology, Medical College and Children's Hospital of Wisconsin, 999 North, 92nd Street, Suite C330, Milwaukee, WI 53226, USA; [b] Department of Biochemistry, Medical College and Children's Hospital of Wisconsin, 999 North, 92nd Street, Suite C330, Milwaukee, WI 53226, USA
* Corresponding author.
E-mail address: hmesrobi@mcw.edu

Pediatr Clin N Am 59 (2012) 839–851
doi:10.1016/j.pcl.2012.05.008
0031-3955/12/$ – see front matter pediatric.theclinics.com

opportunities to arrest or slow down the progression of renal functional deterioration. However, renal function can deteriorate by as much as 50% before it can be detected.[3,4] Despite the magnitude of the problem, the renal response to human obstructive uropathy and subsequent disease progression remain poorly understood. This obscurity is compounded by the fact that current methods of diagnosis of renal impairment are insensitive (serum creatinine level) or invasive (tissue biopsy). The early detection and prevention of progressive renal damage are feasible and important strategies with long-term benefits to the individual and society.[1] Urinary tract obstruction leading to hydronephrosis consists of a spectrum of conditions resulting in a range of renal functional impairment. Unilateral ureteropelvic junction obstruction (UPJO) is the most common prenatally detected disease leading to hydronephrosis.[5] The obstructive anatomic lesion leads to varying degrees of hydronephrosis, ranging from no apparent effect on renal function to atrophy (**Fig. 1**). Furthermore, the natural course of hydronephrosis varies from spontaneous resolution to progressive deterioration and may take upwards of 3 years for a kidney to declare itself.[6] The objectives of this article are to update our knowledge regarding the evaluation and management of UPJO in depth and to discuss the emerging value of urinary proteome analysis to the clinical arena.

CLINICAL SCENARIOS
Patient Number 1

A 2-month-old boy presented with a history of prenatally detected left hydronephrosis, which was confirmed postnatally to be consistent with grade IV (see **Fig. 1**C). The anteroposterior diameter (AP) of the left renal pelvis was 2.15 cm. The AP diameter

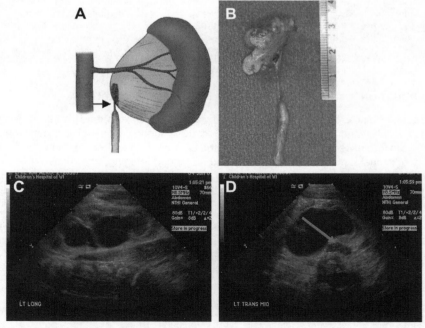

Fig. 1. (*A*) Arrow points to UPJO.1. (*B*) Burned out atrophic kidney UPJO. (*C*) Longitudinal view: grade IV. (*D*) Midtransverse view: AP = 2.15 cm (AP diameter = *blue arrow*).

is by convention a standardized measurement of the degree of hydronephrosis obtained on the midtransverse view (see **Fig. 1** D). Other methods have been described but have not gained widespread use.[7] The workup consisted of a voiding cystourethrogram, which was normal, and a furosemide technetium 99m (^{99m}Tc) mercapto-acetyl-triglycine (MAG 3) renal scan to assess kidney function. MAG-3 is a molecule that is almost exclusively a renal plasma flow agent, excreted by secretion in the proximal tubules and coupled to a radiotracer (^{99m}Tc).[8] Following injection, the radiotracer is followed over the kidneys, and time versus activity curves are generated. The deconvolution of these curves yields a value referred to as percent extraction of the radionuclide for each kidney and another referred to as the $t_{1/2}$. The latter is the time it takes for half of the radiotracer activity to leave the kidney following the administration of a standard dose of Lasix (1 mg/kg). The extraction factor is a surrogate for individual kidney function and the $t\frac{1}{2}$ is the drainage function of the renal pelvis. Surgery is recommended when the percent extraction is reduced to less than 40% for the hydronephrotic kidney and the $t\frac{1}{2}$ exceeds 30 minutes. A 10% or less extraction fraction is usually taken to indicate the presence of a burned-out and nonsalvageable hydronephrotic kidney. Different combinations of the grade of hydronephrosis, the percent extraction, the $t\frac{1}{2}$ can exist and more importantly may change over time. In patient number 1, these values were 49.6% and 10 minutes respectively and, therefore, the authors elected to follow this asymptomatic infant with watchful waiting. Over the following 3 years, the natural course of the disease unfolded and by 27 months of age, the percent extraction had decreased to 39.2% and the $t\frac{1}{2}$ increased to 18.2 minutes (**Fig. 2**). This toddler remained asymptomatic throughout this period. Progression has occurred in 28% of the authors' cohort of 25 patients followed over a period of time averaging 30 months and ranging from 6 to 48.

The course of this real case scenario demonstrates the difficulty in recommending surgery in an asymptomatic infant. It also demonstrates the limits of current imaging

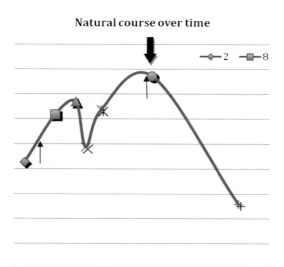

Natural course over time

Fig. 2. Fine arrows point to time at which the MAG-3 renal scans were obtained. Although the AP diameter was increasing and surgery was recommended initially, the parents declined because of absence of symptoms. A pyeloplasty was undertaken at 27 months of age after a MAG-3 renal scan revealed a 10% decrease in function (*thick arrow*).

methods and the least cost-effective method of evaluation and management of this disease.[9] There is a real need for biomarkers that are diagnostic for early functional deterioration and others that are prognostic for disease progression. This patient was found to have intrinsic UPJO at surgery, and a follow-up ultrasound at 9 months demonstrated almost complete resolution of the hydronephrosis. The histology of the ureteropelvic junction revealed a smooth muscle wall comprised of irregular bundles around a narrow lumen. The adjacent renal pelvis demonstrated smooth muscle hypertrophy and mild mononuclear inflammatory cell infiltrates. The kidney biopsy in similar patients reveals glomerular sclerosis, interstitial inflammation, and tubular atrophy with protein casts (**Fig. 3**). In this and an additional 24 patients, urinary specimens were obtained at presentation, during the first year of life, and at surgery. These specimens were subjected to analysis by mass spectrometry (see later discussion). The findings were compared with urine specimens obtained from 21 age-matched control individuals.

Patient Number 2

This 5-week-old boy presented with left grade IV UPJO. The AP diameter of the hydronephrotic kidney was 2.0 cm and a MAG-3 diuretic renal scan revealed a 53.7% extraction and a t½ of 5 minutes. The hydronephrosis did resolve over a 20-month period to a final AP of 0.31 cm. He remained asymptomatic throughout the course of his follow-up. In the authors' experience, resolution of hydronephrosis by ultrasound has been observed as early as 14 months after neonatal presentation and as late as 49 months. Patients in whom the hydronephrosis resolves still require to be followed albeit less intensively. Typically, the authors ask the parents to return patients for follow-up ultrasound studies at 5, 10, and 15 years of age. Delayed emergence of hydronephrosis has been described, and a few will present in adolescence with flank pain.

Patient Number 3

This baby girl presented at 1 month of age with left grade IV hydronephrosis secondary to UPJO. Her renal scan revealed a 48.8% extraction by the hydronephrotic kidney and a t½ of 6.3 minutes. She has now been followed for 3 years with a near stable AP diameter and remains asymptomatic (**Fig. 4**).

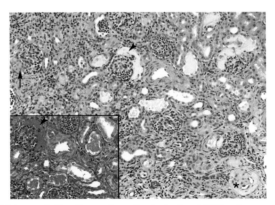

Fig. 3. Biopsy of kidney at the time of pyeloplasty for UPJO; glomerular sclerosis (*black arrow*), crescent formation (*arrowhead*), tubular atrophy (*asterisk*), and protein casts (*inset*) (hematoxylin-eosin).

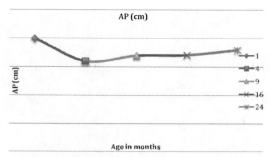

Fig. 4. Chronic hydronephrosis secondary to UPJO.

Because of the lack of a sensitive marker of early kidney function, the authors are planning on following her indefinitely unless the patient develops symptoms or the hydronephrosis resolves or increases. Patients like this little girl represent most of their cohort (58%). Ten percent of this cohort of patients has been shown to loose kidney function over time, which is primarily caused by a loss to follow-up.[10] This group also raises the question whether an opportunity to repair the hydronephrosis is being missed during the first 6 months of life when the kidney is still developing. During this period of time, the tubule lengthens by 3 times and the glomerular filtration rate (GFR) matures by 60%.[11] The concept of renal reserve has been recently introduced as an additional parameter of overall renal function. Renal reserve is defined as the kidney's capacity to increase its basal GFR by at least 20% in response to a protein load.[12] It is different from early functional deterioration (not yet reflected in the serum creatinine) in the presence of a normal contralateral unit. There is considerable evidence in the literature demonstrating that renal pelvic dilation alone activates several responses mediated by stretch and mechanoreceptors with effects on the renal tubule, mesangial cells, and the renal microvasculature.[13]

IMAGING AND GRADING OF HYDRONEPHROSIS

The most common prenatally diagnosed anomaly is an enlarged renal collecting system. The upper urinary tract and bladder can be visualized as early as 15 weeks' gestation. The discovery of a dilated upper urinary tract by itself is not specific. Many are accounted for by physiologic dilation, especially toward the third trimester when the fetal urine output is high. As a minimum, postnatal renal dilation can be antic-ipated if the AP diameter of the fetal renal pelvis exceeds 6 mm at less than 20 weeks' gestation, 8 mm at 20 to 30 weeks' gestation, and greater than 10 mm at more than 30 weeks' gestation.[14] Thus, a neonatal ultrasound study is obtained at or shortly after birth as the initial workup of prenatally discovered hydronephrosis. If confirmed, hydronephrosis is graded according to one of many grading systems. The Society of Fetal Urology (SFU) grading system is the most widely used; not only does it take into consideration the degree of pelviectasis but also the presence or absence of cal-iectasis with and without thinning of the overlying parenchyma (**Fig. 5**).[15]

SFU grades I and II have been shown not to have clinical significance in a large cohort of patients.[16] Therefore, these patients do not require intensive follow-up. The remainder of the discussion focuses on grade III and IV and isolated unilateral disease, which represents the most frequent urinary tract anomaly seen on prenatal sonography. A comprehensive review of the role of sonography as the premier imaging modality in this context can be found in the literature.[17]

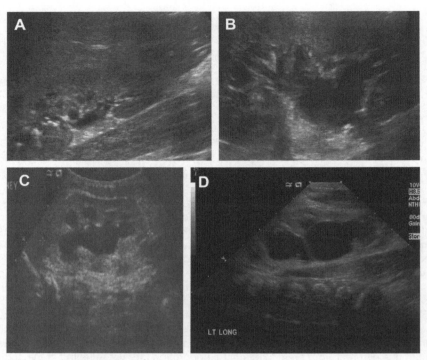

Fig. 5. (*A*) Grade I: separation of renal hilum. (*B*) Grade II: grade I + pelviectasis. (*C*) Grade III: grade II + caliectasis. (*D*) Grade IV: grade III + 50% or more thinning of renal cortex relative to normal.

Routine voiding cystourethrography (VCUG) is indicated to evaluate for the presence of ipsilateral vesicoureteral reflux (VUR). In the presence of bilateral disease or a duplication anomaly on sonography, a VCUG is obtained to look for VUR, an ectopic ureter or ureterocoele, and infravesical obstruction, such as with posterior urethral valves in boys. When a dilated ureter is present, the VCUG may uncover the presence of a refluxing megaureter. A description of the differential diagnosis and the workup in the newborn with prenatal hydronephrosis (with and without oligohydramnios) is provided elsewhere in this issue.

Following the VCUG, a renal nuclear medicine examination is obtained at 6 to 8 weeks' of age (when the kidneys are more mature) as a proxy for individual kidney function and drainage from the hydronephrotic renal pelvis. Currently, a furosemide ^{99m}Tc MAG 3 renal scan is the most popular radionuclide study used for this purpose. MAG 3 is a renal plasma flow agent almost exclusively excreted by secretion in the proximal tubules.[18] There are 2 main parameters that are evaluated: the percent extraction of the tracer by each kidney at 1 to 2 minutes following administration and the time (t½) it takes for half of the tracer activity to drain from the renal pelvis following the administration of a standard dose of furosemide (1 mg/kg). The timing of the furosemide administration may vary depending on the specific objectives of the test. Most imaging experts recommend its administration at 20 minutes into the study or when the collecting system is full with radiotracer activity as seen on a continuous monitor. With respect to t½, a value exceeding 30 minutes indicates the presence of significant obstruction to the drainage function of the kidney. However, a large nonobstructed and dilated collecting system may take that long to drain by virtue of its large capacity alone. Inserting a bladder catheter, maintaining a normal degree of hydration, patient position, and the dosage and timing of the diuretic administered standardizes the study.[19]

Magnetic resonance urography combines both anatomic and functional information in a single test and is capable of providing a comprehensive evaluation of obstructive uropathy.[20] It seems to provide information superior to sonography and diuretic renal scanning individually or combined. It has been described in the preoperative and postoperative setting where it provides superior functional information.[21] It has not been adopted universally, but recent advances promise a bright future.[22]

NATURAL HISTORY OF UPJO

It is precisely the unpredictable natural history of unilateral UPJO that dictates the current standard of evaluation and treatment. The kidney is carefully monitored over time, usually by sonography. This approach is dictated by natural history studies, which have demonstrated spontaneous resolution of hydronephrosis to occur in a well-documented but poorly defined subset of patients (10% of the authors' cohort, case number 2 described previously). Therefore, to avoid unnecessary surgery on the few, serial imaging of the structure and function of the diseased kidney are obtained and all patients are initially followed (historically early surgery was the standard). Approximately 30% of kidneys manifest progression. Surgery is undertaken for decreasing individual percent extraction (detected by nuclear renal scanning), increasing hydronephrosis (detected by renal sonography), pyelonephritis, and occasionally symptoms of pain. Although a 10% decrease in the percent extraction is taken as definitive evidence for a decline in the function of the hydronephrotic kidney, there is no consensus on what percentage increase in the AP diameter represents a significant change. In the authors' opinion and after making sure the bladder is fully decompressed, a 25% increase or more is taken to represent an increase of a sufficient magnitude to further evaluate with a diuretic renal scan or recommend a pyeloplasty. Current clinical or imaging tools are not able to distinguish at presentation or early in infancy between those patients who are likely to progress from those who are likely to undergo spontaneous resolution or remain stable in a chronic state of hydronephrosis. In fact, the latter group composes almost 60% of the cohort of newborns presenting with grade IV hydronephrosis, and indefinite follow-up is mandatory (clinical example number 3). Ironically, early relief of the obstruction at a time when the kidney is still developing may represent the best chance at preserving renal reserve function. The renal reserve function is difficult to measure in the newborn and infant·and is defined as the ability of the GFR to increase by 20% in response to a protein load.[23] Renal reserve has been shown to be decreased in more advanced forms of obstructive uropathy. In addition, the lack of an early biomarkers of glomerular and tubular function, inflammation, oxidative stress and or apoptosis hampers our ability to make better medical decisions regarding the timing of intervention. Although watchful waiting represents the current best strategy, future strategies may rely on urinary biomarkers of disease. There has been a flurry of research in the last 5 years aimed at discovery of proteins in the urine which may be differentially increased or decreased in various disease states-including UPJO (**Fig. 6**). These biomarkers can be used for prognosis, to assess response to treatment, and for early detection of renal pathologic processes, such as inflammation, oxidative stress, and tubular injury or interstitial fibrosis not advanced sufficiently to result in an increase in the serum creatinine or a decrease in percent extraction of radiotracer on a renal scan. In fact, early

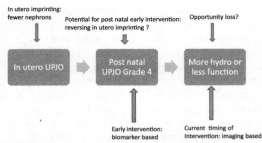

Fig. 6. Biomarker discoveries may facilitate a paradigm shift toward early intervention based on specific biomarkers of early damage.

experience suggests that the urinary proteome may pack in it information heretofore discoverable only by an invasive biopsy of the diseased kidney. In fact, the patient whose biopsy is depicted in **Fig. 3** did have supernormal percent extraction of the radiotracer in the hydronephrotic kidney. He underwent surgery because of a large AP diameter and intrarenal hydronephrosis. How much glomerular or tubular functional damage is required before a decrease in the percent extraction is not known. In fact, recent epidemiologic evidence has resulted in the introduction of the concept of fetal programming as it relates to low birth weight and the discovery of deleterious effects on kidney function.[24] The mechanisms of renal programming in the low-birth-weight baby are not too dissimilar from those operating in UPJO. These mechanisms include the activation of the renin-angiotensin system, reduction in the number of nephrons, increased generation of superoxide, increased sympathetic nerve activity, and other influences on the general vasculature. There is reason to be concerned about the watchful waiting approach to the evaluation and management of newborns and infants with grade IV UPJO. The kidney undergoes significant growth and development during the first year of life. The first 6 months are most crucial; for example, the tubule lengthens by 3 times and the glomerular filtration rate matures by 60%.[25]

URINARY BIOMARKERS OF UPJO

The complement of proteins and peptides found in a cell or environment constitutes a proteome (*prote*in complement of the gen*ome*). Proteomics is the study of the composition, structure, function, and interactions of the proteins directing the activities of cells or found in an environment or special condition (disease). Urinary proteome analysis has been a rapidly growing discipline with applications in biomedical research aimed at the discovery of disease biomarkers[26]; better understanding of physiology and biology[27]; and the discovery of new therapeutic modalities, including pharmacotherapy.[28,29] It is an ideal technology to apply in the context described previously particularly because it allows for the identification of more than 2000 proteins and many more peptides in normal urine. Proteins that are increased or decreased in their level of abundance in disease compared with normal levels become candidate biomarkers. Because a disease like UPJO elicits many different biologic processes, including compensatory and adaptive responses, the sum total of these interactions can be captured in the analysis of the bladder-derived urinary proteome. In contrast to other body fluids or tissues, urinary proteins have been shown to remain stable (up to 6 months at -80° C) and allow the performance of reliable analyses.[30] At least 70% of these urinary proteins originate from the kidney and lower urinary tract, whereas the remaining 30% originates from the circulation. In March of 2006,

Decramer and associates[31] reported on urinary proteome analysis in normal and in newborns and infants with varying degrees of hydronephrosis secondary to UPJO.[31] They used capillary electrophoresis coupled to mass spectrometry (MS) to find significant differences in the urinary proteome pattern between patient groups (different grades of UPJO) and normal individuals. This pioneering study has motivated the authors to embark on a mission to discover and identify specific proteins altered in UPJO by using a whole proteome, identity-based nanospray liquid chromatography-tandem mass spectrometry (LC-MS/MS). This technology allows for the global identification of urinary proteins and associated candidate biomarkers.[32] Although these represent different mass spectrometry technologies, they aim at identifying molecules with different weights and sizes in biologic fluid mixtures, such as urine. The identity of the proteins is derived from matching the output data to known fragmentation patterns of proteins/peptides based on the genome (**Fig. 7**). There are several databases against which the matching is done in an automated fashion.[33] The most important steps are sample collection, storage, and preparation. The Human Kidney and Urine Proteome Project has adopted international guidelines in this regard.[34] Dipstick-negative urine in infants is collected via a bag or catheterization (using sterile technique). In older children, a midstream of random-catch urine other than the first morning urine may be obtained. A total of 2 mL of urine (stored initially in a specimen cup) is sufficient and can be kept at room temperature for up to 4 hours. The specimen is then transferred to a sterile test tube and stored at -80°C until analysis. Sample preparation depends on the objective of the experimentation but should include a purification and depletion or enrichment step, measurement of protein and creatinine concentrations, reduction, alkylation, and trypsin digestion.[35] The resulting peptide mixture is then injected into the mass spectrometer. Each experiment is repeated in triplicate for protein identification and quantification by spectral counting. More advanced methods of quantitative proteomics are selected to validate the results of discovery experiments. For an excellent review, the reader is referred to a recent publication.[36]

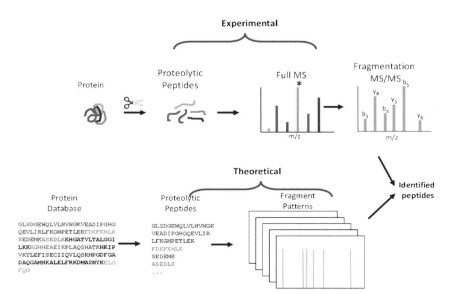

Fig. 7. Mass spectrometry-based protein identification workflow (*asterisk*) fragmentation.

To determine the proteins with significantly different levels of abundance between stable UPJO and normal samples, data from the technical replicates from each sample are combined and compared using Visualize (Software method).[37] The authors rely on the G test (log likelihood ratio test for goodness of fit) to calculate a P value, and the P values are corrected for multiple testing using the Holme-Sidak method based on the number of proteins that passed the filter.[38] Proteins with a normalized P value of .05 or less are sorted into upregulated or downregulated sets based on a log 2 ratio of greater than 1 or less than 1. The output data previously mentioned are analyzed through the use of Ingenuity Pathways Analysis (Ingenuity Systems, Redwood City, California; www.ingenuity.com). A log 2 ratio value of 1 and a P value of .05 cutoffs for each upregulated or downregulated protein are set to identify genes corresponding to proteins whose expressions were significantly differentially regulated in disease specimens compared with normal specimens. The authors' preliminary studies have focused uniquely on patients with grade IV hydronephrosis and confirm the presence of statistically significant differential levels of abundance of several urinary proteins and polypeptides between normal and UPJO.[39] **Table 1** is an illustration of a few urinary proteins. The results strongly point to the presence of inflammation, apoptosis, tubular fibrosis, and oxidative stress in the hydronephrotic kidney even before the emergence of increasing hydronephrosis or decreasing function by imaging. The discovery phase described previously is then validated in several samples derived from a population of patients with various degrees of functional impairment from UPJO. This step is similar to a prospective clinical trial and is intended to reflect the full variation of the targeted population. Western blotting and multiple reaction monitoring are the 2 leading technologies for validation studies.

SURGICAL TREATMENT AND RESULTS

Anderson and Hynes[40] first described the standard repair of UPJO in 1949. The procedure consisted of a flank incision, exposure of the UPJO, and excision of the diseased

Table 1
Illustration of function and origin of select urinary proteins increased in bladder-derived urine of infants presenting with grade IV UPJO

Entrez Gene Name	Location	Function
Alpha-2-macroglobulin	Extracellular space	Fibrosis (member of TGFβ family)
Actin, alpha 2	Cytoplasm	Renal interstitial fibrosis marker
Annexin A1, A5	Plasma membrane	Apoptosis, inflammatory response
Beta-2-microglobulin	Plasma membrane	Apoptosis (FDA)
Clusterin	Extracellular space	Renal tubular injury (FDA)
Capping protein (actin filament), gelsolinlike	Nucleus	Inflammatory response
Heat shock protein 90 kDa alpha	Cytoplasm	Proximal tubular injury
Myeloperoxidase	Cytoplasm	Oxidative stress response
Actin, beta	Cytoplasm	NRF2-mediated oxidative stress
Neutrophil gelatinase associated lipocalin	Extracellular space	Tubular injury (necrosis)
S100 calcium-binding protein A8	Cytoplasm	Chemotaxis
Epidermal growth factor	Extracellular space	Cell growth and development

Abbreviations: FDA, Food and Drug Administration; NRF2, nuclear factor 2; TGFβ, transforming growth factor-β.

segment with a generous portion of adjacent hydronephrotic renal pelvis. This procedure was followed by reanastomosis of the ureter to the renal pelvis and resulted in a dependent and ample junction. Additional surgical procedures were described in response to specific anatomic variants,[41] such as a high insertion of the ureter into the renal pelvis. Patients are discharged after an average of a 2-day hospital stay. A 95% success rate is now attained. Within the past decade, laparoscopic or robot-assisted laparoscopic pyeloplasty have gained wider use in the treatment of UPJO with similar results but with the additional benefit of a shorter length of stay, less postoperative pain, and the absence of a flank incision.[42,43] These techniques are discussed elsewhere in this issue.

REFERENCES

1. Black C, Sharma P, Scotland G, et al. Early referral strategies for management of people with markers of renal disease: a systematic review of the evidence of clinical effectiveness, cost-effectiveness and economic analysis. Health Technol Assess 2010;14(21):1–184.
2. Roth KS, Koo HP, Spottswood SE, et al. Obstructive uropathy: an important cause of chronic renal failure in children. Clin Pediatr 2002;45:309–14.
3. Gilbertson DT, Liu J, Xue JL, et al. Projecting the number of patients with end-stage renal disease in the United States to the year 2015. J Am Soc Nephrol 2005;16(12):3736–41.
4. McRory W. Measurement of renal function, developmental nephrology, chapter 3. Cambridge (MA): Harvard University Press; 1972. p. 95–100.
5. McKenna PH. Epidemiology: incidence and prevalence. In: Congenital urinary tract obstruction. State of the art strategic planning workshop. Bethesda (MD): National Institutes of Health; 2002. p. 8.
6. Fefer S, Ellsworth P. Prenatal hydronephrosis. Edited by Mesrobian and Pan. Pediatr Clin North Am 2006;53:429–47.
7. Imaji R, Dewan PA. Calyx to parenchyma ratio in pelviureteric junction obstruction. BJU Int 2002;89:73–7.
8. Grenier N, Hauger O, Cimpean A, et al. Update of renal imaging. Semin Nucl Med 2006;36(1):3–15.
9. Mesrobian HG. The value of newborn urinary proteome analysis in the evaluation and management of ureteropelvic junction obstruction: a cost-effectiveness study. World J Urol 2009;27(3):379–83.
10. Eskild-Jensen A, Munch Jorgensen T, Olsen LH, et al. Renal function may not be restored when using decreasing differential function as the criterion for surgery in unilateral hydronephrosis. BJU Int 2003;92:779–82.
11. Hunley TE, Valentina K, Ichikawa I. Glomerular circulation and function. In: Avner ED, Harmon WE, Niaudet P, et al. Pediatric nephrology. 6th edition; 2009 Chapter 2. p. 31–64.
12. Musso CG, Reynaldi J, Martinez B, et al. Renal reserve in the oldest old. Int Urol Nephrol 2011;43(1):253–6.
13. Quinlan MR, Docherty NG, William R, et al. Exploring mechanisms involved in renal tubular sensing of mechanical stretch following ureteric obstruction. Am J Physiol Renal Physiol 2008;295:F1–11.
14. Siemens DR, Prouse KA, MacNeily AE, et al. Antenatal hydronephrosis: thresholds of renal pelvic diameter to predict insignificant postnatal pelvicaliectasis. Tech Urol 1998;4(4):198–201.

15. Fernbach SK, Maizels M, Conway JJ. Ultrasound grading of hydronephrosis: introduction to the system used by the Society for Fetal Urology. Pediatr Radiol 1993;23:478–80.

16. Bulent O, Zanetta VC, Retik AB, et al. Predicting factors for complete resolution of uretero-pelvic junction obstruction like hydronephrosis: results from 1,568 children. Abstract # 16, section on urology annual meeting. Boston: NCE; 2011.

17. Sty JR, Pan CG. Genitourinary imaging techniques. Pediatr Clin North Am 2006; 53:339–46.

18. Trejtnar F, Laznicek M. Analysis of renal handling of radiopharmaceuticals. Q J Nucl Med 2002;46(3):181–94.

19. Conway JJ, Maizels M. The "well tempered renogram". J Nucl Med 1992;33: 2047–51. Available at: http://www.ncbi.nlm.nih.gov.proxy.lib.mcw.edu/pubmed/ 1432172. Accessed May 10, 2012.

20. Grattan-Smith JD, Little SB, Jones RA. MR urography evaluation of obstructive uropathy. Pediatr Radiol 2008;38:S49–69.

21. Kirsch AJ, McMann LP, Jones RA, et al. Magnetic resonance urography for evaluating outcomes after pediatric pyeloplasty. J Urol 2006;176:1755–61.

22. Leyendecker JR, Clingan MJ. Magnetic resonance urography update-are we there yet? Semin Ultrasound CT MR 2009;30:246–57.

23. Ansari MS, Surdas R, Barai S, et al. Renal function reserve in children with posterior urethral valve: a novel test to predict long-term outcome. J Urol 2011;185:2329–33.

24. Dotsch J, Plank C, Amann K. Fetal programming of renal function. Pediatr Nephrol 2012;27:513–20.

25. Dotsch J. Renal and extra renal mechanisms of perinatal programming after intrauterine growth retardation. Hypertens Res 2009;32(4):238–41.

26. Haubitz M, Wittke S, Weissinger EM, et al. Urine protein patterns can serve as diagnostic tools in patients with IgA nephropathy. Kidney Int 2005;67: 2313–20.

27. Rossing K, Mishak H, Rossing P, et al. The urinary proteome in diabetes and diabetes-associated complications: new ways to assess disease progression and evaluate therapy. Proteomics Clin Appl 2008;2(7–8):997–1007.

28. Pisikun T, Johnstone R, Knepper MA. Discovery of urinary biomarkers. Mol Cell Proteomics 2006;5(10):1760–71.

29. Kentsis A, Monigatti F, Dorff K, et al. Urine proteomics for profiling of human disease using high accuracy mass spectrometry. Proteomics Clin Appl 2009; 3(9):1052–61.

30. Thongboonkerd V. Practical points in urinary proteomics. J Proteome Res 2007; 6(10):3881–90.

31. Decramer S, Wittke S, Ross MM, et al. Predicting the clinical outcome of congenital unilateral ureteropelvic junction obstruction in newborn by urinary proteome analysis. Nat Med 2006;12:398–400.

32. Mesrobian HG, Halligan DB, Wakim TB, et al. Discovery of candidate urinary biomarkers in ureteropelvic junction obstruction: a whole proteomic approach. J Urol 2010;184:709–14.

33. UniProt Consortium. The Universal Protein Resource (UniProt). Nucleic Acids Res 2008;36(Database issue):D190–5.

34. Available at: http://hkupp.kir.jp/Urine%20collectiion%20Documents.htm. Accessed May 10, 2012.

35. Shama PM, Olivier M. Methods and approaches for the comprehensive characterization and quantification of cellular proteomes using mass spectrometry. Physiol Genomics 2008;33:3–11.

36. Selevsek N, Matondo M, Sanchez Carbayo M, et al. Systematic quantification of peptides/proteins in urine using selected reaction monitoring. Proteomics 2011; 11:1135–47.
37. Halligan BH, Greene A. Visualize: a free and open source multifunction tool for proteomics data analysis. Proteomics 2011;11:1058–63.
38. Hendrickson EL, Xia Q, Wang T, et al. Comparison of spectral counting and metabolic stable isotope labeling for use with quantitative microbial proteomics. Analyst 2006;131(12):1335–41.
39. Mesrobian HG, Mitchell ME, See WA, et al. Candidate urinary biomarker discovery in ureteropelvic junction obstruction: a proteomic approach. J Urol 2010;184(2):709–14.
40. Anderson JC, Hynes W. Retrocaval ureter: a case diagnosed preoperatively and treated successfully by a plastic operation. Br J Urol 1949;21:209.
41. Mesrobian HG. Bypass pyeloplasty: description of a procedure and initial results. J Pediatr Urol 2009;5:34–6.
42. Casale P. Robotic pyeloplasty in the pediatric population. Curr Opin Urol 2009;19: 97–101.
43. Karsli C, El-Hout Y, Lorenzo AJ, et al. Physiological changes in transperitoneal versus retroperitoneal laparoscopy in children: a prospective analysis. J Urol 2011;186(Suppl 4):1649–52.

Update on the Management of Disorders of Sex Development

Rodrigo L.P. Romao, MD[a], Joao L. Pippi Salle, MD, PhD[a],*,
Diane K. Wherrett, MD[b]

KEYWORDS

- Disorders of sex development • Management • Genital ambiguity • Genital surgery

KEY POINTS

- Patients with disorders of sexual development (DSDs) should be assessed and treated in a multidisciplinary clinic.
- Most patients with DSDs present early in life with genital ambiguity.
- A comprehensive assessment of infants with genital ambiguity allows proper gender assignment within a few days.
- DSD encompasses a wide range of diagnoses and clinical scenarios.
- The timing and nature of genital surgery remain controversial topics.

INTRODUCTION

The management of children with ambiguous genitalia remains controversial. Conditions associated with genital ambiguity lack a consistent terminology, and there is a variable approach to diagnosis and management. In 2006, a consensus statement was published in an attempt to standardize the nomenclature and approach, defining these conditions as disorders of sex development (DSDs). After a multidisciplinary meeting held in Chicago that included endocrinologists, surgeons, geneticists, psychologists, and representatives from advocacy groups, it was agreed on that traditional terms, such as intersex, true, and pseudohermaphroditism, and any expression that could give rise to an idea of a third gender should be abandoned. DSDs were categorized under 3 main subgroups according to karyotype (XX, XY, and sex chromosome for mosaic karyotypes). The consensus also acknowledged the integral role of psychosocial support and the management of these patients guided by a multidisciplinary team.[1–3]

[a] Division of Urology, Department of Surgery, The Hospital for Sick Children, University of Toronto, 555 University Avenue, Toronto, ON, Canada M5G 1X8; [b] Division of Endocrinology, Department of Paediatrics, The Hospital for Sick Children, University of Toronto, 555 University Avenue, Toronto, ON, Canada M5G 1X8
* Corresponding author.
E-mail address: pippi.salle@sickkids.ca

Pediatr Clin N Am 59 (2012) 853–869
doi:10.1016/j.pcl.2012.05.020
0031-3955/12/$ – see front matter © 2012 Published by Elsevier Inc.

pediatric.theclinics.com

This consensus statement has been well accepted by the medical and patient community worldwide.[4–7] Despite having diverse diagnoses under its umbrella, the DSD classification has allowed the subject to be addressed in a more scientific way with direct participation of patient support groups.

The embryologic development of the external genitalia (EG) is well understood. The fetal EG remains undifferentiated until 6 to 7 weeks' gestation. The sex-determining region in the Y chromosome (SRY) is the main factor driving the development of the bipotential gonad into a testicle. The Sertoli cells secrete anti-Müllerian hormone (AMH), which in turn will inhibit the development of Müllerian structures (fallopian tubes, uterus, cervix, upper third of the vagina). Subsequently, Leydig cells produce testosterone, which binds to the nuclear androgen receptor to virilize the internal genitalia of the fetus. Testosterone is converted to dihydrotestosterone, a more potent androgen that stimulates the differentiation of the EG into male anatomy (development of the phallus into a penis, fusion of labioscrotal folds to form scrotum, and so forth) by acting on the androgen receptor. Most DSD conditions will result from inadequate androgen action (either excessive or insufficient) or gonadal dysfunction, which clinically will translate into either virilization of the female fetus or undermasculinization of the male one.

CLASSIFICATION

The current DSD classification follows the patients' karyotype and 3 main groups are recognized: 46XY DSD, 46XX DSD, and sex chromosome DSD (mosaic karyotype, most commonly 45X/46XY). Further identification of the source of the problem (ie, gonad structure/function, androgen pathway, and receptor, and so forth) will lead to a specific diagnosis.[2,3,8–11] The most common causes of DSD divided by karyotype are depicted in **Table 1**.

Most patients with DSDs present in the neonatal period with genital ambiguity. Clinical scenarios that should trigger evaluation for DSDs are overt genital ambiguity, virilized female EG (ie, enlarged clitoris, posterior labial fusion, and inguinal/labial mass), undervirilized male EG (bilateral undescended testicles, micropenis, association of hypospadias, and undescended testicles). Although the consensus advocates for a full DSD workup for patients with perineal hypospadias and bilateral descended testicles,[1,2] the authors' group has been moving away from that practice because a review of their own data showed that the large cohort of such patients with well-developed phallus and scrotum was uniformly assigned the male sex and found not to harbor any Müllerian structures. It is important to avoid using the term ambiguous genitalia and lengthy delays in sex assignment for such patients because this is a significant source of stress for parents.[12]

A significant proportion (10%–20%) of patients can present later in life[8,11] (childhood or even young adulthood) and for those, the absence of ambiguity is the rule. Reasons for the referral of female patients include palpable gonad within an inguinal hernia; absent, delayed, or incomplete puberty; virilization; and primary amenorrhea. In teenagers, breast development, gross cyclic hematuria, and sometimes simply infertility flag the possibility of DSD. In pediatric medicine, as karyotype has become more common, discordance between genital appearance and karyotype ordered for issues unrelated to gender assignment is another reason for referral to DSD clinics.[8,11]

APPROACH TO THE NEWBORN WITH GENITAL AMBIGUITY
History

Newborns with genital ambiguity should be evaluated on an urgent basis. The first challenge is to define which patients actually have ambiguous genitalia as opposed

Table 1
DSD classification and most common diagnoses

	XX DSD	XY DSD	Sex Chromosome DSD
Disorders of gonadal development	Ovotesticular DSD XX sex reversal (testicular DSD) Gonadal dysgenesis	Pure gonadal dysgenesis Partial gonadal dysgenesis Ovotesticular DSD Gonadal regression or vanishing testis syndrome	45X/46XY Mixed gonadal dysgenesis Ovotesticular DSD

Disorders related to androgen synthesis or action	Androgen excess
	(a) Maternal
	   i Luteoma
	   ii Exogenous (medications)
	(b) Fetoplacental
	   i Aromatase deficiency
	(c) Fetal
	   i Congenital adrenal hyperplasia (21-hydroxylase deficiency most common)
		Androgen action
		Androgen insensitivity syndrome
		
		Androgen synthesis
		LH receptor mutation
		17-beta hydroxysteroid dehydrogenase deficiency
		5-alpha reductase deficiency
		Male CAH (eg, 3-beta deficiency)	

Abbreviations: CAH, congenital adrenal hyperplasia; LH, luteinizing hormone.

to minor genital abnormalities (eg, mild clitoral enlargement or isolated distal hypospadias) and, therefore, avoid overinvestigation. After identifying one of the scenarios listed in the previous section, the first step is to request an evaluation by an expert in DSD who works as part of a multidisciplinary team. Even before the first assessment is initiated, some general principles should be kept in mind: one should refrain from making comments or statements based on the appearance of the EG alone, every newborn infant should receive a male or female gender assignment after a thorough and timely investigation; a long-term care plan should be discussed in the setting of a multidisciplinary, holistic, patient-centered clinic using the best level of evidence available; family concerns should be addressed promptly, openly, and confidentially by professionals with the best communication skills, without withholding detailed information.[1–3]

A detailed history should focus on a family history of DSD, parental consanguinity, unexplained infant deaths, maternal ingestion of drugs (particularly progestagens and steroids[1]), use of assisted reproductive technologies, and results of prenatal tests. A history of maternal virilization during pregnancy points toward the possibility of aromatase deficiency and, rarely, maternal androgen secreting tumors, such as luteomas.[1,2,13] During the first interview, care should be taken to ascertain the degree of knowledge parents might already have about their baby's condition and DSD. A careful perinatal history focused on the evidence of prematurity, intrauterine growth retardation, or other signs of placental insufficiency should also be obtained because an association of those conditions with undervirilization of the male genitalia has been described.[14,15] Because the parents may not know details of a family history of DSD, it is important to ask about a history of hypospadias, amenorrhea, and infertility.

Physical Examination

Physical examination should initially focus on general findings and potentially life-threatening problems, like the presence of severe dehydration that can be associated with salt-wasting congenital adrenal hyperplasia (CAH), which usually happens after 1 to 2 weeks of life, followed by the inspection for signs of dysmorphic features or associated anomalies. The examination of the EG starts with the careful inspection of the phallic structure, noting length, breadth, and amount of erectile tissue; number of orifices in the perineum and their topography, rugation, pigmentation, and fusion of the labioscrotal folds; and the position and patency of the anus (girls with cloacal anomalies often have some degree of genital ambiguity). Asymmetry is also an important sign to look for because some DSD conditions, like ovotesticular DSD and mixed gonadal dysgenesis, will produce virilization on only one side of the genitalia.[16]

Virilized female genitalia will usually exhibit variable degrees of clitoromegaly, pigmentation, and rugation of the labial skin and labial fusion; depending on the degree of virilization, only one opening other than the anus will be visible in the perineum representing an urogenital sinus (UGS). The Prader classification provides a useful standardization for such findings ranging from 1 (mild clitoromegaly) through to 5 (complete virilization with UGS opening up at the tip of the phallus) - **Fig. 1.**

Male undervirilization is portrayed by variable degrees of hypospadias (urethral opening in the ventral aspect of the penile shaft), which can also be associated with bifid scrotum, penile ventral curvature, and penoscrotal transposition.

In either case, it is important to palpate the phallus for the presence of corpora (erectile tissue) and measure its stretched dorsal length, which can be compared with normalized data.[17]

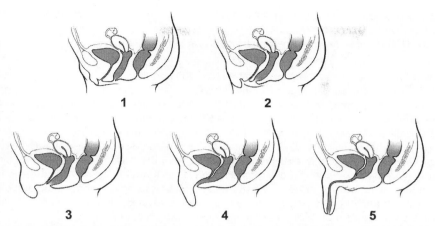

Fig. 1. A sagittal view of the virilized external genitalia corresponding to the Prader classification. Prader 1 corresponds to mild clitoromegaly with separate openings for vagina and urethra. Praders 2 through 4 depict the progression from mild to severe virilization. Prader 5 depicts the most extensive degree of virilization, with enlarged phallus and long urogenital sinus (common channel), which resembles the male urethra.

Even in patients with normal-appearing male genitalia, a penis shorter than 2.0 to 2.5 cm with a narrow breadth should be considered a micropenis and warrants further investigation.

Following the examination of the EG itself, palpation of gonads is a key step in the initial assessment. Gonads can be palpated within the scrotum or labioscrotal folds, inguinal canal, or nonpalpable. The status of the gonads on palpation bears a particularly important weight on the initial diagnostic thought process.

Diagnostic Tests

The most important initial diagnostic tests in the DSD workup are karyotype, pelvic ultrasound to evaluate the presence of Müllerian structures, and serum levels of sodium, potassium, and 17-hydroxyprogesterone (17-OHP) after day 3 of life. A thorough history and physical examination (especially gonad palpation[1,2,8,16]) coupled with the results of the aforementioned tests will allow patients to be situated within the DSD umbrella and receive a final diagnosis based on pathophysiology in most cases. Other serum biochemistry tests frequently used are androgens (testosterone, dihydrotesterone, androstenedione), cortisol, gonadotrophins, and AMH levels. In infants older than 3 to 6 months or if a defect of androgen production is suspected, it may be necessary to perform a stimulation test with human chorionic gonadotropin (hCG) to reliably estimate the gonadal production of androgens.

Pathology reports from gonadal biopsies or removal may be helpful in formulating a more complete diagnosis but such procedures are rarely performed in young newborns or infants right at the outset.

Despite the rapid incorporation of knowledge from genetic studies in recent years, particularly for 46XY DSD, genetic testing is currently not widely available and its ability to add benefit to the initial approach of ambiguous genitalia is uncertain.[4] Nonetheless, increasing availability of such testing can be valuable for defining a molecular cause and supporting genetic counseling for families.

DIAGNOSIS AND MANAGEMENT OF MOST COMMON DSD CONDITIONS/UP-TO-DATE REVIEW OF CONTROVERSIAL ISSUES
46 XX DSD (Former Female Pseudohermaphroditism)

CAH

CAH remains by far the most common 46 XX DSD and the most frequent DSD overall.[3,8–11] The pathophysiology of CAH involves an enzymatic defect in the adrenal cortisol synthesis pathway, which leads to the accumulation of precursors and excessive production of androgens (**Fig. 2**). The EG shows variable degrees of virilization with bilateral *nonpalpable* gonads. Müllerian structures are identified on ultrasound and 17-OHP is elevated in the most common form of the disease (21-alpha hydroxylase–CYP21 deficiency, see diagram). About 75% of the patients will have the salt-wasting form of CAH, which can present with a life-threatening salt-losing crisis in the first or second week of life,[1,18] characterized by severe hyponatremic dehydration. Newborn screening for 21-hydroxylase deficiency is available in many countries and allows the diagnosis of CAH before a significant salt-wasting event.

Medical management Glucocorticoid replacement with the goals of replenishing the lack of cortisol and suppressing excessive androgen production by means of negative feedback on release remains the mainstay of medical therapy for CAH. Hydrocortisone is the preferred drug in children because of its short half-life and it should be administered as crushed tablets.[18,19] Typical dosages are in the range of 10 to 15 $mg/m^2/d$, with lower-range dosages in toddlers and higher in adolescents.

In adults, longer-acting and more potent drugs, such as dexamethasone or prednisone, are favored because growth suppressive effects are less relevant.[18,19]

Treatment with glucocorticoids is not physiologic because normal release follows a circadian rhythm. Most protocols recommend a larger dose in the morning and attempts at using programmed infusion or modified-release forms of the medications to mimic the circadian rhythm are largely experimental.[18] Currently, bilateral adrenalectomy is not part of the standard of care and should be considered only in cases of

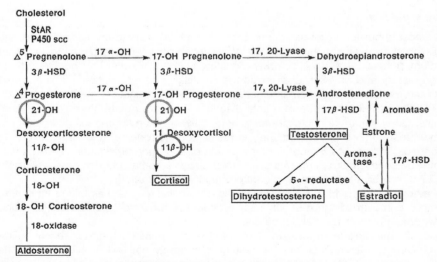

Fig. 2. The androgen pathway and the mechanism of virilization caused by the most common form of CAH (21-OH deficiency). Note that diagnosis is provided by accumulation of 17-OH progesterone and enzymatic defect leads to overproduction of androgens.

failed medical management, particularly in women with salt-wasting CAH and infertility, when compliance to medical treatment is not an issue.[18]

Approximately three-quarters of the CAH population will have the classic salt-wasting form of the disease and also require mineralocorticoid replacement in the form of fludrocortisone.

Therapy is monitored through the determination of morning blood levels of 17-OHP and androstenedione; 17-OHP reflects adrenocorticotropic hormone suppression, and complete normalization usually reflects overtreatment leading to hypercortisolism, which is also deleterious. In children, height and weight should be recorded in each follow-up visit and a bone age should be performed yearly.[18,19] Patients with salt-wasting CAH also require sodium, potassium, and renin monitoring.

A stress dose of steroids should be given in cases of febrile illness, dehydration, surgery, and trauma. Emotional or mental stress and minor illnesses do not require a stress dose.[18]

Gender assignment The DSD consensus supports female gender assignment for patients with XX CAH because more than 90% of those patients identify themselves as women,[2,3] and the presence of normal female internal genitalia offers the potential for fertility. Furthermore, the incidence of gender dysphoria in women with CAH was shown to be around 5%, which, despite being a higher rate than what is found in the general population, was deemed to be acceptable to support a uniform female sex of rearing assignment in this population.[20] However, recent publications have questioned this practice for markedly virilized patients (namely Prader 5 and some Prader 4) and suggested that male gender assignment should be entertained in this particular situation.[21] The topic is controversial, and at this stage it is reasonable to state that the most patients with XX CAH should be assigned the female gender. In the authors' experience, 65 of 70 (93%) patients with XX DSD were assigned the female gender. Three patients with CAH referred after puberty and previously raised as boys underwent hysterectomy, bilateral gonadectomies, and hypospadias repair.[11]

Surgery The timing and magnitude of the surgical treatment of CAH has been a subject for intense debate in recent years. Surgical treatment of girls with CAH involves feminizing genitoplasty, in the form of clitoroplasty and labioplasty, and vaginoplasty, which may be performed at the same time or not, with the goal of exteriorizing the vagina and creating 2 separate openings for the urethra and vagina. As a general rule, the more virilized the patient, the higher the vagina inserts in the common channel (UGS), which is technically more demanding for repair. Most investigators agree that feminizing genitoplasty should be offered routinely in infancy for patients with significant virilization (Prader 3 or higher) and performed by surgeons experienced with the procedure, preferably in centers that offer multidisciplinary care.[2,18,22] In recent years, ethicists and patient support groups have come forward to call a moratorium on any genital surgery in infancy, arguing that patients should be able to give informed consent before undergoing such procedures.[23] However, consequences of this policy to patients and families have not been properly addressed either.

Issues around timing and type of repairs are truly unsettled. Some investigators think that vaginoplasty should be done early along with the clitoroplasty and labioplasty, especially because flaps from the UGS could be useful in the repair of a high vagina. Others state that deferring at least the latter until puberty would be more logical, given that a significant proportion of patients require vaginal dilatation at that time, if they have had early surgery. The level of evidence for either approach is limited at best. Long-term outcome studies are extremely scarce. Although some studies suggest poor cosmetic and functional results of genitoplasty done in infancy[24,25] with a high reintervention rate in adulthood,[26] other publications indicate that adult patients with CAH who had surgery early in life score similarly to those with other surgical and nonsurgical chronic medical conditions in quality of life, and physical and mental health tests[22,26]; moreover, recent surveys completed by adult patients with CAH suggest that most women favor surgery before adolescence.[27,28]

The authors' view is that the surgical treatment of CAH has evolved substantially in recent years. The surgical technique for clitoroplasty is now fairly well standardized across specialized centers and foresees preservation of the neurovascular bundle to maintain clitoral sensitivity.[29] The authors' group has described a corporal-sparing clitoroplasty whereby no tissue is ablated from the clitoris, preserving all sensation-bearing structures. Earlier results are encouraging,[30] but longer follow-up is required. In the last 2 decades, techniques for vaginoplasty have changed significantly. The addition of total and partial UGS mobilization[31,32] as well as the anterior sagittal transrectal approach for high urogenital sinuses[33,34] show promising early results. Thus, it does not seem fair to extrapolate results from feminizing genitoplasty and vaginoplasty performed decades ago without these options to the range of procedures that are offered today in centers with expertise.

The authors' group offers feminizing genitoplasty with concurrent vaginoplasty in infants with severe virilization (Prader 3 or more), which is ideally performed between 3 and 9 months of life. The decision to proceed with surgery only happens after discussion with the family and all members of the multidisciplinary team. In families who opt for surgery, corporal-sparing clitoroplasty is offered and explained, but the final decision always lies with the family. The technique for vaginoplasty depends on the length of the common channel and level of insertion of the vagina in it, which is determined by the combination of genitogram and cystoscopy/vaginoscopy.

Prenatal treatment Prenatal treatment of fetuses at risk for CAH with dexamethasone remains highly controversial. The possibility of reliably determining fetal sex with noninvasive techniques (cell-free fetal Y DNA detected in maternal blood) as early as 4 weeks after conception holds promise because it could allow significant reduction in unnecessary exposure to dexamethasone from 7 in 8 to 3 in 4 (female only) fetuses.[35] A recent systematic review[36] concluded that most studies on prenatal treatment are observational with low methodological quality. Although the data suggest that prenatal treatment is successful in reducing virilization with no significant short-term side effects to the fetus or the mother, some degree of behavioral changes in children exposed to dexamethasone during pregnancy have been suggested and need to be investigated further before making any firm recommendations.[37] Prenatal treatment of CAH should still be regarded as experimental and discussed with families on an individual basis, with a clear explanation of the risks and benefits.[18,36,37]

XY DSD (Former Male Pseudohermaphroditism)

The success rate in establishing the precise pathophysiology and cause of 46 XY DSD is far lower than in XX DSD.[3] XY DSD encompasses a wide range of diagnoses and genital ambiguity is not necessarily present. Furthermore, gender assignment discordant to karyotype (ie, female assignment) is significant in this group (up to 33% in the authors' experience[11]).

Fig. 3 illustrates the pathway of androgen synthesis and action that will lead to virilization of the external genitalia and potential mechanisms for disruption that will cause either undervirilization or no virilization whatsoever (ie, complete female genital appearance).

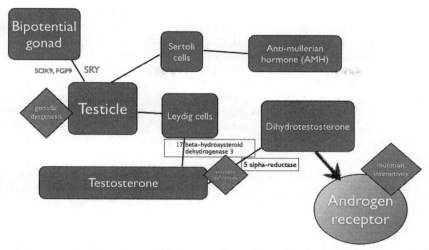

Fig. 3. The mechanism of virilization of the external genitalia. Diamond-shaped boxes depict potential sources of disruption leading to DSD.

Most patients with XY DSD of unknown cause will be labeled as having partial androgen insensitivity syndrome (PAIS). PAIS and the other most common XY DSD diagnoses are highlighted later with the most up-to-date information on management.

PAIS

PAIS is defined by the presence of variable degrees of undervirilization with normal androgen production, normal testicular histology, and the absence of Müllerian structures (ie, normal AMH production). Traditionally, androgen signaling or receptor abnormalities have been hypothesized but molecular confirmation is infrequent.[3,4] Recent advances in the understanding of genetic and environmental factors leading to PAIS, as well as gender assignment and surgical options, are highlighted later.

Cause In patients with PAIS, the identification of a mutation in the androgen receptor has been reported with a frequency of around 50% in recent publications.[4] On analyzing a large cohort of patients with XY DSD and normal testosterone production, Fernandez-Cancio and colleagues[38] identified a mutation in the androgen receptor in 42.5%; furthermore, the investigators described new polymorphisms associated with mutations in the 5-alpha reductase gene (SRD5A2) and suggested that they could be more common than once considered (6.2% in their series), thus explaining variable phenotypes of 46 XY DSD. This finding has been corroborated by other publications that, besides identifying new mutations in SRD5A2, found a higher than previously reported incidence of mutations in XY partially virilized women[39] and a wide spectrum of phenotypes and biologic profiles in patients from diverse geographic and ethnic backgrounds.[40] Patients with mutations in 17-beta hydroxysteroid dehydrogenase can present in a similar way. The genes, steroidogenic factor 1 (SF-1) and mastermindlike domain-containing 1 (MAMLD1), have also been linked to PAIS phenotypes.[4]

Environmental endocrine-disruptor chemicals have been related to the rising incidence of hypospadias, cryptorchidism, and male infertility in the general population.[41]

The comprehension of the interaction between environmental and known and yet-to-be-discovered genetic factors associated with male undervirilization will provide the tools needed by clinicians to establish prognostic criteria in many XY DSD situations.

Gender assignment In the past, severely undervirilized XY patients were offered feminizing surgery, gonadectomy, and hormonal replacement as part of the optimal gender approach, which was based on the assumption that sex of rearing would overrule chromosomal or gonadal sex.[1,16,42] Although most long-term outcome studies suggest that patients with XY DSD are usually satisfied and lead a well-adjusted sexual life regardless of their sex assignment,[42] partially virilized XY women demonstrate the highest rates of gender dysphoria and the need for reassignment among all patients with DSD, as well as dissatisfaction with surgical interventions.[43] Therefore, the authors' group supports the recent trend of assigning the male gender to XY patients with at least one functional testicle and reasonable penile tissue on palpation.[21,44]

Surgery In terms of surgical management, most undervirilized boys will require hypospadias repair with or without orchidopexy. There is no controversy that orchidopexy should be performed in the first year of life and the surgical approach is well standardized.[45]

The surgical management of severe proximal hypospadias still generates a lot of debate. It is difficult to perform high-quality research that is powerful enough to generate broad conclusions; a recent systematic review of the literature on hypospadias treatment from the last 20 years concluded that the current management of severe hypospadias is based on weak evidence, and even the definition of severe hypospadias is not the same between centers.[46] Questions are still largely unanswered, such as the ideal timing for surgery, type of surgery (1- vs 2-stage repair), ideal technique for curvature correction, and functional outcomes after puberty.

The authors' group favors complete correction of severe hypospadias in 2 operations, with the repair being completed ideally before the age of toilet training. For patients with severe ventral curvature, the urethral plate is transected, and the preputial skin is used to graft the ventral surface and is then tubularized after 6 to 8 months, as described by Bracka.[47]

Complete androgen insensitivity syndrome

Patients with complete androgen insensitivity syndrome (CAIS) do not present with genital ambiguity. CAIS is caused by a complete androgen receptor defect, which is transmitted following an X-linked pattern. The complete absence of androgen action precludes any virilization of the external genitalia. Patients with CAIS are usually diagnosed in infancy or childhood when a testicle is palpated or found in the groin during an assessment or exploration for an inguinal hernia in an otherwise female-appearing patient. Another possible clinical presentation is primary amenorrhea at puberty. They usually have a male-typical androgen profile, no identifiable Müllerian structures, and there is consensus around a female gender assignment. A case report of male reassignment in adulthood has been published recently in a patient with CAIS.[48]

Traditionally, these patients would undergo gonadectomy right after diagnosis, because of an increased risk for germ cell malignancies, followed by lifelong hormonal replacement to induce pubertal changes and maintain female secondary sexual characteristics. The exact risk of malignancy in patients with CAIS is not well known but is clearly more than that in the general population.[49] Because the gonads are not dysgenetic and most patients with testicles in situ will experience spontaneous puberty, a case has been made for delaying gonadectomy at least until puberty is complete.[50] Furthermore, recent reports challenge the need to perform gonadectomy at all because there have been anecdotal reports of loss of libido following gonadectomy, concerns about long-term hormonal replacement, and even the potential of the gonads harboring viable germ cells that could be used for fertility purposes in the future with advanced technology.[49] Appropriate follow-up modalities and screening intervals for gonadal tumors have not been delineated because most patients have undergone gonadectomy at the time of diagnosis or after the completion of puberty.

Patients with CAIS usually have a short blind-ending vagina; procedures that may be required to ensure proper intercourse range from simple dilatations to more complex reconstructive procedures, like sigmoid vaginoplasty,[51] and they should be offered, if necessary, when patients are ready to begin sexual life. Despite being well adjusted as women based on long-term follow-up studies,[52] high rates of dissatisfaction with sexual activity have been reported in this patient population, underscoring the importance of long-term psychological support.[43]

Complete or partial gonadal dysgenesis

The clinical presentation of XY gonadal dysgenesis is variable. At the most severe end of the spectrum is pure or complete gonadal dysgenesis, also known as Swyer syndrome, whereby patients are phenotypically female with normal Müllerian structures and bilateral streak gonads. These patients usually present in adolescence for primary amenorrhea. Partial gonadal dysgenesis is a spectrum that is determined by the ability of the dysgenetic testicle to produce AMH and testosterone; therefore, undervirilization with the presence of internal Müllerian structures can be seen as well as a normal male phenotype presenting later to an infertility clinic.[1] Testosterone levels will usually be less than expected values in accordance with testicular function and with variable response to stimulation tests.

DAX1, SOX9, and GATA4 are examples of genes that have been implicated in gonadal dysgenesis. Wilms tumor–related gene on chromosome 11p13 (WT1) mutations are known to be associated with syndromes that present with XY DSD and an increased risk for Wilms tumors, such as Denys-Drash and Frasier. Furthermore, WT1 mutations have been identified in up to 7.5% of patients with severe hypospadias and at least one undescended testicle in a recent publication, highlighting the importance of testing and then screening this subset of patients for renal tumor or nephropathy.[53] Recently, a new WT1 mutation has been identified in a patient with pure gonadal dysgenesis and Wilms tumor.[4] Nevertheless, fewer than half of the patients with gonadal dysgenesis portend an identifiable genetic cause.[1]

For patients with pure gonadal dysgenesis, early gonadectomy is advised[54] because of the high risk of malignancy and female gender assignment is a consensus. Surgical management and gender assignment for patients with partial gonadal dysgenesis follow the same principles for mixed gonadal dysgenesis, which are explained in a separate section.

CAH in XY patients, 5-alpha reductase deficiency, and other androgen biosynthesis defects

Males with CAH caused by CYP 21 deficiency do not present with genital ambiguity. The main concern is impaired fertility associated with testicular adrenal rest tumors.[18,55] The less common 3-beta hydroxysteroid dehydrogenase and 17-alpha hydroxylase deficiencies can produce variable degrees of undervirilization, exacerbated at puberty.

Patients with 5-alpha reductase deficiency, which is characterized by a high testosterone/5-alpha dihydrotestosterone ratio, and 17-beta hydroxysteroid dehydrogenase deficiency will frequently present with significant undervirilization or even a female phenotype.[1,40] However, it is well accepted that patients with these disorders tend to identify in adulthood as men in more than 50% of the cases. That fact, coupled with the potential for fertility, justifies the formal recommendation for male gender assignment given by the consensus in patients with such conditions unless the phenotype is completely female.[2,16]

Sex Chromosome DSD

This category encompasses patients with Turner (45X) and Klinefelter (47XXY) syndromes and their variants and patients with mosaic karyotypes. The most common DSD mosaic karyotype is 45X/46XY and the most common diagnosis associated with it is mixed gonadal dysgenesis (MGD).[8,11] Patients with MGD generally present with genital ambiguity, asymmetrical EG, and, not uncommonly, inguinal hernias. They usually have a streak gonad on one side and a dysgenetic testicle on the other. It is not uncommon to see evidence of virilization only on the side where the testicle is present and Müllerian structures on the side of the streak gonad. The degree of virilization is variable and compatible with the ability of the dysgenetic testicle to produce testosterone. Similarly, to ovotesticular DSD, the clinical presentation and hormonal profile are widely variable. Gender assignment is also challenging and multifactorial (nearly 50/50 between male and female patients in the authors' series[11]).

Ovotesticular DSD

Ovotesticular DSD replaced the term true hermaphroditism and is defined by the presence of normal ovarian tissue containing follicles and normal testicular tissue containing tubules in the same individual. The tissues can be present within the same gonad (ovotestis) or independently (ovary and testicle). The occurrence of ovotesticular DSD is rare.[8,11] Patients with this entity usually present with genital ambiguity and asymmetry of the external genitalia. Associated inguinal hernia is common. The most common karyotype is 46 XX (about 60% of the cases), followed by mosaicism containing a Y chromosome (25%) and XY (15%).[56] Gender assignment decisions are individualized based on the appearance of the external genitalia, hormonal profile and response to hCG and are usually split equally between the male and female gender.[56] Surgical treatment will entail the removal of discordant gonadal tissue and other structures to the sex of rearing. The same controversy presented before in terms of the timing of surgery exists, and psychosocial support to patients and families is paramount as in any other type of DSD.

The multidisciplinary DSD clinic at The Hospital for Sick Children in Toronto has cared for 183 patients in the last 10 years. XY DSD was more common (93 of 184 [51%]) followed by XX DSD (70 of 184 [38%]) and sex chromosome DSD (20 of 184 [11%]). The most common specific diagnoses were CAH (62/183–34%), PAIS (52/183–28%), and MGD (19/183–10%). The final diagnoses for all patients in the authors' series are depicted in **Table 2**.

The most controversial topics in the initial management of the most prevalent DSD diagnoses are highlighted in **Box 1**.

MULTIDISCIPLINARY APPROACH AND PSYCHOSOCIAL SUPPORT

DSDs represent a broad complex field that requires the interaction of multiple disciplines with a diverse knowledge base. One of the most significant contributions of the consensus was to bring such an assortment of professionals and patients' representatives to the same table to improve the care of patients with these difficult conditions. Some literature on the multidisciplinary aspect of care has been generated after the consensus.[57,58] Multidisciplinary care for patients with DSD, although, in the authors' view, challenging at times given the range of opinions within different specialists, should be seen as standard and focused on the patients' best interests.[57]

Table 2
Cause of DSD in the authors' series based on karyotype

	XY DSD	XX DSD	Sex-Chromosome DSD	Total
CAH	3	57	2	62
PAIS	52	0	0	52
MGD	1	0	18	19
CAIS	13	0	0	13
PGD	11	0	0	11
MIS deficiency	3	0	0	3
Ovotesticular DSD	0	3	0	3
Pure urogenital sinus	0	3	0	3
17-beta hydroxysteroid dehydrogenase deficiency	2	0	0	2
Testosterone synthesis deficiency	2	0	0	2
5-alfa reductase deficiency	3	0	0	3
Hypogonadotropic hypogonadism	3	0	0	3
Clitoral hypertrophy	0	4	0	4
Male sex reversal	0	1	0	1
Clitoral fibroma	0	1	0	1
Maternal luteoma	0	1	0	1
Total	93	70	20	183

Abbreviations: MIS, Müllerian-inhibiting substance; PGD, pure gonadal dysgenesis.

Box 1
Summary of the most controversial topics related to DSD diagnoses with the highest prevalence

Current most significant controversial issues

CAH

- Role of prenatal treatment
- Gender assignment in severely virilized patients (eg, Prader 5)
- Timing of feminizing genitoplasty and, foremost, vaginoplasty

Male undervirilization (ie, PAIS)

- Timing of hypospadias repair
- Determining which patients have severe enough undervirilization to warrant female gender assignment

MGD

- Systematic approach to gender assignment
- Same aforementioned issues with timing of genital surgery when needed

CAIS

- Timing of gonadectomy

Essentially, the roles in the multidisciplinary clinic should be well established: geneticists and genetic counselors have a key participation in incorporating new methods for improved etiologic diagnosis, aiding insight into pathophysiological mechanisms and counseling; endocrinologists and surgeons/urologists are responsible for central aspects of patient management; gynecologists are key in the follow-up of teenage girls and issues related to sexuality and fertility. The participation of patient support groups, in a constructive fashion,[59] in forums of discussion and decisions about DSD should be encouraged. Finally, lifelong psychosocial support cannot be underrated and is mandatory for every patient with DSD. This support can be provided by a range of those with expertise in pediatric mental health, including social workers, psychologists, or psychiatrists (ideally all 3). They provide support and guidance to families coping with the difficult period before the decision about sex of rearing through the normal developmental transitions of childhood and adolescence and support the move into adult care. They also provide links to peer support whether it is through connecting families, facilitating contacts with patient support groups, or running groups for adolescents with DSDs. The benefits of such support cannot be underestimated. The clinic group may also include child life specialists, ethicists, and nurses. The multidisciplinary clinic ideally should also focus on the transition from child into adulthood and research aspects both at the basic science (genetics and molecular biology) and clinical (long-term outcomes) level.

Links for patients and families:

http://www.accordalliance.org (all DSDs)
http://www.caresfoundation.org (CAH)
http://www.aisdsd.org (women with CAIS and other DSDs)
http://heainfo.org (hypospadias and epispadias)
http://www.aboutkidshealth.ca/En/HowTheBodyWorks/
SexDevelopmentAnOverview/SexualDifferentiation

REFERENCES

1. Ahmed SF, Rodie M. Investigation and initial management of ambiguous genitalia. Best Pract Res Clin Endocrinol Metab 2010;24(2):197–218.
2. Lee PA. Consensus statement on management of intersex disorders. Pediatrics 2006;118(2):e488–500.
3. Hughes IA. Disorders of sex development: a new definition and classification. Best Pract Res Clin Endocrinol Metab 2008;22(1):119–34.
4. Houk CP, Lee PA. Update on disorders of sex development. Curr Opin Endocrinol Diabetes Obes 2012;19(1):28–32.
5. Pasterski V, Prentice P, Hughes IA. Consequences of the Chicago consensus on disorders of sex development (DSD): current practices in Europe. Arch Dis Child 2010;95(8):618–23.
6. Hughes IA, Nihoul-Fékété C, Thomas B, et al. Consequences of the ESPE/LWPES guidelines for diagnosis and treatment of disorders of sex development. Best Pract Res Clin Endocrinol Metab 2007;21(3):351–65.
7. Davies JH, Knight EJ, Savage A, et al. Evaluation of terminology used to describe disorders of sex development. J Pediatr Urol 2011;7(4):412–5.
8. Parisi MA, Ramsdell LA, Burns MW, et al. A gender assessment team: experience with 250 patients over a period of 25 years. Genet Med 2007;9(6):348–57.
9. Göllü G, Yildiz RV, Bingol-Kologlu M, et al. Ambiguous genitalia: an overview of 17 years' experience. J Pediatr Surg 2007;42(5):840–4.

10. Ocal G, Berberoğlu M, Siklar Z, et al. Disorders of sexual development: an overview of 18 years experience in the pediatric endocrinology department of Ankara University. J Pediatr Endocrinol Metab 2010;23(11):1123–32.

11. Romao R, Bägli D, Lorenzo A, et al. Patterns of presentation, diagnosis and gender assignment in a Canadian multidisciplinary clinic of disorders of sex development (DSD). Can Urol Assoc J 2011;5(3 Suppl 1):S3–114.

12. Romão RL, Bägli DJ, Lorenzo AJ, et al. Should proximal hypospadias with bilaterally descended gonads be considered a disorder of sex development (DSD)? Abstract presented at the American Urological Association meeting. Washington DC, May 15, 2011. p. 1–2.

13. Spitzer RF, Wherrett D, Chitayat D, et al. Maternal luteoma of pregnancy presenting with virilization of the female infant. J Obstet Gynaecol Can 2007;29(10):835–40.

14. Gatti JM, Kirsch AJ, Troyer WA, et al. Increased incidence of hypospadias in small-for-gestational age infants in a neonatal intensive-care unit. BJU Int 2001; 87(6):548–50.

15. Yinon Y, Kingdom JCP, Proctor LK, et al. Hypospadias in males with intrauterine growth restriction due to placental insufficiency: the placental role in the embryogenesis of male external genitalia. Am J Med Genet A 2010;152A(1):75–83.

16. Mieszczak J, Houk CP, Lee PA. Assignment of the sex of rearing in the neonate with a disorder of sex development. Curr Opin Pediatr 2009;21(4):541–7.

17. Cohee L. Endocrinology: Table 10–19: mean stretched penile length. In: Tschudy M, Arcara K, editors. The Harriet Lane handbook. 19th edition. Philadelphia: Elsevier; 2012.

18. Speiser PW, Azziz R, Baskin LS, et al. Congenital adrenal hyperplasia due to steroid 21-hydroxylase deficiency: an Endocrine Society clinical practice guideline. J Clin Endocrinol Metab 2010;95(9):4133–60.

19. Claahsen-van der Grinten HL, Stikkelbroeck NM, Otten BJ, et al. Congenital adrenal hyperplasia–pharmacologic interventions from the prenatal phase to adulthood. Pharmacol Ther 2011;132(1):1–14.

20. Dessens AB, Slijper FM, Drop SL. Gender dysphoria and gender change in chromosomal females with congenital adrenal hyperplasia. Arch Sex Behav 2005; 34(4):389–97.

21. Houk CP, Lee PA. Approach to assigning gender in 46, XX congenital adrenal hyperplasia with male external genitalia: replacing dogmatism with pragmatism. J Clin Endocrinol Metab 2010;95(10):4501–8.

22. Warne G, Grover S, Hutson J, et al. A long-term outcome study of intersex conditions. J Pediatr Endocrinol Metab 2005;18(6):555–67.

23. D'Alberton F. Disclosing disorders of sex development and opening the doors. Sex Dev 2010;4(4–5):304–9.

24. Creighton SM, Minto CL, Steele SJ. Objective cosmetic and anatomical outcomes at adolescence of feminising surgery for ambiguous genitalia done in childhood. Lancet 2001;358(9276):124–5.

25. Crouch NS, Minto CL, Laio LM, et al. Genital sensation after feminizing genitoplasty for congenital adrenal hyperplasia: a pilot study. BJU Int 2004;93(1):135–8.

26. Stikkelbroeck NM, Beerendonk CC, Willemsen WNP, et al. The long-term outcome of feminizing genital surgery for congenital adrenal hyperplasia: anatomical, functional and cosmetic outcomes, psychosexual development, and satisfaction in adult female patients. J Pediatr Adolesc Gynecol 2003;16(5):289–96.

27. Wisniewski AB, Migeon CJ, Malouf MA, et al. Psychosexual outcome in women affected by congenital adrenal hyperplasia due to 21-hydroxylase deficiency. J Urol 2004;171(6 Pt 1):2497–501.

28. Nordenskjöld A, Holmdahl G, Frisén L, et al. Type of mutation and surgical proce-dure affect long-term quality of life for women with congenital adrenal hyper-plasia. J Clin Endocrinol Metab 2008;93(2):380–6.
29. Kogan SJ, Smey P, Levitt SB. Subtunical total reduction clitoroplasty: a safe modi-fication of existing techniques. J Urol 1983;130(4):746–8.
30. Pippi Salle JL, Braga LP, Macedo N, et al. Corporeal sparing dismembered clitoroplasty: an alternative technique for feminizing genitoplasty. J Urol 2007; 178(4 Pt 2):1796–800 [discussion: 1801].
31. Ludwikowski B, Oesch Hayward I, Gonzalez R. Total urogenital sinus mobiliza-tion: expanded applications. BJU Int 1999;83(7):820–2.
32. Rink RC, Metcalfe PD, Kaefer MA, et al. Partial urogenital mobilization: a limited proximal dissection. J Pediatr Urol 2006;2(4):351–6.
33. Di Benedetto V, Di Benedetto A. Introduction of the anterior sagittal trans-ano-rectal approach (ASTRA) as a technical variation of the Passerini-Glazel clitoro-vaginoplasty: preliminary results. Pediatr Med Chir 1997;19(4):273–6 [in Italian].
34. Pippi Salle JL, Lorenzo AJ, Jesus LE, et al. Surgical treatment of high urogenital sinuses using the anterior sagittal transrectal approach: a useful strategy to opti-mize exposure and outcomes. J Urol 2012;187(3):1024–31.
35. Hill M, Finning K, Martin P, et al. Non-invasive prenatal determination of fetal sex: translating research into clinical practice. Clin Genet 2011;80(1):68–75.
36. Mercè Fernández-Balsells M, Muthusamy K, Smushkin G, et al. Prenatal dexa-methasone use for the prevention of virilization in pregnancies at risk for classical congenital adrenal hyperplasia because of 21-hydroxylase (CYP21A2) defi-ciency: a systematic review and meta-analyses. Clin Endocrinol (Oxf) 2010; 73(4):436–44.
37. Lajic S, Nordenström A, Hirvikoski T. Long-term outcome of prenatal dexametha-sone treatment of 21-hydroxylase deficiency. Endocr Dev 2011;20:96–105.
38. Fernández-Cancio M, Audí L, Andaluz P, et al. SRD5A2 gene mutations and poly-morphisms in Spanish 46, XY patients with a disorder of sex differentiation. Int J Androl 2011;34(6 Pt 2):e526–35.
39. Berra M, Williams EL, Muroni B, et al. Recognition of 5α-reductase-2 deficiency in an adult female 46XY DSD clinic. Eur J Endocrinol 2011;164(6):1019–25.
40. Maimoun L, Philibert P, Cammas B, et al. Phenotypical, biological, and molecular heterogeneity of 5α-reductase deficiency: an extensive international experience of 55 patients. J Clin Endocrinol Metab 2011;96(2):296–307.
41. Giwercman A, Giwercman YL. Environmental factors and testicular function. Best Pract Res Clin Endocrinol Metab 2011;25(2):391–402.
42. Migeon CJ, Wisniewski AB, Gearhart JP, et al. Ambiguous genitalia with perineo-scrotal hypospadias in 46, XY individuals: long-term medical, surgical, and psychosexual outcome. Pediatrics 2002;110(3):e31.
43. Köhler B, Kleinemeier E, Lux A, et al. Satisfaction with genital surgery and sexual life of adults with XY disorders of sex development: results from the German Clin-ical Evaluation Study. J Clin Endocrinol Metab 2012;97(2):577–88.
44. Barthold JS. Disorders of sex differentiation: a pediatric urologist's perspective of new terminology and recommendations. J Urol 2011;185(2):393–400.
45. Hutson JM, Clarke MC. Current management of the undescended testicle. Semin Pediatr Surg 2007;16(1):64–70.
46. Castagnetti M, El-Ghoneimi A. Surgical management of primary severe hypospa-dias in children: systematic 20-year review. J Urol 2010;184(4):1469–74.
47. Manzoni G, Bracka A, Palminteri E, et al. Hypospadias surgery: when, what and by whom? BJU Int 2004;94(8):1188–95.

48. T'Sjoen G, De Cuypere G, Monstrey S, et al. Male gender identity in complete androgen insensitivity syndrome. Arch Sex Behav 2011;40(3):635–8.
49. Deans R, Creighton SM, Liao L-M, et al. Timing of gonadectomy in adult women with compete androgen insensitivity syndrome (CAIS): patient preferences and clinical evidence. Clin Endocrinol (Oxf) 2012;76(6):894–8.
50. Papadimitriou DT, Linglart A, Morel Y, et al. Puberty in subjects with complete androgen insensitivity syndrome. Horm Res 2006;65(3):126–31.
51. Munoz JA, Swan KG. Disorders of sexual differentiation: surgical challenges of vaginal reconstruction in complete androgen insensitivity syndrome (CAIS). Am Surg 2010;76(2):188–92.
52. Pappas KB, Wisniewski AB, Migeon CJ. Gender role across development in adults with 46, XY disorders of sex development including perineoscrotal hypospadias and small phallus raised male or female. J Pediatr Endocrinol Metab 2008;21(7):625–30.
53. Köhler B, Biebermann H, Friedsam V, et al. Analysis of the Wilms' tumor suppressor gene (WT1) in patients 46, XY disorders of sex development. J Clin Endocrinol Metab 2011;96(7):E1131–6.
54. Capito C, Leclair M-D, Arnaud A, et al. 46, XY pure gonadal dysgenesis: clinical presentations and management of the tumor risk. J Pediatr Urol 2011;7(1):72–5.
55. Falhammar H, Filipsson Nyström H, Ekström U, et al. Fertility, sexuality and testicular adrenal rest tumors in adult males with congenital adrenal hyperplasia. Eur J Endocrinol 2011;164(2):285–93.
56. Matsui F, Shimada K, Matsumoto F, et al. Long-term outcome of ovotesticular disorder of sex development: a single center experience. Int J Urol 2011;18(3):231–6.
57. Brain CE, Creighton SM, Mushtaq I, et al. Holistic management of DSD. Best Pract Res Clin Endocrinol Metab 2010;24(2):335–54.
58. Jürgensen M, Kleinemeier E, Lux A, et al. Psychosexual development in children with disorder of sex development (DSD)–results from the German Clinical Evaluation Study. J Pediatr Endocrinol Metab 2010;23(6):565–78.
59. Lee PA, Houk CP. The role of support groups, advocacy groups, and other interested parties in improving the care of patients with congenital adrenal hyperplasia: pleas and warnings. Int J Pediatr Endocrinol 2010;2010:563640.

Management of Disorders of Sex Development: Editorial Commentary

David E. Sandberg, PhD

KEYWORDS

- Disorders of sex development • Health-related quality of life • Multidisciplinary
- Psychosocial • Psychosexual • Disclosure

KEY POINTS

- As new genomic technologies have rapidly become an integral part of the diagnostic tools at the disposal of the clinician, and as the cost of DNA sequencing has plummeted, the diagnostic approach to many congenital disorders has shifted dramatically, and disorders of sex development (DSD) are no exception.
- Expectations of the family and health care providers regarding the somatic sex of the child are increasingly driven by advances in technology.
- For the previous half-century, much of the medical literature on the treatment of children with DSD has focused on gender.
- Questions about surgery to normalize genital appearance and function can arise shortly after birth.
- As in other chronic pediatric conditions, accurate diagnosis and delivering appropriate medical and surgical treatment are central aspects of best practices in the clinical management of DSD.
- The update by Romao and colleagues elsewhere in this issue effectively acquaints the reader with major changes in diagnostic nomenclature and clinical management strategies for DSD. This commentary expands on several of the topics explored, with special emphasis on the psychosocial aspects of care for persons affected by DSD and their families.

This editorial commentary was written in response to the article written by Romao RL, Pippi Salle JL, Wherrett DK, entitled, "Update on the management of disorders of sex development (DSD)" in *Pediatric Clinics of North America* (59:4), August 2012.

Disclosure: The author's research is supported, in part, by grants from the Eunice Kennedy Shriver National Institute of Child Health and Human Development (R01HD053637 and R01HD068138). The content is solely the responsibility of the author and does not necessarily represent the official views of the Eunice Kennedy Shriver National Institute of Child Health and Human Development or the National Institutes of Health.

Division of Child Behavioral Health, Department of Pediatrics & Communicable Diseases and Program for Disorders of Sex Development, University of Michigan, 1500 East Medical Center Drive, Ann Arbor, MI 48109-5318, USA

E-mail address: dsandber@med.umich.edu

DSD NOMENCLATURE

In 2005, the Lawson Wilkins Pediatric Endocrine Society (LWPES) and the European Society for Pediatric Endocrinology (ESPE) convened a conference to review clinical management practices in intersex and data from long-term health-related and gender-related outcomes research and to identify key areas for future research. Invited conference participants included 48 clinicians and scientists specializing in this field and 2 participants serving as patient advocates. The *Consensus Statement on Management of Intersex Disorders*, published in 2006, recommended elimination of confusing and potentially stigmatizing terms such as intersex, pseudohermaphroditism, hermaphroditism, and sex reversal to refer to these conditions.[1] Further, the conference summary (hereafter referred to as the Consensus Statement) incorporated all variations in sex development under 1 umbrella term, disorders of sex development (DSD), defined as "congenital conditions in which development of chromosomal, gonadal, or anatomic sex is atypical." This move allowed for the shedding of the simplifying notion that gonads are the only parameter defining sex.

As noted by Romao and colleagues elsewhere in this issue DSD are subcategorized based on sex chromosomes: sex chromosome DSD, XY, DSD and XX, DSD. There remains some uncertainty regarding the boundaries for these categories. Perhaps most contentious is the inclusion of Klinefelter syndrome (47,XXY) and Turner syndrome (45,X), and their variants, within the category of sex chromosome DSD. In 2007, ESPE published its own classification of pediatric endocrine diagnoses.[2] The category of DSD appeared and with the same subcategories first introduced in the Consensus Statement. However, this classification scheme excluded from sex chromosome DSD "disorders of gonadal differentiation that do not result in sex reversal/virilised female infant/undervirilised male." Specific examples of conditions excluded were Klinefelter syndrome and Turner syndrome, both of which were instead classified under the general category of syndromes with endocrine features (subcategory of chromosomal abnormalities).

The principle guiding exclusion from sex chromosome DSD (ie, "disorders of gonadal differentiation that do not result in sex reversal/virilised female infant/undervirilised male") implies that atypical genital appearance is the sine qua non of DSD. If we follow the argument that Turner and Klinefelter syndromes should not be classified as DSD because the external genitalia are typical, then we should also exclude from DSD women with XY pure gonadal dysgenesis (who have typical external genitalia), males who are XX caused by a translocation of SRY, who often have typical male genitals, and even individuals with complete androgen insensitivity syndrome (CAIS), who appear at birth with typical female genitalia.

In addition, the nomenclature adopted in the Consensus Statement was designed to overturn the practice of classifying DSD exclusively based on the characteristics of the gonads, which did not reflect the various parameters influencing sex development. The definition of DSD now includes not only the gonads and the genitals but also the sex chromosomes as a parameter. Excluding Klinefelter syndrome from the subcategory of sex chromosome DSD because it does not result in undervirilized males is questionable and depends on one's definition of undervirilized. Suggesting that small, dysgenetic testes, which do not support spermatogenesis (a major male function) are not undervirilized seems to be a subjective interpretation.

The classification of hypospadias as a DSD is also not without debate. Despite the inclusive definition of DSD as "congenital conditions in which development of chromosomal, gonadal, or anatomic sex is atypical," the Consensus Statement itself seems to waver when it comes to hypospadias: "Criteria that *suggest* [italics added] DSD include … isolated perineal hypospadias, or mild hypospadias with undescended testis.[1] Although Romao and colleagues report moving away from evaluating such cases as DSD, recent reports suggest that hypospadias (mild and severe) can be associated with endocrine dysfunction in a few cases and that those with severe hypospadias and an undescended testis may be at higher risk for impaired spermatogenesis.[3,4]

Romao and colleagues suggest that labeling hypospadias as DSD may evoke needless distress for parents. Although there may be truth to this claim, a recent systematic review of sexual adaptation in adult men who underwent hypospadias repair in childhood suggests they are less satisfied with sexual functioning and less likely to experience intimate relationships compared with control groups, despite positive, objectively assessed, cosmetic results.[5] The Consensus Statement calls for persons with DSD to be cared for by multidisciplinary teams that include mental health providers with qualifying expertise in DSD. If patients with hypospadias are not seen in such clinics, then folding endocrine surveillance and behavioral health services into the treatment plan should be considered.

GENETIC DIAGNOSIS

In contrast to the views of Romao and colleagues, there is good reason to be more optimistic regarding the promise of genetic diagnosis in DSD. As new genomic technologies have rapidly become an integral part of the diagnostic tools at the disposal of the clinician, and as the cost of DNA sequencing has plummeted, the diagnostic approach to many congenital disorders has shifted dramatically, and DSD is no exception. Ordering a regular karyotype may not any longer be a first-tier test, because sex chromosomes can be rapidly and routinely detected by interphase fluorescent in situ hybridization. A follow-up test, comparative genomic hybridization microarray, detecting copy number variants (microdeletions and microduplications) is now proposed to replace regular cytogenetics approaches for the diagnosis of DSD.[6] Next-generation sequencing is poised to tackle additional diagnostic challenges of DSD, with the already increasing clinical use of whole exome sequencing.[7] It could be argued that the long diagnostic process of DSD, involving a combination of karyotype, endocrine testing, genital imaging, and molecular sequencing, could be drastically reduced by the use of these novel genomic technologies.

PRENATAL ASCERTAINMENT OF DSD

Romao and colleagues accurately report that most cases of DSD are detected in the newborn period; however, these conditions are increasingly identified prenatally. Expectations of the family and health care providers regarding the somatic sex of the child are increasingly driven by advances in technology; for example, remarkably clear ultrasonographic images[8] and genetic testing that can noninvasively and reliably ascertain fetal chromosomal sex between 7 and 12 weeks[9] are widely available in industrialized countries. Discordance between prenatal test findings (eg, genital appearance by ultrasonography and karyotype) can initiate the DSD counseling process even at this early stage. Evidence from studies of prenatal diagnostic counseling suggests that termination of a pregnancy is dependent on the professional background of the health care provider delivering postdiagnostic counseling.[10–12] There is substantial variation in health care providers' knowledge regarding DSD. Because these conditions are rare and, historically, understudied and misunderstood, parents are at risk of receiving outdated or incomplete information unless major efforts are made in the context of interdisciplinary care teams.

Beyond diagnosis, the prenatal period has seen efforts at medical intervention to avert phenotypic changes associated with DSD; a case in point, described by Romao and colleagues, is prenatal suppression of adrenal androgens that masculinize the genitalia in 46,XX congenital adrenal hyperplasia (CAH). CAH comprises a family of autosomal-recessive disorders involving impaired synthesis of cortisol. If a woman has previously had a child with CAH and again becomes pregnant with the same partner, the fetus has a 1 in 4 chance of acquiring the genotype associated with CAH. Suppression of fetal adrenal androgens in CAH is achievable by administering glucocorticoids (dexamethasone [DEX]) during the pregnancy.[13] The goal is to reduce genital masculinization of female offspring and obviate reconstructive surgery and presumed distress associated with the birth of a child with atypical genitalia.

Beyond the facts provided in the target article, this topic is worthy of additional discussion to better inform the reader about the nature of the controversy. Criticism of this intervention centers around several issues: first, as noted, the treatment is experimental and, yet, not characteristically delivered in the context of a clinical trial with necessary human subject oversight as called for in CAH practice guidelines[14,15]; second, to be effective, DEX treatment must be initiated between gestational weeks 6 and 7 and before it can be determined whether the fetus carries the CAH gene mutation. Treatment continues until chorionic villi sampling can be used for genotyping. If the fetus is 46,XY or 46,XX without the CAH genotype, then treatment is discontinued. Accordingly, 7 of 8 fetuses (all 46,XY and 3 of 4 46,XX) gain no benefit from the treatment but are exposed to potential risks; third, the safety of prenatal DEX for outcomes such as metabolism, cognitive function, and behavioral-emotional adaptation is in question based on animal experimental and human clinical research[16–22]; fourth, prenatal treatment does not change the need for lifelong glucocorticoid replacement therapy, the need for careful medical monitoring, or the risk of life-threatening salt-losing crises if treatment adherence is poor. Concern over prenatal DEX treatment has been expressed by bioethicists, who have questioned whether treatment introduced to normalize genital anatomy is confounded with the goal of making gender-role behavior and sexual orientation more typical.[14]

Opportunities for systematic research and theory development that examine the influence of timing of diagnosis (prenatal vs later) on treatment choices (eg, gender assignment, genital surgery, and so forth) and health-related quality of life (HRQoL) outcomes for patients and families are as yet untapped.

GENDER ASSIGNMENT

For the previous half-century, much of the medical literature on the treatment of children with DSD has focused on gender, including patient gender identity, gender role, and sexual orientation.[23] (Gender identity refers to a sense of oneself as boy/man or girl/woman; gender role refers to behaviors or traits that show sex-related variation in a culture at one point in time; sexual orientation refers to sexual arousal to individuals of the same sex [homosexual], opposite sex [heterosexual], or both sexes [bisexual]). Beginning in the 1950s, the standard of care as it emerged primarily out of Johns Hopkins University assumed that making a child's body look gender-typical would facilitate consistent rearing of the child in the assigned gender.[24] As this system spread beyond Hopkins to become a standard of care, some advocated withholding personal medical histories and other important medical information from patients so as not to potentially challenge the sense of gendered self.[24,25]

The heavy clinical focus on gender identity, gender role, and sexual orientation (ie, psychosexual differentiation) reflected the weight of interest coming from researchers examining the effects of early sex hormone exposure on sex-dimorphic brain development and sexual differentiation of behavior in a variety of animal species[26–28] as well as sexologically oriented clinical researchers.[29] This clinical work represented a natural extension of animal experimental research showing that early sex hormone exposure during sensitive periods of brain development has permanent (ie, organizational) effects of brain structure and physiology.[30] Persons with DSD were accordingly seen by some researchers as experiments of nature, natural models for the study of the roles of sex chromosomes and hormones on sexual differentiation of human brain and behavior. What few longitudinal studies existed therefore tended to focus on gender-related outcomes to the exclusion of patients' quality of life. Thus, psychological outcome studies considered whether patients identified as girls/women or boys/men, and whether they were attracted to males or females (or both), but not whether they experienced emotional equanimity, satisfying peer and romantic relations, or how they functioned in various roles across the life span. A recent systematic review of behavioral outcomes in CAH quantifies this bias.[31]

An important guidance in the Consensus Statement directs health care providers to view outcomes in DSD more broadly. For example, it states that "Quality of life encompasses falling in love, dating, attraction, ability to develop intimate relationships, sexual functioning, and the opportunity to marry and raise children, regardless of biologic indicators of sex." Similarly, providers are encouraged to recognize that "The focus should be on interpersonal relationships and not solely on sexual function and activity.[1(pe493)]

GENITAL SURGERY

Questions about surgery to normalize genital appearance and function can arise shortly after birth. Surgeons have the responsibility to describe to families surgical options and the range of possible consequences from infancy to adulthood.[1] Although there seems to be consensus on some types of genital surgery (eg, neonatal surgery in case of severe virilization in female-assigned children or ultimate gonadectomy in female-reared children with partial androgen insensitivity [PAIS] and complete androgen insensitivity syndrome [CAIS]), decisions remain that are not obvious. Controversies regarding types of surgery and their timing remain unresolved. This situation is readily apparent in conditions commonly diagnosed late, such as Mayer-Rokitansky-Küster-Hauser syndrome[32] or CAIS,[33] in which older girls/women need to decide whether they will opt for vaginal surgery or dilation to create a vagina and when it is optimal to proceed based on psychological readiness.

If there is not enough evidence from outcome studies that unequivocally show superiority of one approach over another, then choices depend on individual characteristics and detailed discussions with the patient (and, as applicable, the parents) regarding perceptions of advantages and disadvantages of the various choices. The goals of genital surgery and, in particular their consequences for sexual function and satisfaction need to be explicitly addressed. Naturally, the clinician who provides this counseling should feel comfortable when speaking about sexuality. Systematic decision-support tools, as developed for a variety of conditions (see the Foundation for Informed Medical Decision Making http://informedmedicaldecisions.org/), would be valuable, but have yet to be developed for DSD.

INFORMATION MANAGEMENT

Information management refers to 2 processes: first, the sharing of information about the DSD between clinicians, the parents and the child and second, the sharing of information about the condition by the child or family with the wider social environment. Both processes are activated to varying degrees once families are aware that their child has a DSD; this may begin with a prenatal diagnosis.

The first process often requires more than just presenting information in a clear manner. Some of the information potentially carries strong emotional implications. This is commonly the case with information about karyotype and gonadal status, especially when these results are discordant with the gender of assignment. To learn that the condition implies infertility may also pose challenges for coping. The second process, involving education of those beyond the affected person and parents, requires careful balancing of the potential advantages and disadvantages. It is still an open question whether sharing information about the DSD with the wider social environment has positive or negative consequences for the child. Living a normal life with a secret could be harmful, just as living a life without secrets but with an increased risk of stigmatization or rejection. The advice given to parents remains largely based on clinicians' personal opinions on what would be preferable, considering their evaluation of the family, the child, and their wider social and cultural context. Research on the effects of timing, type of information (and a potential interaction of the two), the way of conveying information, and the influence of cultural, family, and child factors on how the information is managed is virtually nonexistent. Nevertheless, clinicians can find guidance in the general pediatric literature concerning physician-parent communication, especially as it relates to the sharing of bad news.[34]

Initial statements to parents should provide support and information. With regard to gender, health care providers should counsel families on differences between gender identity, gender role, and sexual orientation,[35] including general, evidence-based statements on the psychosexual development of individuals born with the child's particular condition.[36–39] The process (and not a single event) of educating the parents and the affected person requires a flexible individualized approach. Medical education and counseling for children and their families is a continuing process of gradually increasing complexity that takes into account health literacy[40] and emotional readiness. Fostering open communication between the parents and child is a high priority.[41–43] This iterative process should be planned with the parents from the time of diagnosis.[1,34,44]

SEXUALITY

When entering puberty, some adolescents with DSD may develop anxieties. Repeated genital examinations and medical photography, treatment by clinicians experienced as disrespectful, or an atypical genital appearance are particularly anxiety provoking.[45,46] After entering puberty, some feel increasingly uncertain about their masculinity/femininity, sexual adequacy, or sexual orientation. They often postpone initiating intimate relationships because of such insecurities and fear of rejection. Sexual problems occur more often in DSD than non-DSD groups.[47,48] For instance, the sexual lives of women with CAH differ from control groups in terms of timing of psychosexual milestones (delayed), sexual experiences (fewer), sexual activity and imagery (less), sexual motivation (less), partnership and marriage (less), and sexual self-image (less favorable)[49–51] and the sexual orientation of women with CAH is more often homosexual compared with the general population.[51,52] In 1 study, sexual problems, primarily low sexual desire and inability to become sexually aroused and experience orgasm, were reported by women with CAIS, whereas most women with PAIS feared to have sexual contact and had experienced dyspareunia or fear of becoming hurt through sexual contact. In the latter group, an increase of nonheterosexuality was also found.[48]

Comprehensive sex education together with timely preparation for romantic and sexual relationships can contribute to a positive HRQoL. Adolescents should have the opportunity to discuss their concerns repeatedly, and in private, with a mental health clinician.

FINAL THOUGHTS

As in other chronic pediatric conditions, accurate diagnosis and delivering appropriate medical and surgical treatment are central aspects of best practices in the clinical management of DSD; nevertheless, and potentially more than in other congenital conditions, the affected person's HRQoL and adaptation of the family also depend on the extent to which health care providers attend to psychosocial aspects of the condition. Psychology, particularly research in developmental psychology, provides a road map.

A commonly adopted model for understanding HRQoL outcomes in DSD is one in which assigning the right diagnosis and providing the best medical or surgical treatment(s) are viewed as the exclusive predictors of positive HRQoL. A linear model in which outcomes are hypothesized to be directly determined by biologic factors or medical/surgical interventions proves to be an oversimplification that leaves substantial variability in end points unaccounted for. Moreover, an exclusive focus on biologic and medical/surgical aspects of DSD limits theory development and impedes innovation in clinical management strategies. Instead, and consistent with commonly adopted paradigms in developmental psychology, psychopathology, and theory in gender development,[43,44] conceptual models that consider the potential influences of moderating and mediating variables are more likely to be robust in accounting for variability in DSD outcomes.[53,54] In addition to this approach, more accurately reflecting the complexity of psychological development, it offers the benefit of studying DSD within the mainstream of theory development and behavioral health intervention research.

In cases in which gender assignment is in question, or gender reassignment is under consideration, decision making needs to be informed by evidence from both developmental and clinical psychology. The necessity of psychological counseling also emerges in the context of decisions about the timing of interventions, education of the patient and others about medical history (ie, disclosure), management of potential psychosocial or educational problems that emerge for the child, or when parents need support in understanding the cause of the child's condition and its implications. The importance of these aspects of care is reflected by the increasing participation of mental health professionals in multidisciplinary DSD teams, as called for in the Consensus Statement.[1,55,56]

ACKNOWLEDGMENTS

The author acknowledges and thanks Peggy T. Cohen Kettenis PhD, Alice Dreger PhD, Melissa Gardner MA, and Eric Vilain MD PhD for ideas and conversations reflected here.

REFERENCES

1. Lee PA, Houk CP, Ahmed SF, et al. Consensus statement on management of intersex disorders. Pediatrics 2006;118(2):e488-500.
2. Wit JM, Ranke MB, Kelnar CJ. ESPE classification of paediatric endocrine diagnoses. Disorders of sex development (DSD). Horm Res 2007;68(Suppl 2):21-6.
3. Moriya K, Mitsui T, Tanaka H, et al. Long-term outcome of pituitary-gonadal axis and gonadal growth in patients with hypospadias at puberty. J Urol 2010; 184(4 Suppl 1):1610-4.
4. Ogata T, Wada Y, Fukami M. MAMLD1 (CXorf6): a new gene for hypospadias. Sex Dev 2008;2(4-5):244-50.
5. Rynja SP, de Jong TP, Bosch JL, et al. Functional, cosmetic and psychosexual results in adult men who underwent hypospadias correction in childhood. J Pediatr Urol 2011;7(5):504-15.
6. Arboleda V, Fleming A, Vilain E. Disorders of sex development. In: Weiss R, Refetoff S, editors. Genetic diagnosis of endocrine disorders. London: Elsevier; 2010. p. 227-43.
7. Biesecker LG. Opportunities and challenges for the integration of massively parallel genomic sequencing into clinical practice: lessons from the ClinSeq project. Genet Med 2012;14(4):393-8.
8. Chitayat D, Glanc P. Diagnostic approach in prenatally detected genital abnormalities. Ultrasound Obstet Gynecol 2010;35(6):637-46.
9. Devaney SA, Palomaki GE, Scott JA, et al. Noninvasive fetal sex determination using cell-free fetal DNA. JAMA 2011;306(6):627-36.
10. Marteau TM, Nippert I, Hall S, et al. Outcomes of pregnancies diagnosed with Klinefelter syndrome: the possible influence of health professionals. Prenat Diagn 2002;22(7):562-6.
11. Abramsky L, Hall S, Levitan J, et al. What parents are told after prenatal diagnosis of a sex chromosome abnormality: interview and questionnaire study. BMJ 2001; 322(7284):463-6.
12. Girardin CM, Van Vliet G. Counselling of a couple faced with a prenatal diagnosis of Klinefelter syndrome. Acta Paediatr 2011;100(6):917-22.
13. Evans MI, Chrousos GP, Mann DW, et al. Pharmacologic suppression of the fetal adrenal gland in utero. Attempted prevention of abnormal external genital masculinization in suspected congenital adrenal hyperplasia. JAMA 1985;253(7):1015-20.
14. Dreger A, Feder E, Tamar-Mattis A. Preventing homosexuality (and uppity women) in the womb? Bioethics Forum. 2010. Available at: http://www.thehastingscenter. org/Bioethicsforum/Post.aspx?id=4754&blogid=140&terms=dreger+and+%23 filename+*.html. Accessed July 15, 2010.
15. Speiser PW, Azziz R, Baskin LS, et al. Congenital adrenal hyperplasia due to steroid 21-hydroxylase deficiency: an Endocrine Society clinical practice guideline. J Clin Endocrinol Metab 2010;95(9):4133-60.
16. Matthews S. Antenatal glucocorticoids and the developing brain: mechanisms of action. Semin Neonatol 2001;6(4):309-17.
17. Murphy KE, Hannah ME, Willan AR, et al. Multiple courses of antenatal corticosteroids for preterm birth (MACS): a randomised controlled trial. Lancet 2008; 372(9656):2143-51.
18. Lajic S, Nordenström A, Hirvikoski T. Long-term outcome of prenatal treatment of congenital adrenal hyperplasia. Endocrine development. In: Flück C, Miller W, editors. Disorders of the human adrenal cortex. Basel (Switzerland): Karger; 2008. p. 82-98.

19. Huang W, Beazley L, Quinlivan J, et al. Effect of corticosteroids on brain growth in fetal sheep. Obstet Gynecol 1999;94(2):213–8.

20. Hirvikoski T, Lindholm T, Lajic S, et al. Gender role behaviour in prenatally dexamethasone-treated children at risk for congenital adrenal hyperplasia–a pilot study. Acta Paediatr 2011;100(9):e112–9.

21. Hirvikoski T, Nordenstrom A, Lindholm T, et al. Cognitive functions in children at risk for congenital adrenal hyperplasia treated prenatally with dexamethasone. J Clin Endocrinol Metab 2007;92(2):542–8.

22. Trautman PD, Meyer-Bahlburg HF, Postelnek J, et al. Effects of early prenatal dexamethasone on the cognitive and behavioral development of young children: results of a pilot study. Psychoneuroendocrinology 1995;20(4):439–49.

23. Meyer-Bahlburg HF. Hormones and psychosexual differentiation: implications for the management of intersexuality, homosexuality and transsexuality. Clin Endocrinol Metab 1982;11:681–701.

24. Karkazis K. Fixing sex: intersex, medical authority, and lived experience. Durham (NC): Duke University Press; 2008.

25. Dreger A. 'Ambiguous sex'–or ambivalent medicine? Ethical issues in the treatment of intersexuality. Hastings Cent Rep 1998;28(3):24–35.

26. Collaer ML, Hines M. Human behavioral sex differences: a role for gonadal hormones during early development? Psychol Bull 1995;118(1):55–107.

27. Hines M. Abnormal sexual development and psychosexual issues. Baillieres Clin Endocrinol Metab 1998;12(1):173–89.

28. Berenbaum SA, Beltz AM. Sexual differentiation of human behavior: effects of prenatal and pubertal organizational hormones. Front Neuroendocrinol 2011; 32(2):183–200.

29. Money J, Ehrhardt AA. Man and woman, boy and girl: the differentiation and dimorphism of gender identity from conception to maturity. Baltimore (MD): Johns Hopkins University Press; 1972.

30. McEwen BS. Steroid hormones: effect on brain development and function. Horm Res 1992;37(Suppl 3):1–10.

31. Stout SA, Litvak M, Robbins NM, et al. Congenital adrenal hyperplasia: classification of studies employing psychological endpoints. Int J Pediatr Endocrinol 2010;2010:11. Available at: http://www.ijpeonline.com/content/2010/1/191520. Accessed June 1, 2012.

32. Liao LM, Doyle J, Crouch NS, et al. Dilation as treatment for vaginal agenesis and hypoplasia: a pilot exploration of benefits and barriers as perceived by patients. J Obstet Gynaecol 2006;26(2):144–8.

33. Ismail-Pratt IS, Bikoo M, Liao LM, et al. Normalization of the vagina by dilator treatment alone in complete androgen insensitivity syndrome and Mayer-Rokitansky-Kuster-Hauser syndrome. Humanit Rep 2007;22(7):2020–4.

34. Strauss RP, Sharp MC, Lorch SC, et al. Physicians and the communication of "bad news": parent experiences of being informed of their child's cleft lip and/ or palate. Pediatr 1995;96(1):82–9.

35. Zucker KJ. Intersexuality and gender identity differentiation. J Pediatr Adolesc Gynecol 2002;15(1):3–13.

36. Cohen-Kettenis PT. Gender change in 46, XY persons with 5α-reductase-2 deficiency and 17β-hydroxysteroid dehydrogenase-3 deficiency. Arch Sex Behav 2005;34(4):399–410.

37. Dessens AB, Slijper FM, Drop SL. Gender dysphoria and gender change in chromosomal females with congenital adrenal hyperplasia. Arch Sex Behav 2005; 34(4):389–97.

38. Mazur T. Gender dysphoria and gender change in androgen insensitivity or micropenis. Arch Sex Behav 2005;34(4):411–21.
39. Meyer-Bahlburg HF. Gender identity outcome in female-raised 46, XY persons with penile agenesis, cloacal exstrophy of the bladder, or penile ablation. Arch Sex Behav 2005;34(4):423–38.
40. Committee on Health Literacy, Institute of Medicine, Nielsen-Bohlman L, et al. Health literacy: a prescription to end confusion. Washington, DC: The National Academies Press; 2004.
41. Money J. Sex errors of the body: dilemmas, education, counseling. Baltimore: The Johns Hopkins Press; 1968.
42. Money J. Sex errors of the body and related syndromes: a guide to counseling children, adolescents, and their families. Baltimore (MD): Paul H. Brookes; 1994.
43. Meyer-Bahlburg HF. Gender assignment and psychosocial management. In: Martini L, editor. Encyclopedia of endocrine diseases. Elsevier; 2004. p. 125–34.
44. Carmichael P, Ransley P. Telling children about a physical intersex condition. Dialogues Pediatr Urol 2002;25(6):7–8.
45. Creighton S, Alderson J, Brown S, et al. Medical photography: ethics, consent and the intersex patient. BJU Int 2002;89(1):67–71.
46. Money J, Lamacz M. Genital examination and exposure experienced as nosocomial sexual abuse in childhood. J Nerv Ment Dis 1987;175(12):713–21.
47. Ismail I, Creighton S. Surgery for intersex. Rev Gynaecol Pract 2005;5(1):57–64.
48. Schönbucher V, Schweizer K, Rustige L, et al. Sexual quality of life of individuals with 46, XY disorders of sex development. J Sex Med 2010. DOI:10.1111/j.1743–6109.2009.01639.x.
49. Kuhnle U, Bullinger M, Schwarz HP. The quality of life in adult female patients with congenital adrenal hyperplasia: a comprehensive study of the impact of genital malformations and chronic disease on female patients life. Eur J Pediatr 1995; 154(9):708–16.
50. Slijper F, van der Kamp H, Brandenbrug H, et al. Evaluation of psychosexual development of young women with congenital adrenal hyperplasia: a pilot study. J Sex Educ Ther 1992;18:200–7.
51. Zucker KJ, Bradley SJ, Oliver G, et al. Psychosexual development of women with congenital adrenal hyperplasia. Horm Behav 1996;30(4):300–18.
52. Hines M, Brook C, Conway GS. Androgen and psychosexual development: core gender identity, sexual orientation, and recalled childhood gender role behavior in women and men with congenital adrenal hyperplasia (CAH). J Sex Res 2004; 41(1):75–81.
53. Baron RM, Kenny DA. The moderator-mediator variable distinction in social psychological research: conceptual, strategic, and statistical considerations. J Pers Soc Psychol 1986;51:1173–82.
54. Rose BM, Holmbeck GN, Coakley RM, et al. Mediator and moderator effects in developmental and behavioral pediatric research. J Dev Behav Pediatr 2004; 26:58–67.
55. Pasterski V, Prentice P, Hughes IA. Consequences of the Chicago consensus on disorders of sex development (DSD): current practices in Europe. Arch Dis Child 2010;95(8):618–23.
56. Ahmed SF, Achermann JC, Arlt W, et al. UK guidance on the initial evaluation of an infant or an adolescent with a suspected disorder of sex development. Clin Endocrinol 2011;75(1):12–26.

Urolithiasis in Children
Medical Approach

Lawrence Copelovitch, MD

KEYWORDS

- Urolithiasis • Nephrolithiasis • Renal calculi • Hypercalciuria • Hyperoxaluria
- Hypocitraturia • Cystinuria • Children

KEY POINTS

- The incidence and prevalence of childhood urolithiasis has been increasing over the last decade.
- The majority of renal calculi in children are comprised of either calcium oxalate or calcium phosphate and are often associated with a metabolic abnormality.
- Idiopathic hypercalciuria and hypocitraturia are the most frequently reported metabolic abnormalities.
- Given the high risk of recurrences in children with idiopathic hypercalciuria and hypocitraturia and the importance of excluding rare but treatable conditions such as primary hyperoxaluria and cystinuria a comprehensive metabolic evaluation is indicated in all children.

INTRODUCTION

Urolithiasis is a fairly common disease in adults with an estimated prevalence of 3% to 5%.[1] In economically developed countries, urolithiasis has been regarded as an uncommon condition in children. The estimated incidence in the United States from the 1950s to the 1970s is approximately 1% to 2% that of adults.[2,3] More recent studies from the United States suggest an increase in the incidence and prevalence,[4,5] with one study demonstrating a nearly 5-fold increase in the incidence in the last decade.[4] Reports regarding gender predisposition have varied, with some studies suggesting equal prevalence and others indicating a greater risk among boys.[6] Race and geography seem to play a vital role in the prevalence and cause of pediatric stone disease. In certain regions, such as Southeast Asia, the Middle East, India, and Pakistan, calculi are endemic. Calculi are particularly uncommon in children of African descent. The endemic calculi observed in developing nations are often confined to the bladder and comprise predominantly ammonium acid, urate, and uric acid, and seem to correlate

Division of Nephrology, Department of Pediatrics, The Children's Hospital of Philadelphia, 34th Street and Civic Center Boulevard, Philadelphia, PA 19104, USA
E-mail address: Copelovitch@email.chop.edu

Pediatr Clin N Am 59 (2012) 881–896
doi:10.1016/j.pcl.2012.05.009
0031-3955/12/$ – see front matter © 2012 Elsevier Inc. All rights reserved.

with a decreased availability of dietary phosphates. In the United States, urolithiasis seems to be more common in Caucasian children from the Southeastern region. Over the last 3 decades the cause of childhood urolithiasis in the United Kingdom has shifted from predominantly infectious to metabolic in nature.[7] Most calculi in the United States are found in the kidneys or ureters, comprise either calcium oxalate or calcium phosphate, and often associated with a metabolic abnormality.[8]

PATHOPHYSIOLOGY

Urolithiasis is associated with an identifiable metabolic abnormality in approximately 40% to 50% of children.[7–10] The major metabolic abnormalities include: hypercalciuria, hyperoxaluria, hypocitraturia, cystinuria, and hyperuricosuria. Hypercalciuria or hypo-citraturia are the most frequently reported abnormalities in children.[4,7] In the United States approximately 40% to 65% of calculi comprises calcium oxalate, 14% to 30% of calcium phosphate, 10% to 20% of struvite, 5% to 10% of cystine, and 1% to 4% of uric acid.[8,11] Rarely, stones may also comprise xanthine, or 2,8-dihydroxyadenine.

The initiation and growth of calculi requires the supersaturation of certain ions in the urine. The most important determinants of urine solubility and the likelihood of ion supersaturation (crystallization) are the total urine volume, the concentration of the stone-forming ions, the concentration of inhibitors of crystallization, the concentration of promoters of crystallization, and the urine pH. All types of calculi are less likely to form in dilute urine. Citrate, magnesium, pyrophosphate, certain glycosaminoglycans, nephrocalcin, and phytates all act to inhibit crystallization of calcium oxalate and calcium phosphate. Citrate acts as an inhibitor for the formation of calcium stones and binds to urinary calcium, thereby forming a soluble complex, which decreases the availability of free ionic calcium necessary for calcium oxalate or calcium phosphate crystallization. Citrate also acts as a direct inhibitor of calcium crystal aggregation and growth.[12,13] Conversely, the presence of uric acid promotes calcium oxalate crystallization, which exemplifies the process of epitaxy, in which the crystal base of one material allows the growth of a second mineral that it is in the same crystalline orientation. Urine pH is important in that certain crystals such as cystine (pH <7.5) and uric acid (pH <6.0) are more likely to aggregate in acid urine whereas calcium phosphate (pH >6) is more likely to precipitate in alkaline urine. Calcium oxalate solubility is not appreciably affected by changes in urinary pH within the physiologic range.

Crystals in the urine usually form on the surface of a nidus that allows nucleation, growth, and aggregation of a stone particle at much lower concentrations than would be required otherwise. Any source of uroepithelial damage (eg, infection, foreign body, or Randall plaques) can serve as a nidus. Randall plaques comprise calcium phosphate crystals, which originate in the basement membrane in the thin loops of Henle. As the crystals aggregate they fuse into plaques in the interstitium and finally extrude through the uroepithelium of the renal papillae. Here they form a nidus and are thought to be critical in the formation of most cases of idiopathic calcium oxalate calculi. As a result, calcium oxalate calculi, either as monohydrate (whewellite) or as dihydrate (weddellite), are often admixed with small amounts of calcium phosphate, which form the initial nidus of the stone. Stones comprising predominantly calcium phosphate (brushite) are less common and seem to originate from plugging of the inner medullary collecting ducts.[14]

Genitourinary anomalies (hydronephrosis, duplex ureter, posterior uretheral valves, and bladder exstrophy) are found in approximately 30% of children with urolithiasis.[11] Functional or anatomic obstruction predisposes children to stone formation by promoting stasis of urine and infection. Only 1% to 5% of children with urologic abnormalities develop calculi,[15] suggesting a concomitant metabolic abnormality in patients with both urologic abnormalities and calculi. To emphasize this point, a study of 22 children with ureteropelvic junction obstruction and noninfectious calculi demonstrated that 15 (68%) had at least 1 concomitant metabolic abnormality, with hypercalciuria being the most common.[16] Although infection is commonly associated with kidney stones, it is unlikely to be causative of non–struvite calculi. Although an important source of calculi in children, struvite stones will not be discussed further in this review because the only medical therapy centers on appropriate antibiotic treatment.

METABOLIC ABNORMALITIES
Hypercalciuria

Hypercalciuria is found in approximately 30% to 50% of stone-forming children.[8,9] Hypercalciuria is not a single entity but a condition associated with many causes (**Box 1**). The most common cause in children and adults is idiopathic hypercalciuria. Idiopathic hypercalciuria is defined as hypercalciuria that occurs in the absence of hypercalcemia in patients in whom no other cause can be identified. The gene (or genes) responsible for familial idiopathic hypercalciuria has not been identified, but appear to be transmitted in an autosomal dominant fashion with incomplete penetrance. Approximately 4% of asymptomatic healthy children demonstrate evidence of idiopathic hypercalciuria,[17] and 40% to 50% of those children have a positive family history of urolithiasis.[18] Hypercalciuria is formally defined as calcium excretion of greater than 4 mg/kg/d in children older than 2 years. In many children, a 24-hour urine collection is not practical and a urine calcium to creatinine ratio is used to estimate daily calcium excretion (**Table 1**). In school-aged children, a calcium to creatinine ratio of 0.2 mg/mg or less is considered normal, although higher values are reported in younger children.

When hypercalciuria is observed, several conditions must be excluded before establishing a diagnosis of idiopathic hypercalciuria. By definition the patient should be normocalcemic. In patients with hypercalcemic hypercalciuria, the possibility of hyperparathyroidism and hypervitaminosis D should be investigated and, when clinically indicated, a diagnosis of prolonged immobilization, sarcoidosis, malignancy, juvenile idiopathic arthritis, corticosteroid excess, adrenal insufficiency or William syndrome should be considered. Children with hypocalcemic hypercalciuria should be evaluated for hypoparathyroidism and autosomal, dominant hypocalcemic hypercalciuria (gain of function mutation in the calcium-sensing receptor). Although the vast majority of patients with normocalcemic hypercalciuria will ultimately be diagnosed with idiopathic hypercalciuria, other associated conditions, such as prematurity, diuretic exposure (furosemide and acetazolamide), anticonvulsant usage (topiramate and zonisamide), the ketogenic diet, Dent disease, Bartter syndrome, familial hypomagnesemia with hypercalciuria and nephrocalcinosis (FHHNC), distal renal tubular acidosis (dRTA), hereditary hypophosphatemic rickets with hypercalciuria (HHRH), and possibly medullary sponge kidney should be excluded and considered during the initial evaluation.

Genetic conditions associated with normocalcemic hypercalciuria

Dent disease is an X-linked inherited condition caused by a mutation in the *CLCN5* gene. The condition is characterized by low-molecular-weight proteinuria, nephrocalcinosis, hypercalciuria, nephrolithiasis, and chronic kidney disease. The clinical presentation is often insidious with many patients remaining asymptomatic throughout childhood; however, signs and symptoms of nephrocalcinosis and hypercalciuria are not uncommon in childhood. The defect is in proximal tubular function, and

---

Box 1
Clinical disorders associated with hypercalciuria

Hypercalcemia

Hyperparathyroidism

Hypervitaminosis D

Immobilization

Sarcoidosis

Malignancy

Juvenile idiopathic arthritis

Corticosteroid excess

Adrenal insufficiency

Williams syndrome

Idiopathic hypercalcemia of infancy

Hypocalcemia

Hypoparathyroidism

Autosomal dominant hypocalcemic hypercalciuria

Normocalcemia

Acquired

Prematurity

Furosemide

Topiramate

Ketogenic diet

Genetic

Idiopathic

Dent disease

Bartter syndrome

Familial hypomagnesemia with hypercalciuria and nephrocalcinosis

Primary distal renal tubular acidosis (dRTA)

Hereditary hypophosphatemic rickets with hypercalciuria

Other

Medullary sponge kidney

Secondary dRTA

Glycogen-storage disease type I

---

occasionally glucosuria, aminoaciduria, metabolic acidosis, and hypophosphatemia may all occur as part of an associated partial Fanconi syndrome. In a minority of patients, the Dent phenotype results from a mutation in the *OCRL* gene (Dent 2), which is also involved in the oculocerebrorenal syndrome of Lowe.

Bartter syndrome is an autosomal recessive condition characterized by renal salt wasting, hypokalemia, metabolic alkalosis, hypercalciuria, and normal serum

Table 1 Normal values for urinary solute excretion			
Metabolite	Age	Random (mg/mg)	24-h (All Ages)
Calcium	0–6 mo	<0.8	<4 mg/kg/d
	7–12 mo	<0.6	
	>24 mo	<0.21	
Oxalate	0–6 mo	<0.26	<50 mg/1.73 m^2
	7–24 mo	<0.11	
	2–5 y	<0.08	
	5–14 y	<0.06	
	>16 y	<0.03	
Citrate	0–5 y	>0.2–0.42	>180 mg/gm Males, >300 mg/gm Females
	>5 y		
Cystine	>6 mo	<0.075	<50 mg/1.73 m^2
Uric acid	>2 y	0.56 mg/dL GFR[a]	<815 mg/1.73 m^2

[a] Equation 1: Urine uric acid (mg/dL) × Plasma creatinine (mg/dL)/Urine creatinine (mg/dL).

magnesium levels. Children younger than 6 years typically present with salt craving, polyuria, dehydration, emesis, constipation, and failure to thrive. Severe polyhydramnios, prematurity, and occasionally sensorineural deafness are the hallmark features. Mutations in the *SLC12A, KCNJ1,* and *BSND* genes (Bartter syndrome type I, type II, and type IV, respectively) typically result in severe dysfunction of the thick ascending limb (TAL) of the loop of Henle in the neonatal period (neonatal Bartter syndrome). Mutations in the *ClCKB* gene (Bartter syndrome type III) usually cause milder TAL dysfunction and often present outside the neonatal period (classic Bartter syndrome).

FHHNC often presents in childhood with seizures or tetany caused by hypomagnesemia. Other clinical manifestations include frequent urinary tract infections (UTI), polyuria, polydipsia, failure to thrive, nephrolithiasis, and progressive renal failure.[19] FHHNC is an autosomal recessive condition caused by mutations in either the *CLDN-16* or *CLDN-19* genes. Homozygous *CLDN*-16 or -19 mutations are associated with impaired tight junction integrity in the TAL, urinary magnesium and calcium wasting, and resultant hypomagnesemia. Patients usually develop the characteristic triad of hypomagnesemia, hypercalciuria, and nephrocalcinosis. Profound visual impairment characterized by macular coloboma, significant myopia, and horizontal nystagmus can been seen in association with *CLDN-19* mutations.[20]

Primary dRTA is an inherited condition characterized by systemic acidosis as a result of the inability of the distal tubule to adequately acidify the urine. Failure to thrive, polyuria, polydipsia, hypercalciuria, hypocitraturia, nephrocalcinosis, renal calculi, and hypokalemia are common presenting signs in infancy. Primary dRTA may be a dominant (*SLC4A1* gene) or a recessive condition (*ATP6V1B1* or *ATP6V0A4* genes). The inability to secrete H$^+$ ions from the α-intercalated cells of the distal tubule is caused by either a defective vacuolar H$^+$-ATPase (*ATP6V1B1* or *ATP6V0A4* genes) or a defective Cl$^-$/HCO3$^-$ anion exchanger-1 (*SLC4A1* gene). Sensorineural hearing loss may be found in patients with *ATP6V1B1* mutations.

HHRH is a rare, autosomal recessive disorder caused by mutations in the *SLC34A3* gene, resulting in loss-of-function of the type IIc sodium phosphate cotransporters of the proximal tubule. The decreased renal phosphate reabsorption can result in profound hypophosphatemia, normocalcemia, rickets, and bone pain. Hypercalciuria and nephrolithiasis are also commonly observed and may be the result of a hypophosphatemia-induced stimulation of 1,25-dihydroxyvitamin D synthesis. The increased synthesis purportedly causes increased gastrointestinal absorption of calcium and excessive urinary calcium losses in the face of normal serum calcium levels.[21]

Hyperoxaluria

Oxalate is an end product of the metabolic pathways for glyoxylate and ascorbic acid and is primarily excreted by the kidneys. The vast majority (80%–85%) of daily urinary oxalate excretion is derived from normal metabolic homeostasis, and the remainder (10%–15%) is from dietary intake. Daily urine oxalate excretion is generally less than 50 mg/d/1.73 m^2 of body surface area. The impracticality of performing 24-hour urine collections in very young patients requires the use of a random urine oxalate to creatinine ratio, which can be used to estimate oxalate excretion (see **Table 1**). Increased urinary oxalate excretion may be caused by an inherited metabolic disorder (primary hyperoxaluria [PH]) or, more commonly, as a secondary phenomenon caused by increased oxalate absorption or excessive intake of oxalate precursors.

PH

PH type I and II are relatively rare, autosomal recessive disorders of endogenous oxalate production. Overproduction of oxalate by the liver causes excessive urinary oxalate excretion with resultant nephrocalcinosis and nephrolithiasis. The calcium oxalate deposition results in progressive renal damage; however, the clinical presentation can vary from end-stage renal failure in the neonate to occasional stone passage into adulthood. Because of the clinical variability, the diagnosis is often overlooked and only realized after the loss of a transplanted kidney.[22]

PH type I is caused by mutations in the *AGXT* gene, which result in a functional defect of the hepatic peroxisomal enzyme alanine–glyoxylate aminotransferase (AGT). The deficit leads to accumulation of glyoxylate, glycolate, and oxalate in the urine.Pyridoxine is an essential cofactor for proper AGT activity and, rarely, profound vitamin B6 deficiency can mimic PH type I. PH type II is caused by mutations in the *GRHPR* gene with resultant deficient glyoxylate reductase–hydroxypyruvate reductase enzyme activity. Excessive amounts of oxalate and L-glyceric acid are excreted by the kidney.[23] PH type II is somewhat milder compared with PH type I but is not benign. Recently, a third variant, PH type III has been described in 8 families with hyperoxaluria and mutations in the *DHDPSL* gene.[24] The exact mechanism by which hyperoxaluria occurs in PH type III is yet to be fully elucidated.

Secondary hyperoxaluria

In secondary hyperoxaluria, there is either a dietary exposure to large amounts of oxalate (or oxalate precursors) or an underlying disorder that causes increased absorption of dietary oxalic acid from the intestinal tract. Gastrointestinal absorption varies inversely with dietary calcium intake, and, as a result, calcium-deficient diets may increase oxalate absorption and hyperoxaluria.[25] Oxalate is a byproduct of ascorbic acid metabolism, and high doses of vitamin C have also been associated with hyperoxaluria. Increased dietary absorption is usually characterized by fat malabsorption or a chronic diarrheal disorder. Among secondary causes of hyperoxaluria, those attributable to gastrointestinal disease are inflammatory bowel disease, celiac disease, exocrine pancreatic insufficiency (cystic fibrosis), biliary tract disease, and small bowel resection or short bowel syndrome. The pathogenesis in these conditions results from the presence of free fatty acids that bind calcium in the intestinal lumen resulting in more unbound oxalate, which is free to be absorbed.

Hypocitraturia

Citrate is normally present in the urine and regulated through a process of both absorption and metabolism at the level of the proximal tubule. Hypocitraturia is generally defined as a citrate to creatinine ratio of less than 180 mg/gm in men and less than 300 mg/gm in women on a 24-hour collection (see **Table 1**). Intracellular acidosis of the proximal tubule, caused by either metabolic acidosis or hypokalemia results in an increased citrate absorption in the proximal tubule and resultant hypocitraturia. As a result, the ketogenic diet, certain medications (topiramate, zonisamide, and acetazolamide), dRTA, and chronic diarrhea are commonly associated with hypocitraturia. Given that an incomplete dRTA can occur in the absence of an overt systemic acidosis or hypokalemia, the condition can often be overlooked in the face of hypocitraturia if provocative acid-load testing is not readily available. Despite these known associations, most cases of hypocitraturia are idiopathic although a diet rich in animal protein and low in vegetable fiber and potassium seems to promote lower citrate excretion.[26,27]

Cystinuria

Cystinuria is an autosomal recessive disorder caused by mutations in either the *SLC3A1* or the *SLC7A9* genes, resulting in a disordered amino acid transport in the proximal tubule.[28] Cystinuria is characterized by urinary hyperexcretion of cystine and the dibasic amino acids lysine, ornithine, and arginine. Normal individuals excrete less than 50–60 mg of cystine/d/1.73 m^2 of body surface area, whereas patients who are homozygous for cystinuria often excrete greater than 400 mg/d/1.73 m^2 of body surface area.[7] Patients typically present with renal colic and urolithiasis in the second or third decade of life; however, they may present as early as infancy with staghorn calculi. The poor solubility of cystine in the urine causes precipitation in the collecting system, which, if left untreated, usually results in recurrent episodes of calculi and long-term risk for renal failure. Associated UTI's are common, and combined cystine and struvite calculi have been observed.[29]

In cystinuria, the disordered cystine transport primarily results from dysfunction of the heteromeric amino acid transporter (rBAT/$b^{0,+}$AT), comprising heavy (rBAT) and light ($b^{0,+}$AT) subunits. Cystinuria was originally classified into type I and non–type I (types II and III) based on the urinary cystine concentration pattern of obligate heterozygotes and the presumed mode of inheritance. Type I follows the classic autosomal recessive inheritance with heterozygotes showing normal cystine excretion. In contrast, non–type I (type II and III) heterozygotes demonstrate moderate or high excretion of urinary cystine. Types II and III differ in that type III homozygotes show a nearly normal increase in cystine plasma levels after oral cystine administration.[30] It is now clear that homozygous mutations in the *SLC3A1* gene, which encodes rBAT is associated with type I cystinuira, and homozygous mutations in the *SLC7A9* gene, which encodes $b^{0,+}$AT accounts for most cases of type II and III. A more recent classification system has been developed, which designates patients who are homozygous for the *SLC3A1* mutations as cystinuria type A, patients who are homozygous for the *SLC7A9* mutations as type B, and those who have a mutation in both the *SLC3A1* and *SLC7A9* genes as type AB.[31]

Hyperuricosuria

Uric acid excretion is greater in children than in adults, with the highest urinary fractional excretion (Fe) found in neonates (Fe 30%–50%) and levels reaching adult values (Fe 8%–12%) in adolescence.[32] Hyperuricosuria is defined as uric acid excretion of greater than 815 mg/d/1.73 m^2 of body surface area. When adjusted for glomerular filtration rate (GFR), relative uric acid excretion is fairly constant after 2 years of age (see **Table 1**). In children who are not yet trained to use toilet but older than of 2 years, hyperuricosuria can be defined as greater than 0.56 mg/dL of GFR on a spot urine collection. This value may be calculated using Equation 1:

$$\text{Urine uric acid (mg/dL)} \times \text{Plasma creatinine(mg/dL)/Urine creatinine(mg/dL)} \quad (1)$$

Hyperuricosuria in the setting of low urinary pH is the greatest risk factor for uric acid stone formation. Hyperuricosuria associated with significant hyperuricemia is usually associated with inherited disorders of purine metabolism (see section on Inherited disorders of purine metabolism), lymphoproliferative disorders, and polycythemia. Rarely, a condition known as hereditary renal hypouricemia characterized by low serum uric acid, hyperuricosuria, nephrolithiasis, and exercise-induced acute renal failure has been observed. Mutations in either the *SLC22A12* or the *SLC2A9* genes, both of which encode urate transporters expressed in the proximal tubule, are known to be causative.[28] Other causes of hyperuricosuria include excessive purine intake (animal protein, anchovies, and mussels), hemolysis, uricosuric medications (probenecid, salicylates, and losartan), cyanotic congenital heart disease, melamine toxicity, and idiopathic (familial). There is also a phenomenon primarily observed in adults called hyperuricosuric calcium oxalate urolithiasis in which hyperuricosuria seems to be the principle contributor to the development of calcium oxalate stones with either no or minimal uric acid content (epitaxy).

Inherited disorders of purine metabolism
Phosphoribosyl pyrophosphate synthetase superactivity (PRPSS) is an X-linked condition caused by mutations in the *PRPS1* gene. The overactive PRPSS is associated with excessive purine production. The subsequent purine degradation results in hyperuricemia, gout, hyperuricosuria, and uric acid nephrolithiasis. Some affected individuals have neurodevelopmental abnormalities, particularly sensorineural deafness.[33] Hypoxanthine-guanine phosphoribosyl transferase (HPRT) deficiency is an X-linked inborn error of purine metabolism caused by mutations in the *HPRT1* gene associated with overproduction of uric acid. Complete deficiency of HPRT activity is associated with the Lesch-Nyhan syndrome, characterized by mental retardation, spastic cerebral palsy, choreoathetosis, uric acid calculi, and self-injurious behavior. Children with partial HPRT deficiency can be phenotypically similar to patients with complete deficiencies or may have more subtle or mild neurologic symptoms. Renal stones, uric acid nephropathy, renal obstruction, or gout may be the first presenting signs of the disease.[28]

CLINICAL PRESENTATION

The classic adult presentation of acute, severe flank pain, which radiates to the groin is uncommon in children, particularly in children younger than 5 years. Although adolescents present similarly to adult patients, younger children have varied presentations including nonspecific pain localized to the abdomen, flank, or pelvis. In infants, symptoms of stones may be confused with colic pain. Macroscopic or microscopic hematuria can occur in up to 90% of children with urolithiasis.[34] Ureteral stones are much more likely to cause obstruction that leads to pain. Renal stones may be found incidentally and remain present for years without causing symptoms. Approximately 10% of calculi can present with dysuria and urinary frequency and are usually localized to the lower urinary tract. UTI may also complicate nephrolithiasis, although pyuria may also be present without bacteriuria or infection. Rarely, a urethral stone can present with acute urinary obstruction.[11,35]

MEDICAL HISTORY AND PHYSICAL EXAMINATION

Obtaining a thorough medical history followed by careful examination is essential for establishing an accurate diagnosis. Information pertaining to a family history of calculi, hematuria, and renal failure can be essential in identifying those patients at highest risk for inherited metabolic or genetic conditions (eg, cystinuria, primary hyperoxaluria, and Dent disease). A focused dietary history with special emphasis on fluid and salt intake, vitamin (C, D) mineral supplementation, and special diets (eg, ketogenic diet) is indicated in every patient. Eliciting a detailed medication history with special emphasis on corticosteroids, diuretics (furosemide and acetazolamide), protease inhibitors (indinavir), and anticonvulsants (topiramate and zonisamide) can be instructive. Children with a history of prematurity, urinary tract abnormalities, UTIs, intestinal malabsorption (eg, Crohn's disease, bowel resection, and cystic fibrosis), and prolonged immobility are all at special risk for calculi formation. Detailed physical examination of the child for dysmorphic features (William syndrome), rickets (Dent disease and HHRH), tetany (FHHNC and autosomal dominant hypocalcemic hypercalciuria), and gout (HPRT deficiency, PRPSS) can be helpful.

EVALUATION
Imaging

The first step involved in the evaluation of urolithiasis is detection of the calculus. The sensitivity of plain abdominal radiography in the detection of calculi is approximately 45% to 58%; although many stones are radiopaque, radiography alone is insufficient in the evaluation of a patient with suspected urolithiasis.[36] In addition, calculi comprising uric acid, cystine, xanthine, or indinavir are usually radiolucent. Ultrasonography (US) has the ability to detect 90% of calculi confined to the kidney; however, the sensitivity for detecting ureteral calculi and smaller calculi (<5 mm) is poor.[5] Nonetheless, because radiation exposure is not without risk, US remains the initial study of choice in the assessment of calculi in children. Noncontrast computed tomography remains the gold standard and is indicated in children with persistent symptoms of urolithiasis and a nondiagnostic US. In patients with hypercalciuria in whom medullary sponge kidney is suspected, an intravenous pyelogram can be considered.

Metabolic Investigations

When urinary calculi develop during childhood, the risk of life-long stone formation is significant, with approximately 16% to 20% having recurrences within 3 to 13 years.[10,37] Furthermore, children with an identifiable metabolic abnormality have an up to 5-fold increased risk of having a recurrence as compared with children with no identifiable metabolic disorder.[10] As a result, all children should undergo a comprehensive initial evaluation. Whenever possible, analysis should begin with an infrared spectroscopy or radiograph diffraction analysis of a passed stone. If a cystine or struvite stone is found, the analysis will be diagnostic.

Serum and urine studies should be obtained in patients in whom stone analysis could not be performed or for those with either calcium or uric acid-based stones. A serum creatinine level is essential to evaluate for possible acute kidney injury or chronic kidney disease. Serum calcium, phosphorous, bicarbonate, magnesium, and uric acid levels are effective in screening for hypercalcemia- and hypocalcemia-associated calculi (discussed earlier), hyperuricemia, HHRH, Bartter syndrome, dRTA, and FHHNC. Unlike in adults, primary hyperparathyroidism is rare in children and an intact parathyroid hormone level is not an essential part of the initial evaluation unless there is evidence of hypercalcemia and hypophosphatemia. A 25-hydroxyvitamin D level should be evaluated in all patients with hypercalcemia. A spot urine beta-2 microglobulin (low-molecular-weight protein) is a useful screening test for Dent disease and should be considered in men and possibly carrier women if there are recurrent calcium-based calculi in the setting of proteinuria or a family history of renal failure, focal segmental glomerulosclerosis, or recurrent calculi.

A 24-hour urine collection should be analyzed for calcium, oxalate, uric acid, sodium, citrate, creatinine levels, volume, pH, and cystine (cyanide-nitroprusside screening test). Results must be evaluated with respect to weight, body surface area, and creatinine level to be properly interpreted in children. Urine creatinine excretion (normal 15–25 mg/kg/d) is useful in assessing the adequacy of the urine collection. Supersaturations for calcium oxalate, calcium phosphate, and uric acid can be calculated from computer models based on the results of the urine collection. There is ongoing controversy as to whether a single 24-hour urine collection at the time of diagnosis is sufficient for proper evaluation[38] or whether 2 separate collections yield a greater number of specific diagnoses.[39] Several commercial companies, including Litholink, Mission, Dianon, and Urocor offer these 24-hour urine stone chemistry profiles. Although less precise, when children are not yet trained to use toilet, the evaluation may be performed by measuring the ratio of calcium, uric acid, citrate, and oxalate levels to creatinine level in a random urine sample. Repeat urine testing should be performed several weeks to months after a change in diet or after the initiation of a medication. Microscopic urinalysis for crystalluria is generally not diagnostic unless hexagonal crystals (cystine) or coffin lid–shaped triple phosphate crystals (struvite) are observed.

MEDICAL MANAGEMENT
Acute Management

The first goal of medical management should be directed toward control of the acute complications. Pain associated with the passage of a stone is often severe and should be treated promptly with narcotic analgesics (morphine sulfate) and/or nonsteroidal antiinflammatory drugs (Ketorolac). If the patient is vomiting or unable to drink, parenteral hydration should be used to maintain a high urine flow rate. In the absence of oligoanuric renal failure or a complete obstruction, an intravenous infusion rate of 1.5 to 2 times maintenance is recommended. Agents that may promote the passage of stones and reduce symptoms (medical expulsive therapy), such as alpha-adrenergic blockers (tamsulosin) and calcium-channel blockers (nifedipine), have shown promising results in adults with distal ureteral calculi.[40] Although studies in children are limited, 1 prospective study showed that in children with distal ureteral calculi who were treated with tamsulosin, there was a greater stone expulsion rate and decreased time to stone expulsion when compared with controls.[41] Urine should be strained for several days to recover any gravel or calculi passed for analysis. Because UTIs often present concomitantly in children with calculi, a urine culture should be obtained and empiric antibiotic therapy initiated if a UTI is suspected.

Preventative Measures

Fluid
Fluid intake is a critical component of stone prevention by effectively reducing the concentration of lithogenic factors, including calcium, oxalate, uric acid, and cystine. Although high daily fluid intake reduces the risk of recurrent stone formation,[42] the exact prescription is unknown. Most clinicians recommend intake at least equal to calculated maintenance rates in children and no less than 2 to 2.5 L in adolescents and adults. Even higher fluid intake levels (1.5–2 L/m^2) may be recommended for

children with cystinuria or PH. Increased intake requirements may be required during periods of increased insensible water loss. Regarding fluids other than water, reports suggest that fluids that increase urinary pH and citrate excretion such as orange juice, lemonade, and black currant juice, as well as those that increase urinary volume such as coffee, tea, beer, and wine, reduce the risk of calcium stone formation.[43] Conversely, grapefruit juices seem to increase the risk of calcium-based stones.[43,44] Whether cola drinks increase lithogenic potential or not remains controversial.[43,44]

Sodium

The association between sodium intake and calcium stone formation has been reported but has not been confirmed in all studies.[44] Increased sodium intake is known to promote calciuria by competing for reabsorption at the level of the renal tubules. A low salt diet corresponding to less than 2 to 3 mEq/kg/d in children or less than 2.4 g/d in adolescents or adults is generally recommended for patients with hypercalciuria or calcium-containing stones. A low salt diet may also reduce urinary cystine excretion in patients with cystinuria.

Calcium

Until recently, higher calcium intake was thought to increase the risk of stone formation; however, there is substantial evidence now that a higher calcium containing diet is associated with a reduced risk of stone formation.[45] A potential mechanism that might explain this paradox is that higher calcium intake effectively binds dietary oxalate in the gut, thereby reducing intestinal absorption and eventual urinary oxalate excretion. The current recommendation for stone formers is to curtail excess calcium intake, but calcium restriction is not recommended, in part, because of the long-term risk of osteoporosis. Excess consumption of vitamin D with or without calcium supplements can also induce excessive urinary calcium excretion.

Animal protein

There is compelling evidence for a role of dietary animal proteins (meat, fish, and poultry) in calcium oxalate stone formation. The metabolism of sulfur-containing amino acids in animal meat generates an acid load in the form of sulfuric acid. As a result, excessive dietary animal protein intake causes increased urinary calcium excretion and reduced urinary citrate excretion and pH. Vegetable and dairy protein sources do not seem to carry the same lithogenic potential. The consumption of excessive amounts of dietary animal protein also results in increased purine intake, increased uric acid production, and may contribute to both uricosuria and more acidic urine. In patients with cystinuria, there is little evidence to support the dietary restriction of proteins high in cystine content; however, reducing animal protein intake might be helpful by increasing urinary pH. Children with calculi are recommended not to eat excessive amounts of protein but should aim for 100% of the daily recommended allowance for age to supply adequate substrate for growth and nutrition.

Oxalate

The role of dietary oxalate in stone formation is controversial because only approximately 10% to 20% of urinary oxalate excretion is derived from the diet. As a precautionary measure, most clinicians recommend limiting dietary oxalate ingestion in calcium oxalate stone formers who demonstrate evidence of hyperoxaluria. Foods that contain high levels of oxalate include certain nuts (almonds, peanuts, cashews, walnuts, and pecans), spinach, soy beans, tofu, rhubarb, beets, sweet potatoes, wheat bran, okra, parsley, chives, black raspberries, star fruit, green tea, and chocolate. Vitamin C supplements have been associated with increased risk of calcium oxalate stone formation because oxalate is a byproduct of ascorbic acid metabolism and therefore, these supplements should be discontinued in calcium oxalate stone formers with hyperoxaluria.[46]

Potassium/citrate

Potassium-rich foods such as fruits and vegetables usually contain large amounts of citrate, which are protective against the formation of calcium oxalate stones. In many studies, a diet high in potassium is protective against urolithiasis.[45] In addition, a potassium-restricted diet can cause increased urinary calcium excretion and overt hypokalemia, leading to hypocitraturia. One recent study suggests that chronically low potassium intake in the absence of overt hypokalemia may also result in low urinary potassium and citrate levels.[47] As a result, a diet containing potassium-rich fruits and vegetables can theoretically increase urinary citrate excretion directly because of the citrate content found in those foods and indirectly through the dietary potassium content.

Others

Magnesium complexes with oxalate and may prevent enteric oxalate absorption as well as decrease calcium oxalate supersaturation in the urine. In some studies, higher dietary magnesium has been associated with a lower risk of stone formation in men,[46] and supplementation may be helpful in the treatment of children with secondary hyperoxaluria. Carbohydrate ingestion has been associated with hypercalciuria, and sucrose ingestion has been found to be associated with urolithiasis.[45] Phyate, a dietary factor found in many high fiber-containing foods (cereals, legumes, vegetables, and nuts), seems to bind calcium avidly and may inhibit the formation of calcium oxalate stones.

Medications

Pharmacotherapy is recommended for children in whom fluid and dietary therapy is ineffective in controlling the formation of stones, or for those with primary hyperoxaluria, cystinuria, or a known genetic condition associated with normocalcemic hypercalciuria (see previous section on Genetic conditions associated with normocalcemic hypercalciuria).

Diuretics

A thiazide diuretic is often required for children with hypercalciuria who do not respond to a restricted sodium diet. The usual recommendation is hydrochlorothiazide 1 to 2 mg/kg/d (adult 25–100 mg/d). Amiloride can be added for its potassium-sparing effect as well as for its ability to independently reduce calcium excretion. Alternatively, potassium citrate could be provided to mitigate the effects of potassium depletion. Thiazide diuretics have also been used in an attempt to reduce calcium excretion in patients with Dent disease, FHHNC, and PH.

Alkali agents

Treatment with either potassium citrate (2–4 mEq/kg/d, adults 30–90 mEq/d)[48] or potassium-magnesium citrate[49] has been shown to reduce the recurrence of calcium oxalate stone formation in patients with low or normal citrate excretion. Sodium citrate is generally considered less ideal because it is associated with increased sodium delivery to the nephron. Treatment is considered safe with only minor gastrointestinal side effects; however, one potential concern is that over-treatment with alkali may increase the risk of calcium phosphate stone formation by increasing the urinary pH to greater than 6.5, thereby decreasing the calcium phosphate supersaturation product. Potassium citrate is also used to alkalinize the urine in patients with Dent disease, FHHNC, dRTA, uric acid lithiasis (goal of urine pH >6.5), cystinuria (goal of urine pH >7), and hyperoxaluria.

Thiol-containing agents

These agents are used exclusively for patients with cystinuria in whom fluid and dietary modifications as well as urinary alkalinization are ineffective in preventing stone recurrences or dissolving preexisting stones. The 2 most common agents are D-penicillamine and α-mercaptopropionylglycine (tiopronin). Cystine is formed as a dimer of cysteine and these agents work by reducing the disulfide bond that bridges the 2 molecules of cysteine. The thiol group combines with cysteine to form a more soluble cysteine-drug product combination, which is be excreted. D-penicillamine has a large number of adverse side effects, including febrile reactions, gastrointestinal discomfort, liver dysfunction, impaired taste, bone marrow suppression, trace metal deficiencies, membranous glomerulopathy, myasthenia gravis, and skin eruptions (elastosis perforans serpiginosa). The incidence of adverse effects for α-mercaptopropionylglycine is similar but may be slightly less. Monitoring of liver enzymes, complete blood count, urinalysis, and copper and zinc levels should be performed regularly. Special assays (solid-phase assay or high performance liquid chromatography) can readily distinguish between urinary cystine and cysteine-drug complexes and may help in guiding long-term medical therapy.

Allopurinol

The mainstay of therapy for most children with uric acid calculi is a combination of high urine flow rate and alkalinization of the urine. Allopurinol (4–10 mg/kg/d, adult maximum 300 mg/d) is indicated conditions in which there is both hyperuricemia and hyperuricosuria, such as PRPSS or HPRT deficiency. Inhibition of xanthine dehydrogenase by allopurinol may lead to the accumulation and urinary excretion of xanthine. Rarely, a secondary xanthinuria with xanthine calculi is observed in children on long-term therapy. Allopurinol may also be the agent of choice for treating hyperuricosuric calcium oxalate urolithiasis if there is no concomitant evidence of hypercalciuria, hyperoxaluria, or hypocitraturia.[50]

Pyridoxine

Pyridoxine is an important cofactor of AGT. Approximately 10% to 30% of children with PH type I are pyridoxine sensitive (>30% reduction of urinary oxalate excretion). In particular, patients who are homozygous for Gly170Arg or Phe152Ile mutations are more likely to respond and have preserved renal function over time with adequate treatment.[42] In patients with suspected PH type I, treatment should be initiated (2–5 mg/kg/d) and titrated upward (8–10 mg/kg/d) until a diagnosis can be made and response assessed. Large doses of pyridoxine have been known to induce sensory neuropathies. There is currently no evidence to suggest that pyridoxine supplementation is beneficial in the treatment of other forms of hyperoxaluria unless a true pyridoxine deficiency is present.

REFERENCES

1. Stamatelou KK, Francis ME, Jones CA, et al. Time trends in reported prevalence of kidney stones in the United States: 1976-1994. Kidney Int 2003;63(5):1817–23.
2. Bass NH, Emmanuel B. Nephrolithiasis in childhood. J Urol 1966;95:749–53.
3. Troup CW, Lawnicki CC, Bourne RB, et al. Renal calculus in children. J Urol 1972; 107(2):306–7.

4. VanDervoort K, Wiesen J, Frank R, et al. Urolithiasis in pediatric patients: a single center study of incidence, clinical presentation and outcome. J Urol 2007;177(6): 2300–5.

5. Palmer JS, Donaher ER, O'riordan MA, et al. Diagnosis of pediatric urolithiasis: role of ultrasound and computerized tomography. J Urol 2005;174: 1413–6.

6. Cameron MA, Sakhaee K, Orson WM. Nephrolithiasis in children. Pediatr Nephrol 2005;20:1587–92.

7. Coward RJ, Peters CJ, Duffy PG, et al. Epidemiology of paediatric renal stone disease in the UK. Arch Dis Child 2003;88(11):962–5.

8. Milliner DS, Murphy ME. Urolithiasis in pediatric patients. Mayo Clin Proc 1993; 68:241–8.

9. Stapleton FB, McKay CP, Noe NH. Urolithiasis in children: the role of hypercalciuria. Pediatr Ann 1987;16:980–92.

10. Pietrow PK, Pope JC IV, Adams MC, et al. Clinical outcome of pediatric stone disease. J Urol 2002;167:670–3.

11. McKay CP. Renal stone disease. Pediatr Rev 2010;31(5):179–88.

12. Nicar MJ, Hill K, Pak CY. Inhibition by citrate of spontaneous precipitation of calcium oxalate in vitro. J Bone Miner Res 1987;2:215–20.

13. Meyer JL, Smith LH. Growth of calcium oxalate crystals. II. Inhibition by natural urinary crystal growth inhibitors. Invest Urol 1975;13(1):36–9.

14. Evan A, Lingeman J, Coe FL, et al. Randall's plaque: pathogenesis and role in calcium oxalate nephrolithiasis. Kidney Int 2006;69:1313–8.

15. Wenzl JE, Burke EC, Stickler GB, et al. Nephrolithiasis and nephrocalcinosis in children. Pediatrics 1968;41(1):57–61.

16. Husmann DA, Milliner DS, Segura JW. Ureteropelvic junction obstruction with concurrent renal pelvic calculi in the pediatric patient: a long-term followup. J Urol 1996;156:741–3.

17. Kruse K, Kracht U, Kruse U. Reference values for urinary calcium excretion and screening for hypercalciuria in children and adolescents. Eur J Pediatr 1984; 143(1):25–31.

18. Coe FL, Parks JH, Moore ES. Familial idiopathic hypercalciuria. N Engl J Med 1979;300(7):337–40.

19. Hou J, Goodenough DA. Claudin-16 and claudin-19 function in the thick ascending limb. Curr Opin Nephrol Hypertens 2010;19(5):483–8.

20. Konrad M, Schaller A, Seelow D, et al. Mutations in the tight-junction gene claudin 19 (CLDN19) are associated with renal magnesium wasting, renal failure, and severe ocular involvement. Am J Hum Genet 2006;79:949–57.

21. Lorenz-Depiereux B, Benet-Pages A, Eckstein G, et al. Hereditary hypophosphatemic rickets with hypercalciuria is caused by mutations in the sodium-phosphate cotransporter gene SLC34A3. Am J Hum Genet 2006;78:193–201.

22. Spasovski G, Beck BB, Blau N, et al. Late diagnosis of primary hyperoxaluria after failed kidney transplantation. Int Urol Nephrol 2010;42(3):825–9.

23. Hoppe B, Beck BB, Milliner DS. The primary hyperoxalurias. Kidney Int 2009; 75(12):1264–71.

24. Belostotsky R, Seboun E, Idelson GH, et al. Mutations in DHDPSL are responsible for primary hyperoxaluria type III. Am J Hum Genet 2010;87(3):392–9.

25. Polinsky MS, Kaiser BA, Baluarte JB. Urolithiasis in childhood. Pediatr Clin North Am 1987;34(3):683–710.

26. Kok DJ, Iestra JA, Doorhenbos CJ, et al. The effects of dietary excesses in animal protein and in sodium composition on the composition and the crystallization

kinetics of calcium oxalate monohydrate in the urines of healthy men. J Clin Endocrinol Metab 1990;71:861–7.

27. Hess B, Michel R, Takkinen R, et al. Risk factors for low urinary citrate in calcium nephrolithiasis: low vegetable fiber and low urine volume to be added to the list. Nephrol Dial Transplant 1994;9:642–9.

28. Online Mendelian Inheritance in Man. Available at: http://www.ncbi/nlm.nih.gov/entrez. Accessed January 14, 2012.

29. Evans WP, Resnick MI, Boyce WH. Homozygous cystinuria–evaluation of 35 patients. J Urol 1982;127:707.

30. Rosenberg LE, Downing SE, Durant JL, et al. Cystinuria: biochemical evidence for three genetically distinct diseases. J Clin Invest 1966;45:365–71.

31. Dello Strologo L, Pras E, Pontesilli C, et al. Comparison between SLC3A1 and SLC7A9 cystinuria patients and carriers: a need for a new classification. J Am Soc Nephrol 2002;13:2547–53.

32. Cameron JS, Moro F, Simmonds HA. Gout, uric acid and purine metabolism in paediatric nephrology. Pediatr Nephrol 1993;7:105–18.

33. Becker MA, Puig JG, Mateos FA, et al. Inherited superactivity of phosphoribosyl-pyrophosphate synthetase: association of uric acid production and sensorineural deafness. Am J Med 1988;85:383–90.

34. Bartosh SM. Medical management of pediatric stone disease. Urol Clin North Am 2004;31:575–87.

35. Stapleton FB. Nephrolithiasis in children. Pediatr Rev 1989;11(1):21–30.

36. Mandeville JA, Gnessin E, Lingeman JE. Imaging evaluation in the patient with renal stone disease. Semin Nephrol 2011;31(3):254–8.

37. Diamond DA, Menon M, Lee PH, et al. Etiological factors in pediatric stone recurrence. J Urol 1989;142(2):606–8.

38. Castle SM, Cooperburg MR, Sadetsky N, et al. Adequacy of a single 24-hour urine collection for metabolic evaluation of recurrent nephrolithiasis. J Urol 2010;184:579–83.

39. Parks JH, Goldfisher E, Asplin JR, et al. A single 24-hour collection is inadequate for the medical evaluation of nephrolithiasis. J Urol 2002;167:1607–12.

40. Moe OW, Pearle MS, Sakhaee K. Pharmacotherapy of urolithiasis: evidence from clinical trails. Kidney Int 2001;79:385–92.

41. Mokhless I, Zahran AR, Youssif M, et al. Tamsulosin for the management of distal ureteral stones in children: a prospective randomized study. J Pediatr Urol 2011. [Epub ahead of print].

42. Borghi L, Meschi T, Amato F, et al. Urinary volume, water and recurrences in idiopathic calcium nephrolithiasis: a 5-year randomized prospective study. J Urol 1996;155(3):839–43.

43. Borghi L, Meschi T, Maggiore U, et al. Dietary therapy in idiopathic nephrolithiasis. Nutr Rev 2006;64(7):301–12.

44. Taylor EN, Curhan GC. Diet and fluid prescription in stone disease. Kidney Int 2006;70:835–9.

45. Curhan GC, Willett WC, Speizer FE, et al. Comparison of dietary calcium with supplemental calcium and other nutrients as factors affecting the risk for kidney stones in women. Ann Intern Med 1997;126(7):497–504.

46. Taylor EN, Stampfer MJ, Curhan GC. Dietary factors and the risk of incipient kidney stones in men: new insights after 14 years of follow up. J Am Soc Nephrol 2004;15(12):3225–32.

47. Domrongkitchaiporn S, Stitchantrakul W, Kochakarn W. Causes of hypocitraturia in recurrent calcium stone formers: focusing on urinary potassium excretion. Am J Kidney Dis 2006;48(4):546–54.

48. Barcelo P, Wuhl O, Servitge E, et al. Randomized double-blind study of potassium citrate in idiopathic hypocitraturic calcium nephrolithiasis. J Urol 1993;150(6):1761–4.

49. Ettinger B, Pak CY, Citron JT, et al. Potassium-magnesium citrate is an effective prophylaxis against recurrent calcium oxalate nephrolithiasis. J Urol 1997; 158(6):2069–73.

50. van Woerden CS, Groothoff JW, Wijburg FA, et al. Clinical implications of mutational analysis in primary hyperoxaluria type I. Kidney Int 2004;66:746–52.

Urolithiasis in Children
Surgical Approach

Candace F. Granberg, MD, Linda A. Baker, MD*

KEYWORDS

- Extracorporeal shock wave lithotripsy • Ureteroscopy
- Percutaneous nephrolithotomy • Stone • Urolithiasis • Pediatric • Child

KEY POINTS

- In children, the choice of stone treatment modality is individualized, considering patient age, stone size, number, location, and anatomic and clinical contributing factors.
- When surgical intervention is warranted for pediatric urolithiasis, extracorporeal shock wave lithotripsy (ESWL) and ureteroscopy (URS) provide effective, safe, minimally invasive outpatient options for less complex cases, each with inherent advantages and disadvantages.
- When faced with complex stone disease, percutaneous nephrolithotomy (PCNL) with or without adjunctive ESWL is useful but carries higher risks.
- Given that stone disease is increasing in children in the United States and, if left untreated, can lead to loss of a kidney or renal function, it is comforting to know that minimally invasive treatments performed by pediatric urologists expert in urolithiasis surgery are effective.

INTRODUCTION

As in adults, the vast majority of urinary stones in children become symptomatic or detected when present within the upper urinary tract (kidneys and ureters). Although a stone may sit in the upper urinary tract for weeks to years, renal colic only ensues when the stone moves to a location that partially or completely obstructs the flow of urine, causing stretch of the kidney, renal pelvis, and possibly ureter. Stones typically become obstructing in 3 locations within the ureter, namely, the ureteropelvic junction (UPJ), the ureterovesical junction (UVJ), and where the ureter crosses the common iliac vessels. Rarely, stones are trapped within the kidney in a renal calyx behind a narrow infundibulum or a calyceal diverticulum (**Fig. 1**). Staghorn calculi, which

Disclosures: None.
Department of Urology, University of Texas Southwestern Medical Center, Children's Medical Center at Dallas, 2350 Stemmons Freeway, Suite D-4300, M.C. F4.04, Dallas, TX 75207, USA
* Corresponding author. Children's Medical Center at Dallas, 2350 Stemmons Freeway, Suite D-4300, M.C. F4.04, Dallas, TX 75207.
E-mail address: linda.baker@childrens.com

Pediatr Clin N Am 59 (2012) 897–908
doi:10.1016/j.pcl.2012.05.019
0031-3955/12/$ – see front matter © 2012 Elsevier Inc. All rights reserved.

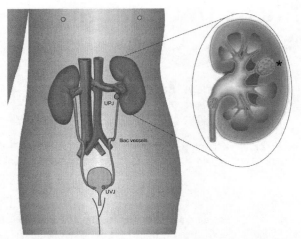

Fig. 1. Typical locations stones tend to become lodged, often requiring surgical intervention. (*Inset*) Occasionally, stones can be lodged in a hydrocalyx obstruced by infundibular stenosis or a calyceal diverticulum (*asterisk*).

partially or completely fill renal calyces and renal pelvis, require surgical therapy because they are unable to pass. Otherwise, for simple renal or ureteral stones, a trial of stone passage may be permitted depending on the size of the stone. Whereas hydration, antiemetics, and analgesics were previously all that was offered during renal colic episodes not complicated by urinary tract infection (UTI), now α_{1A}-adrenergic receptor antagonists, such as tamsulosin, are administered to selectively relax distal ureteral smooth muscle in adults and children. Although not Food and Drug Administration approved for use in children, one recent prospective randomized pediatric trial has shown off-label use of α_{1A}-blockers to have significant efficacy, increasing stone passage rates, decreasing days until stone passage, and providing pain relief during passage of stones less than 12 mm.[1]

If 14 days of α_{1A}-antagonist therapy have not resulted in stone passage, if pain is uncontrolled, if UTI occurs, or if vomiting prevents medication efficacy, then surgical intervention for stone removal is typically required. Fortunately, several surgical approaches are available (**Table 1**) that are minimally invasive, relatively safe, and efficacious; the choice of which approach to use is dictated by the scenario of each patient.

EXTRACORPOREAL SHOCK WAVE LITHOTRIPSY

ESWL is a noninvasive, outpatient technique for the surgical approach to kidney and ureteral stones. Beginning in 1986,[2] ESWL has been routinely used in children and is now widely accepted despite lack of Food and Drug Administration approval for pediatric use. The joint European Association of Urology (EAU)/American Urological Association (AUA) Nephrolithiasis Guideline Panel's "2007 Guideline for the Management of Ureteral Calculi" states, in reference to recommendations for the pediatric patient: "...Treatment choices should be based on the child's size and urinary tract anatomy. The small size of the pediatric ureter and urethra favors the less invasive approach of ESWL."[3] Thus, ESWL remains a first-line treatment option for most pediatric upper tract urinary calculi.

Table 1
Comparison of ESWL, URS, and PCNL in children

	ESWL	Ureteroscopy	PCNL
Typical use	Simple renal or ureteral stones <1–2 cm	Simple renal or ureteral stones <1–2 cm	Staghorn or multiple larger stones
Anesthesia	General	General	General
Service	Outpatient	Outpatient	Inpatient (2–6 days)
Site of entry into body	None, waves pass through skin to stone (extracorporeal)	Through the urethra, bladder, and ureter to the ureter/kidney stone	Tubes are passed through the flank skin into kidney (percutaneous)
Stone removal rate	44%–95%	50%–100%	70%–90%
Need for second surgery	Low–moderate	Low	Moderate–high (planned second PCNL typically done at same hospitalization)
Success depends on spontaneous stone fragment passage	Totally	Partially	~None
Need for ureteral stent postoperatively	Very low	High (usually for 3–5 days postoperatively and removed in office)	High (usually removed before discharge)
Need for nephrostomy tube postoperatively	None	None	High
Complications	0%–18% (Pain, bleeding, sepsis, retention, ureteral obstruction, UTI, ureteral stricture)	0%–8% (Renal colic, gross hematuria, febrile UTI, ureteral stricture, ureteral perforation or ureteral avulsion)	0%–30% (Self-limited urine leak, urine leak requiring stent, fever, hematuria requiring transfusion, colon injury, perforation, sepsis, vascular injury, pneumothorax, and hydrothorax)
Possibility of adjacent organ injury	Very low	None	Low (lung, colon)
Need for blood transfusion	None	None	<5%
Days off from school/work	Up to 7	Up to 14	Up to 20

ESWL Technique

Modern-day lithotriptors use an external generator to create pulses of energy that are subsequently generated into shockwaves. These shockwaves are transmitted through a flexible treatment head covered with gel (for acoustic coupling) that is compressed against the patient's body. Shockwaves travel through the body and are focused at the target (stone), wherein collective force is created to break up the stone. Breakage is accomplished by cavitation, the formation and subsequent collapse of bubbles at the surface of the stone. If successful stone shattering occurs, stone fragments must then be spontaneously passed through the urinary tract and voided per urethra. Unfortunately, spontaneous stone fragment passage is variable.

ESWL is performed using fluoroscopy, ultrasonography, or a combination of fluoroscopy and ultrasonography to localize and target the stone 3-D, thereby correctly positioning the treatment head on the skin to focus the shockwaves on the stone (**Fig. 2**). Anesthetic requirements may be minimized in adults undergoing ESWL, with some tolerating the procedure with only intravenous sedation. Pediatric cases, however, require general anesthesia because patient movement can shift the stone off target, losing stone fragmentation efficacy if not readjusted back on target.

For the majority of ESWL cases, there is no associated UTI and the size of the stone (stone burden) is low. For the remaining cases, however, consideration should be given to placement of a ureteral stent, an internal tube spanning from the renal pelvis

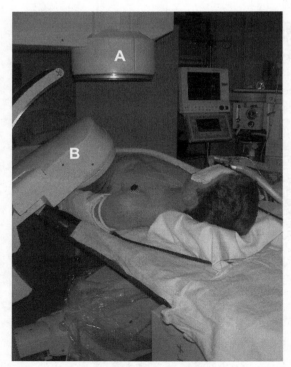

Fig. 2. Typical outpatient lithotripter with fluoroscope (A) and treatment head (B) containing the shockwave generator. Under general anesthesia, the child is laid supine, positioning the kidney within the cutout of the bed such that the stone can be fluoroscopically imaged. The fluoroscopy unit, treatment head and the bed are all computer synchronized so that the child's stone is moved 3-D into the focal point target of the shockwaves.

to the bladder for urine drainage (**Fig. 3**). The EAU/AUA Nephrolithiasis Guideline Panel states, "routine [ureteral] stenting is not recommended as part of ESWL," based on Panel consensus and level III evidence.[3] When treating staghorn stones with ESWL monotherapy, one group reported similar stone-free outcomes in stented versus non-stented children (78% vs 79%); however, unstented children were found to have more major complications (21% vs 0, $P = .035$) and longer hospital stays (6.4 vs 4.6 days, $P = .022$) than stented children.[4] Nevertheless, surgeons may elect to place stents before ESWL in specific scenarios, such as sepsis, obstruction, solitary kidney, and anomalous anatomy, or to facilitate retrograde pyelography for stone localization.

ESWL Outcomes

There is wide variation in reported success rates after ESWL, because some investigators declare that stone fragments less than 4 mm to 5 mm after ESWL are "clinically insignificant residual fragments" and thus success has been achieved, whereas others require complete absence of fragments to be deemed stone-free. Afshar and colleagues[5] evaluated children with small residual fragments (<5 mm) after ESWL and concluded that these fragments were clinically significant, increasing risk for adverse clinical outcomes (either growth of the fragment or clinical symptoms) compared with children who were rendered completely stone-free (odds ratio 3.9; 95% CI, 1.5–9.6). Moreover, use of different imaging modalities (potentially underestimating stone burden) and variable timing at post-ESWL imaging (potentially not allowing all fragments to pass spontaneously) may contribute to variable reporting of success.

Overall stone-free rates for ESWL in children range from as low as 44% after a single session[6] to 95%.[7] Retreatment rates (additional ESWL sessions) have been reported to occur in 10% to 54%.[6,8]

Children have been shown to have a greater propensity for passing stone fragments after ESWL than adults (95% vs 79%, $P = .086$).[7] This may be attributed to the shorter length and greater elasticity of the pediatric ureter. Additionally, multiple studies have

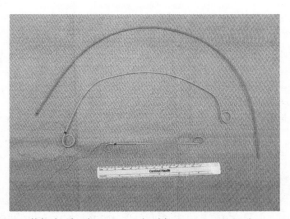

Fig. 3. Ureteral stents (*blue*), also known as double-J stents, come in a range of sizes, 3.0F–12F diameters and 4 cm–24 cm lengths. If desired, the black "dangler" retrieval suture can be left on the double J stent and taped to the genital skin, permitting later removal of the double J stent awake in the office. As double J stents are placed over wires, the orange pusher with metal tip is used by the pediatric urologist for double J stent positioning during the surgery.

demonstrated that successful ESWL outcomes are achieved regardless of stone location, including isolated lower pole stones.[9–11]

As opposed to adults, body mass index does not seem to negatively correlate with stone-free status in children.[9] Skin-to-stone distance (SSD) as measured on noncontrast CT scan has been shown predictive of outcome after ESWL in adults, with SSD greater than 10 cm more likely to fail treatment.[12] The authors' multicenter study evaluated SSD in children, concluding that on univariate analysis SSD was a statistically significant predictor of success but was not significant on multivariate logistic regression.[13]

Certain stone types, including brushite, cysteine, and calcium oxalate monohydrate, are known to be resistant to ESWL due to their hardness. Thus, knowledge of stone composition or suspicion of stone composition based on preoperative CT Hounsfield units may contribute to decision making for treatment. The authors' multicenter study identified stone attenuation of less than 1000 Hounsfield units on noncontrast CT scan as a significant predictor of success with ESWL in children, independent of stone size.[13] Total stone diameter has also been shown the only factor to independently predict stone-free status after ESWL, with age, gender, body mass index, and number and location of stones not predictive.[9]

ESWL Complications

Complications after ESWL in children, tabulated from meta-analysis, include bleeding (5%), pain (18%), retention (2%), sepsis (4%), stricture (1%), ureteral obstruction (2%), and UTI (2%).[3]

The process of cavitation as well as shear forces, although beneficial for stone fragmentation, can cause damage to surrounding tissues. Animal studies have shown that a slower delivery of shock waves significantly decreases renal tissue injury.[14] A prospective study by Fayad and colleagues[15] involved obtaining baseline technetium dimercaptosuccinic acid (DMSA) scan and glomerular filtration rate (estimated using diethylene triamine pentaacetic acid [DTPA]) and comparing with studies obtained 6 months after ESWL. In their cohort, no patient developed renal scarring or statistically significant decrease in renal function. Reisiger and colleagues[16] also showed that treatment with ESWL did not impact renal growth in children.

URETEROSCOPY

The first reported case of URS used in a child was in 1988.[17] Since that time, significant strides have been made in the development of miniaturized instrumentation and improved ancillary equipment. Thus, URS has evolved to become an accepted outpatient option not only for distal calculi but also for proximal ureteral and renal calculi. The choice to proceed with URS is based on both patient and stone characteristics, taking into account anatomic limitations as well as stone burden and location.

URS Technique

To perform URS with stone removal, a broad range of equipment is required in children (**Fig. 4**). Under general anesthesia, cystoscopy is performed and the ureter is accessed with guide wires under fluoroscopic guidance. Retrograde pyeloureterography may be performed to localize the stone(s) and is performed in a gentle fashion to prevent stone migration. An attempt is made to pass instruments into the ureter. If difficulty is encountered from a tight distal ureter, ureteral dilation may be achieved either passively by placing a stent[18] and postponing definitive stone treatment for 1 to 2 weeks or actively by proceeding with dilation using instrumentation. Long-term risks of active

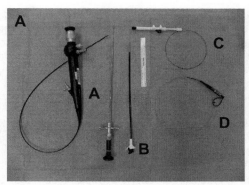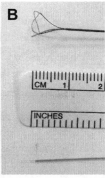

Fig. 4. (*A*) Some of the needed pieces of equipment to perform URS, with stone extraction: A—rigid and flexible ureteroscopes, B—ureteral access sheaths, C—Stone retrieval baskets, and D—holmium:YAG laser. (*B*) Close-up view of stone retrieval basket (*top*) and laser fiber (*bottom*).

dilation are unknown but are postulated to include secondary vesicoureteral reflux or ureteral stricture as a result of mucosal tears and/or ischemia. In one series, 57% (95/167) of ureters could not be accessed, of which 83% were in children less than 10 years of age; after passive dilation, all ureters were then accessed successfully.[19]

If multiple passes of the ureteroscope are anticipated to remove multiple stone fragments, a 9.5-French (F) to 14F ureteral access sheath may be used to minimize ureteral trauma as well as to decrease intrarenal pressure from irrigation fluid.[20] A variety of rigid, semirigid, and flexible ureteroscopes exist, averaging 7.5F, with scope chosen based on stone and patient characteristics as well as surgeon preference.

If stones are too large to be extracted en bloc, holmium:YAG laser is used for fragmentation of stones through the rigid or flexible ureteroscope. Stone removal of large stone fragments is achieved under direct vision with an endoscopic basket while remaining small pieces of stone must be spontaneously passed. The decision to leave a ureteral stent postoperatively is at the surgeon's discretion and may be based on operative time, number of passes with the scope, impacted stone, potential risk of edema, or other factors. Stents left for a short term can be left on a dangler (string) exiting the urethra and can be removed without anesthesia compared with indwelling ureteral stents that require a brief anesthetic for cystoscopic removal.

URS Outcomes

As with ESWL, stone-free rates after URS are subject to the same reporting variability with respect to varying definitions of stone-free status (discussed previously). Success rates range from as low as 50% for intrarenal stones[21] to 97% and 100% for ureteral stones greater than 10 mm and less than 10 mm, respectively, after a single treatment.[19]

Larger stone size and more proximal stone location have been found associated with statistically significantly lower success rates.[21–23] One group found that for lower pole calculi, stone-free rate after URS was 93 versus 33% for stones less than 15 mm and greater than or equal to 15 mm, respectively ($P = .01$).[24]

URS Complications

Overall complication rates range from 0 to 8% in contemporary series and include renal colic, gross hematuria, febrile UTI, ureteral stricture, ureteral perforation, or ureteral avulsion.[19,24–26]

A retrospective review of 642 children found that on univariate analysis, operative time, age, dilation of ureteral orifice, stenting, stone burden, and institutional experience were statistically significant predictive factors for postoperative complications. On multivariate analysis, however, only operative time was shown statistically significant.[25]

PERCUTANEOUS NEPHROLITHOTOMY

The first report of PCNL in pediatric patients was in 1997 by Mor and colleagues,[27] Due to the complexity of the procedure, PCNL is performed during an inpatient hospitalization, ranging from 2 to 5 days' duration. PCNL may be the initial procedure chosen for patients with anatomic abnormalities that preclude ESWL or URS (unable to clear fragments or pass instruments retrograde), known stone composition resistant to ESWL (cystine, brushite, and calcium oxalate monohydrate), or infection stones (struvite). As opposed to in adults, children may undergo ESWL as the primary procedure for staghorn stones; however, if combination therapy (ESWL + PCNL) is chosen for treatment, PCNL should be the last procedure performed in most patients according to the AUA Guideline Panel recommendation.[28] Others have successfully used adjunctive ESWL after PCNL to aid in clearance of remaining fragments.[29,30]

PCNL Technique

General anesthesia and an assembly of equipment are required for PCNL (**Fig. 5**). In the prone position, access to the renal collecting system is obtained directly by placing a needle into the selected calyx through the flank skin. Fluoroscopy is most commonly used to aid in localization for access and subsequent nephrolithotomy; however, use of ultrasound has also been reported.[31]

A percutaneous tract is dilated using one of a variety of techniques based on surgeon preference. Although pediatric instrumentation has been developed such that PCNL can be performed through tracts as small as 11F (mini-perc),[32] adult-sized instruments through tracts up to 30F have been successfully described in infants and children with comparable results.[33] Drawbacks to smaller tract size include difficulty with visualization using smaller scopes and potentially prolonged operative time for fragmentation and removal of larger stones.

Through the tract, rigid and flexible nephroscopy is performed and nephrolithotomy using holmium:YAG laser and/or combination ultrasonic lithotripter plus pneumatic

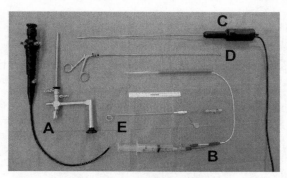

Fig. 5. In addition to the aforementioned pieces of equipment, additional equipment items are needed for PCNL: A—rigid nephroscope and flexible cystoscope, B—balloon dilation system with outer rigid working sheath, C—cyberwand combination ultrasonic lithotripter + pneumatic lithoclast, D—grasping forceps, and E—nephrostomy tube.

lithoclast is performed. The latter tool not only is capable of grinding stone but also has large caliber suction, permitting highly efficient removal of the stone fragments and sand. Thus, patients do not have to spontaneously pass stone fragments postoperatively. In some cases of multiple stones or complex partial or complete staghorn stones, one nephrostomy tract does not permit nephroscopic access to all stone-filled calyces. Additional nephrostomy tracts may be necessary to achieve stone eradication.

The decision to leave a ureteral stent or nephrostomy tube for postoperative drainage is individualized to surgeon and patient situation and has been described after both mini-perc[34] and using standard adult-sized instruments.[33,35] Reporting of postoperative complications, hospital stay, and so forth in tubeless versus nephrostomy tube patients may be biased by those left tubeless possibly having had a less complicated procedure. In most complex cases, the PCNL may require planning of two operative sessions during one hospitalization to completely remove all stones.

PCNL Outcomes

Stone-free rates range from 70% to greater than 90% after PCNL in children.[36–38] This rate has been shown lower for complex (complete or partial staghorn) stones, with complete clearance after a single treatment of only 61%.[33] Stone-free status did not differ when using pediatric or adult-sized instruments.[33]

Although older children (>5 years) have a higher stone burden and tend to need more than one access tract, stone-free outcomes are not different when stratifying by age.[39]

PCNL Complications

Overall, complications after PCNL occur in up to 30% in children in contemporary series.[33,34,40] Given the proximity of the renal vasculature, the colon, the ribs, and the lungs, reported complications include self-limited urine leak, urine leak requiring stent, fever, hematuria requiring transfusion, colon injury, perforation, sepsis, vascular injury, pneumothorax, and hydrothorax. Independent risk factors contributing to complications after PCNL include stone burden and operative time.[40] Supracostal PCNL did not significantly differ from subcostal PCNL with respect to hospital stay, complications, need for additional surgery, or stone-free status.[41]

Comparing postoperative use of nephrostomy tubes, procedures without a tube had shorter operative time, decreased pain, and shorter hospital stay.[34,35] Additionally, a prospective, randomized controlled trial of children less than 14 years of age undergoing tubeless versus standard PCNL found no difference in operative time, transfusion rate, complications, reoperation rate, and hemoglobin drop, although hospital stay and analgesic use were lower in the tubeless cohort.[42]

In some studies, hemoglobin drop and/or transfusion rates seem higher in pediatric patients undergoing PCNL with adult-sized versus pediatric-sized instruments.[33,36,37,43] This difference may not take into account, however, variation in surgical technique, experience, complexity of case, or other factors not identified in a retrospective review rather than simply the size of the instruments used. Other investigators have shown safety of adult-sized instruments with low transfusion rates in children less than 5 years of age.[44]

SUMMARY

When surgical intervention is warranted for pediatric urolithiasis, ESWL and URS provide effective, safe outpatient options for less complex cases, each with inherent advantages and disadvantages. When faced with complex stone disease, PCNL with or without adjunctive ESWL is useful but carries higher risks. Given stone disease is increasing in children in the United States and if left untreated can lead to loss of a kidney or renal function,[45] it is comforting to know that minimally invasive treatments performed by pediatric urologists expert in urolithiasis surgery are effective.

REFERENCES

1. Mokhless I, Zahran AR, Youssif M, et al. Tamsulosin for the management of distal ureteral stones in children: a prospective randomized study. J Pediatr Urol 2011 Nov 16. [Epub ahead of print].
2. Newman DM, Coury T, Lingeman JE, et al. Extracorporeal shock wave lithotripsy experience in children. J Urol 1986;136(1 Pt 2):138–40.
3. Preminger GM, Tiselius HG, Assimos DG, et al. 2007 Guideline for the management of ureteral calculi. Eur Urol 2007;52(6):1610–31.
4. Al-Busaidy SS, Prem AR, Medhat M. Pediatric staghorn calculi: the role of extracorporeal shock wave lithotripsy monotherapy with special reference to ureteral stenting. J Urol 2003;169:629–33.
5. Afshar K, McLorie G, Papanikolaou F, et al. Outcome of small residual stone fragments following shock wave lithotripsy in children. J Urol 2004;172:1600–3.
6. Muslumanoglu AY, Tefekli A, Sarilar O, et al. Extracorporeal shock wave lithotripsy as first line treatment alternative for urinary tract stones in children: a large scale retrospective analysis. J Urol 2003;170:2405–8.
7. Gofrit ON, Pode D, Meretyk S, et al. Is the pediatric ureter as efficient as the adult ureter in transporting fragments following extracorporeal shock wave lithotripsy for renal calculi larger than 10mm? J Urol 2001;166:1862–4.
8. Myers DA, Mobley TB, Jenkins JM, et al. Pediatric low energy lithotripsy with the Lithostar. J Urol 1995;153(2):453–7.
9. McAdams S, Kim N, Ravish IR, et al. Stone size is only independent predictor of shock wave lithotripsy success in children: a community experience. J Urol 2010; 184:659–64.
10. Hammad FT, Kaya M, Kazim E. Pediatric extracorporeal shockwave lithotripsy: its efficiency at various locations in the upper tract. J Endourol 2009;23(2): 229–35.
11. Onal B, Demirkesen O, Tansu N, et al. The impact of caliceal pelvic anatomy on stone clearance after shock wave lithotripsy for pediatric lower pole stones. J Urol 2004;172:1082–6.
12. Pareek G, Hedican SP, Lee FT, et al. Shock wave lithotripsy success determined by skin-to-stone distance on computed tomography. Urology 2005; 66(5):941–4.
13. McAdams S, Kim N, Dajusta D, et al. preoperative stone attenuation value predicts success after shock wave lithotripsy in children. J Urol 2010;184:1804–9.
14. Evan AP, McAteer JA, Connors BA, et al. Renal injury during shock wave lithotripsy is significantly reduced by slowing the rate of shock wave delivery. BJU Int 2007;100(3):624–7.
15. Fayad A, El-Sheikh G, AbdelMohsen M, et al. Evaluation of renal function in children undergoing extracorporeal shock wave lithotripsy. J Urol 2010;184:1111–5.
16. Reisiger K, Vardi I, Yan Y, et al. Pediatric nephrolithiasis: does treatment affect renal growth? Urology 2007;69(6):1190–4.
17. Ritchey M, Patterson DE, Kelalis PP, et al. A case of pediatric ureteroscopic lasertripsy. J Urol 1988;139:1272.

18. Shields JM, Bird VG, Graves R, et al. Impact of preoperative ureteral stenting on outcome of ureteroscopic treatment for urinary lithiasis. J Urol 2009;182: 2768–74.

19. Kim SS, Kolon TF, Canter D, et al. Pediatric flexible ureterosocpic lithotripsy: the Children's Hospital of Philadelphia experience. J Urol 2008;180:2616–9.

20. Singh A, Shah G, Young J, et al. Ureteral access sheath for the management of pediatric renal and ureteral stones: a single center experience. J Urol 2006;175: 1080–2.

21. Tanaka ST, Makari JH, Pope JC, et al. Pediatric ureteroscopic management of intrarenal calculi. J Urol 2008;180:2150–4.

22. Turunc T, Kuzgunbay B, Gul U, et al. Factors affecting the success of ureteroscopy in management of ureteral stone diseases in children. J Endourol 2010; 24(8):1273–7.

23. Jaidane M, Hidoussi A, Slama A, et al. Factors affecting the outcome of ureteroscopy in the management of ureteral stones in children. Pediatr Surg Int 2010;26: 501–4.

24. Cannon GM, Smaldone MC, Wu HY, et al. Ureteroscopic management of lower-pole stones in a pediatric population. J Endourol 2007;21(10):1179–82.

25. Dogan HS, Onal B, Satar N, et al. Factors affecting complication rates of ureteroscopic lithotripsy in children: results of multi-institutional retrospective analysis by Pediatric Stone Disease Study Group of Turkish Pediatric Urology Society. J Urol 2011;196:1035–40.

26. Minevich E, DeFoor W, Reddy P, et al. Ureteroscopy is safe and effective in prepubertal children. J Urol 2005;174:276–9.

27. Mor Y, Elmasry YE, Kellett MJ, et al. The role of percutaneous nephrolithotomy in the management of pediatric renal calculi. J Urol 1997;158(3 Pt 2):1319–21.

28. Preminger GM, Assimos DG, Lingeman JE, et al. AUA report on the management of Staghorn Calculi. 2005. Avilable at: http://www.auanet.org/content/clinical-practice-guidelines/clinical-guidelines.cfm?sub=sc. Accessed May 14, 2012.

29. Mahmud M, Zaidi Z. Percutaneous nephrolithotomy in children before school age: experience of a Pakistani centre. BJU Int 2004;94(9):1352–4.

30. Samad L, Aquil S, Zaidi Z. Paediatric percutaneous nephrolithotomy: setting new frontiers. BJU Int 2006;97(2):359–63.

31. Penbegul N, Tepeler A, Sancaktutar AA, et al. Safety and efficacy of ultrasound-guided percutaneous nephrolithotomy for treatment of urinary stone disease in children. Urology 2012;79(5):1015–9.

32. Jackman SV, Hedican SP, Peters CA, et al. Percutaneous nephrolithotomy in infants and preschool age children: experience with a new technique. Urology 1998;52(4):697–701.

33. Guven S, Istanbulluoglu O, Gul U, et al. Successful percutaneous nephrolithotomy in children: multicenter study on current status of its use, efficacy and complications using Clavien classification. J Urol 2011;195:1419–24.

34. Bilen CY, Gunay M, Ozden E, et al. Tubeless mini percutaneous nephrolithotomy in infants and preschool children: a preliminary report. J Urol 2010;184: 2498–503.

35. Salem HK, Morsi A, Omran A, et al. Tubeless percutaneous nephrolithotomy in children. J Pediatr Urol 2006;3:235–8.

36. Desai MR, Kukreja RA, Patel SH, et al. Percutaneous nephrolithotomy for complex pediatric renal calculus disease. J Endourol 2004;18(1):23–7.

37. Bilen CY, Kocak B, Kitirci G, et al. Percutaneous nephrolithotomy in children: lessons learned in 5 years at a single institution. J Urol 2007;177(5):1867–71.

38. Salah MA, Toth C, Khan AM, et al. Percutaneous nephrolithotomy in children: experience with 138 cases in a developing country. World J Urol 2004;22(4): 277–80.
39. Dogan HS, Kilicarslan H, Kordan Y, et al. Percutaneous nephrolithotomy in children: does age matter? World J Urol 2011;29(6):725–9.
40. Ozden E, Mercimek MN, Yakupoglu YK, et al. Modified Clavien classification in percutaneous nephrolithotomy: assessment of complications in children. J Urol 2011;195:264–8.
41. El-Nahas AR, Shokeir AA, El-Kenawy MR, et al. Safety and efficacy of supracostal percutaneous nephrolithotomy in pediatric patients. J Urol 2008;180:676–80.
42. Aghamir SM, Salavati A, Aloosh M, et al. Feasibility of totally tubeless percutaneous nephrolithotomy under the age of 14 years: a randomized clinical trial. J Endourol 2012;26(6):621–4.
43. Unsal A, Resorlu B, Kara C, et al. Safety and efficacy of percutaneous nephrolithotomy in infants, preschool age, and older children with different sizes of instruments. Urology 2010;76(1):247–52.
44. Nouralizadeh A, Basiri A, Javaherforooshzadeh A, et al. Experience of percutaneous nephrolithotomy using adult-sized instruments in children less than 5 years old. J Pediatr Urol 2009;5:351–4.
45. Bush NC, Xu L, Brown BJ, et al. Hospitalizations for pediatric stone disease in United States, 2002-2007. J Urol 2010;183(3):1151–6.

Issues in Febrile Urinary Tract Infection Management

Martin A. Koyle, MD, FRCS (Eng.)[a],*, Donald Shifrin, MD[b]

KEYWORDS

- Urinary tract infections • Pediatric • Fever • Guidelines • Vesicoureteral reflux
- Renal scarring

KEY POINTS

- Urinary tract infections are common occurrences in the pediatric age group and are a cause of significant morbidity and expense. The understanding of the consequences and sequelae of febrile urinary tract infections, and especially recent analysis of the risk versus benefit of radiologic evaluation of this population, has led to revision of standard protocols initiated by the American Academy of Pediatrics (AAP) in 1999.
- Proper diagnosis of urinary tract infection is considered essential before a child is improperly labeled as having suffered a urinary tract infection.
- A less invasive protocol of radiologic evaluation, with an emphasis on reducing the number of voiding cystourethrograms, has been the major outcome of the revised AAP guidelines.
- Emphasis on prevention of recurrent febrile urinary tract infections by understanding the importance of bowel-bladder dysfunction/dysfunctional elimination-voiding syndromes as a major cause, has also led to therapeutic programs that are centered less around the use of prophylactic antibiotics than has previously been the practice.

INTRODUCTION

Urinary tract infection (UTI) affects approximately 7% to 8% of girls and 2% of boys during the first 8 years of life.[1,2] Febrile UTI (fUTI) is most common in infants and children less than 1 year old, whereas nonfebrile UTI predominates in girls more than 3 years old.[2] It is now the most common serious bacterial infection of childhood. Vesicoureteral reflux (VUR), the abnormal retrograde flow of urine from the bladder to the upper urinary tract, is present in 30% to 40% of symptomatic documented UTIs.[3,4] This association of VUR with fUTI diminishes with increasing age, because lower grades of VUR, in particular, are most likely to resolve spontaneously over time.

An editorial commentary by Dr Thomas Newman, entitled, "Evidence Basis for Individualized Evaluation and Less Imaging in Febrile Urinary Tract Infection: An Editorial Commentary" is based on this article and can be found in *Pediatric Clinics of North America* (59:4), August 2012.
[a] Division of Pediatric Urology, Hospital for Sick Children, University of Toronto, 555 University Avenue, Black Wing, M-299, Toronto, Ontario M5G1X8, Canada; [b] University of Washington School of Medicine, Seattle Children's Hospital, 4800 Sand Point Way NE, Seattle, WA 98105, USA
* Corresponding author.
E-mail address: martin.koyle@sickkids.ca

Pediatr Clin N Am 59 (2012) 909–922
doi:10.1016/j.pcl.2012.05.013
0031-3955/12/$ – see front matter © 2012 Elsevier Inc. All rights reserved.

pediatric.theclinics.com

The most important clinical sequelae of VUR include fUTI/acute pyelonephritis (APN) and, potentially, renal scarring. The severity (higher grades) of VUR and increased frequency of fUTI are directly related to the risk of scarring.[4] APN, defined as inflammation or infection of the kidneys, affects an estimated 60% of children with fUTI. High fever with temperature of 39.5°C or more is the single best predictive parameter.[5,6] The risk of APN increases when bladder infection occurs in patients with VUR, because colonized lower tract urine then has direct retrograde access to the upper tracts.[7] Furthermore, results of the International Reflux Study Committee (IRSC) have shown that successful antireflux surgery reduces the risk of fUTI by a factor of 3.[8] Additional risk factors for APN include other anatomic urologic and neurologic disorders, bowel-bladder dysfunction (BBD), recurrent UTIs, female gender for children more than 1 year old, and certain social situations, especially those that lead to delayed treatment. It is estimated that 15% of all children develop renal scarring after a first UTI, with VUR itself a risk factor for renal scarring.[6,9,10]

However, patients with fUTI may also develop scarring in the absence of VUR. Moreover, most children with VUR and fUTI do not develop acquired (secondary) scars. Despite the finding of chronic photopenic areas on dimercaptosuccinic acid (DMSA) scans that are thought to represent scars, there is controversy as to their ultimate physiologic and clinical significance. A better understanding of which patients are most likely to develop renal scarring, and, of paramount importance, identifying the significance of such scarring in a given individual patient, is essential to enable better management selection.

ISSUES IN PEDIATRIC UTI: DEVELOPMENT OF GUIDELINES

Clinical practice guidelines are developed to help physicians, patients, and their families make sound decisions about specific clinical situations. However, guidelines reflect interpretations of available data, and are thus subjective and tend to differ between different groups of experts. Furthermore, guidelines are most applicable to a large group of patients who fulfill specific clinical criteria rather than to the individual patient; this is particularly problematic in pediatric medicine, in which parents may be more prone to make treatment decisions for their children based on present symptoms and family history rather than what is published in academic journals. It is even more difficult in a tertiary referral practice to follow algorithmic protocols, rather than to individualize care to a patient who is being evaluated for expert care.

The management landscape of fUTI is constantly evolving as past tradition and dogma are questioned, and more is learnt about the pathophysiology and treatment outcomes. As a result, pediatric UTI guidelines are appropriately updated with expanding data and knowledge. In recent years, the UK National Institute for Health and Clinical Excellence (NICE), the American Urological Association (AUA), and the American Academy of Pediatrics (AAP) have updated their pediatric UTI and VUR guidelines. The NICE guidelines, which were published in 2007, were developed to achieve more consistent clinical practice based on accurate diagnosis and effective management.[11] With respect to diagnosis, the NICE guidelines underscore the importance of urine culture in patients with fever without a source (FWS), and they distinguish between upper and lower UTI. The AUA guidelines published in 2010 are specific to VUR, and reflect the limited amount of evidence-based knowledge about this condition.[10] However, these guidelines contribute to the understanding of several issues specifically in patients with UTI and VUR, including the relevance of renal scarring, usefulness of continuous antibiotic prophylaxis (CAP), appropriate use of imaging, and consideration of BBD. The AAP guidelines, which were published in

August 2011, have been long awaited and have led to confusion among practitioners because of major investigational protocol changes that have been made compared with the 1999 guidelines. In particular, the AAP guidelines have been cited for stating that CAP is not useful in preventing recurrent fUTI and that routine voiding cystoureth-rogram (VCUG) is not indicated after first fUTI if ultrasonography results are normal.[12] However, these guidelines were developed for a specific age group (pre–potty-trained infants and children age 2 to 24 months) and they should not be extrapolated to older or younger patients, or to those with complex situations. Key issues in pediatric UTI management are discussed later; where pertinent, a discussion of the guidelines regarding these issues is also presented.

ISSUES IN PEDIATRIC UTI: DIAGNOSIS

Fever in children, especially in young children, is a cause of concern for parents and caregivers and is the most common reason for children to be taken to the doctor or hospital. Of 5.4 million emergency department (ED) visits per year with fever, an esti-mated 6% to 14% have an FWS; UTIs occur in approximately 7% of boys 6 months old or younger and 8% of girls 1 year old or younger with an FWS.[13,14] Thus, testing for the presence of UTI seems to be warranted in this patient population, in particular if certain risk criteria are met. The AAP guideline analyzes risk factors that can be addressed to define the at-risk populations: sex, age, fever greater than 39°C, sus-tained fever of more than 2 days, white more than black race, and uncircumcised status. This analysis is reflected in recent guidelines from major organizations, as summarized in **Box 1**. An important component of diagnosis is proper collection of

---

Box 1
Guidelines on diagnosis of UTI in children

NICE guidelines[a]

- Infants and children presenting with unexplained fever of 38°C or higher should have a urine sample tested after 24 hours at the latest.

- Infants and children with symptoms and signs of UTI should have a urine sample tested for infection.

AAP guidelines[b]

- If a clinician decides that a febrile infant with no apparent source of the fever requires antimicrobial therapy to be administered because of ill appearances or another pressing reason, the clinician should ensure that a urine specimen is obtained for both culture and urinalysis before an antimicrobial agent is administered.

- The first option is for the urine specimen to be obtained through catheterization or suprapubic aspiration, because the diagnosis of UTI cannot be established reliably through culture of urine collected in a bag. The second option is to obtain the urine specimen through the most convenient means and to perform a urinalysis. If the urinalysis suggests a UTI, then a urine specimen should be obtained through catheterization or suprapubic aspiration.

[a] *Data from* National Institute for Health and Clinical Excellence (NICE). Urinary tract infection in children: diagnosis, treatment and long-term management. Clinical guideline 57. 2007. Available at: http://guidance.nice.org.uk/CG54. Accessed December 19, 2011.
[b] *Data from* Roberts KB and the Subcommittee on Urinary Tract Infection, Steering Committee on Quality Improvement and Management. Clinical Practice Guideline. Urinary tract infection: clinical practice guideline for the diagnosis and management of the initial UTI in febrile infants and children 2 to 24 months. Pediatrics 2011;128(3):597.

urine. A clean-catch urine specimen is preferred, when possible, in older, potty-trained patients, although catheterization or suprapubic aspiration (SPA) must be performed in younger patients, especially if a urine sample collected by other means (such as bag collection) is suspicious for the diagnosis of UTI. If the treating physician decides that a febrile infant requires antimicrobial therapy, and the urinary tract is considered a most likely source, then collection bag specimens, by themselves, are not generally considered to be acceptable to support the diagnosis.[4,11,12] The 2011 AAP guidelines recommend that in patients 2 to 24 months old, both a urinalysis with pyuria and/or bacteriuria and a culture with at least 50,000 colony-forming units of a uropathogen per milliliter, are essential to establish a diagnosis of UTI.[12]

ISSUES IN PEDIATRIC UTI: TREATMENT

Once the diagnosis and decision to treat have been made, oral antimicrobial or parenteral treatment may be administered, because they are equally effective. The 2011 AAP guideline states that the route of administration should be based on practical considerations, such as whether the child can retain orally administered fluids and medications.[12] Choice of agent should be based on antimicrobial susceptibility of the isolated uropathogen and may include ceftriaxone, cefotaxime, ceftazidime, gentamicin, tobramycin, or piperacillin for parenteral treatment and amoxicillin plus clavulanic acid, trimethoprim-sulfamethoxazole, sulfisoxazole, or a cephalosporin for oral treatment. The duration of antimicrobial therapy should be 7 to 14 days. The AAP guideline recommends against agents such as nitrofurantoin and others that predominantly are excreted in urine to treat fUTI in infants, because the serum antimicrobial concentration attained is not sufficient to treat pyelonephritis or urosepsis.[12]

ISSUES IN PEDIATRIC UTI FOLLOW-UP: CAP

The goals of follow-up after initial treatment of fUTI are to reduce the risk of developing another fUTI, to prevent renal injury, and to minimize the morbidity of being recurrently ill. The use of CAP to prevent recurrent UTI has been a contentious issue, although it has been a gold standard for 5 decades. The benefit of CAP must be weighed against the risks (eg, development of antibiotic resistance), cost, and inconvenience of therapy.

Several risk factors for recurrent UTI have been proposed in the literature. The risk of experiencing a UTI recurrence seems to depend on general patient characteristics, such as age and gender, as well as certain patient-specific characteristics. One proposed risk factor is high-grade VUR. VUR is commonly classified into 5 grades according to the International Classification of Vesicoureteral Reflux, with grade V being the most severe (**Table 1**).[15] Although higher grade VUR is associated with an increased risk of UTI recurrence, no clear cutoff VUR grade for which CAP is or is not indicated has been established.[16]

BBD can influence VUR outcomes; the AUA guidelines recommend that the presence of BBD should be determined in patients with VUR. Furthermore, these guidelines state that in children older than 1 year with grades I to IV VUR and BBD, and/or in patients with renal cortical abnormalities, CAP is recommended.[10] Even the NICE guidelines suggest that CAP might be appropriate in those with recurrent fUTI rather than after a first episode. In contrast, although the AAP guidelines define some similar risk criteria for determining whether or not to use CAP, they, like the NICE guidelines, do not comment on the importance of BBD.[12] In addition to a lack of anatomic abnormalities such as BBD, factors associated with a low risk of recurrent UTI are listed in **Box 2**. Children possessing these characteristics may be considered to be low-risk patients who are not expected to have another UTI that could lead to

Table 1 VUR grades	
Grade	Description
I	Reflux into a nondilated ureter only
II	Reflux into the renal pelvis and calyces without dilatation
III	Reflux into a mildly to moderately dilated ureter and renal pelvis with no or only slight blunting of fornices
IV	Moderate dilatation and tortuosity of the ureter and renal pelvis, with obliteration of the sharp angle of the fornices but maintenance of papillary impressions in most calyces
V	Gross dilatation and tortuosity of the ureter, renal pelvis, and calyces with loss of papillary impressions

Data from International Reflux Study Committee. Medical versus surgical treatment of primary vesicoureteral reflux: report of the International Reflux Study Committee. Pediatrics 1981;67:392–400.

scarring[10]; such patients would accordingly derive less benefit from CAP compared with high-risk patients.

Six important clinical studies have addressed the usefulness of CAP in preventing fUTI recurrence. The results of 4 of these studies indicated no benefit of CAP versus observation[17-20]; however, few of the patients in these studies had grade IV or V VUR. Thus, because high-grade VUR has been shown to be associated with an increased risk of UTI recurrence, the results of these studies are not considered to be definitive. Moreover, and given that these studies were not North American, circumcision status in boys was not reported. The Australian Prevention of Recurrent Urinary Tract Infection in Children with Vesicoureteric Reflux and Normal Renal Tracts (PRIVENT) study was designed to test the efficacy of CAP in preventing recurrence in children who had had 1 or more fUTIs.[21] A total of 576 children were randomly assigned to receive CAP versus placebo for 12 months. Although the results of this study suggested a benefit of CAP in reducing the incidence of UTI recurrence, this benefit was not convincing: 15 children had to be treated for 12 months to prevent a single UTI. This study also did not have sufficient statistical power to assess risk according to VUR grade.[21] Renal scarring was not studied and it is likely that many more children would have required treatment to prevent a single significant renal scar.

Box 2 Factors associated with a low risk of recurrent UTI
• Lack of anatomic abnormalities (eg, BBD)
• No recent history of prior UTIs
• Circumcised boys
• Absence of scarring
• Completion of toilet training/normal voiding habits
• Older children who can verbalize symptoms well
• Lower grades of VUR
• Normal renal ultrasound or DMSA scan

Data from Peters CA, Skoog SJ, Arant BS Jr, et al. Summary of the AUA guideline on management of primary vesicoureteral reflux in children. J Urol 2010;184(3):1134–44.

The Swedish Reflux Trial is the only clinical trial to specifically evaluate children with higher grade (grade III–V) VUR. This study enrolled 203 children (128 girls, 75 boys) aged 1 to 2 years with VUR.[22] The results indicated that CAP and endoscopic injection (EI) were comparable in reducing fUTI recurrences compared with cohorts who were only observed. Although they were unable to recruit their desired number of patients into the study, they showed, that girls were at risk of developing new scars, with boys seemingly having resilient kidneys to new scars.[23] Thus, the body of literature regarding the usefulness of CAP in preventing UTI recurrence remains unsatisfactory.

The practitioner is placed in the position of determining whether to administer CAP to a given patient, or to consider the benefits versus risks of surveillance; that is, of not using CAP.[24] The potential benefits of not using CAP include cost, bacterial resistance, side effects, and the parental inconvenience of administering it on a daily basis (ie, compliance). In a surveillance protocol, each child (and family) becomes his or her own stress test and pits the risk aversion of VUR against treatment-associated morbidity. The AAP reviewed raw data from the 6 randomized clinical trials mentioned earlier[17–21,23] and compiled a data set of 1091 infants aged 2 to 24 months. They performed a meta-analysis and found no statistically significant benefit of prophylaxis in preventing recurrent fUTI/pyelonephritis in infants without reflux or in those with grades I to IV VUR.[12]

Especially in the presence of documented VUR, if the child does clinically well and renal units remain stable, further invasive imaging (eg, VCUG) becomes superfluous. Regardless, it is imperative to address other overt and covert factors, in particular BBD. The team from pediatric urologist to primary provider to patient and family must completely accept the concept that surveillance does not mean nontreatment. Its success depends on the patient's family being educated about vigilantly watching for signs and symptoms of UTI recurrence and the importance of prompt evaluation and treatment.[24]

The ongoing RIVUR (Randomized Intervention for Children with Vesicoureteral Reflux) study may help identify acquired renal changes in patients receiving CAP versus observation. This multicenter trial sponsored by the US National Institutes of Health/National Institute of Diabetes and Digestive and Kidney Diseases was initiated in 2005 and will close in 2013. The intended enrollment is 600 children aged 2 to 72 months (ie, 6 years) with grade I to IV VUR identified after fUTI or symptomatic UTI, who will be randomized to CAP versus placebo. The primary outcome measure is UTI recurrence; secondary end points include time to UTI recurrence, renal scarring, treatment failure, renal function, resource utilization, and development of antimicrobial resistance in stool flora.[25] The results of this trial are expected to further contribute to the body of data regarding the use of CAP in children with fUTI.

ISSUES IN PEDIATRIC UTI FOLLOW-UP: IMAGING

Imaging studies traditionally have been performed to provide information about how to best evaluate and manage children with fUTI. The primary goal of imaging has been to identify the presence of risk factors, such as VUR and preexisting renal damage, and thus to determine whether or not further testing or medical or surgical therapeutic intervention is indicated.[10] Several types of imaging modalities are performed in pediatric urology; each is associated with its own benefits and limitations/risks.

Renal-bladder ultrasonography (RUS) enables assessment of anatomic features, such as the renal architecture, size discrepancy, dilatation, and some scarring. However, it cannot be used to reliably detect low-grade/moderate-grade VUR or APN, and it can miss renal scarring. Compared with other imaging modalities, RUS is noninvasive, with no radiation risks, although it still is associated with costs. RUS, as recommended in the 2011 AAP guideline, is recommended as the initial screening study after fUTI, particularly in younger patients (**Boxes 3** and **4; Table 2**).[10–12] Based on the patient peculiarities and the results of the RUS, further studies might be indicated for that patient.

VCUG enables complete examination of the bladder and urethra and has been the gold standard study to evaluate for VUR and to grade it appropriately. Because VUR is the most commonly associated urologic finding in infants and children, initial VCUG in all patients with fUTI, or what has been termed the bottom-up approach to evaluation, has been traditional in most North American pediatric urologic and primary care practices. The requirement for catheterization and the use of fluoroscopy is associated with the inherent radiation exposure and the inconvenience and discomfort of placing a catheter. Catheterization can even introduce bacteria and lead to iatrogenic UTI. Moreover, most cases of VUR that are uncovered with VCUG are of lower grade and it is known from routine maternal-fetal ultrasonography studies in the past quarter of a century that many cases of renal scarring result from embryogenic mishaps and represent congenital dysplasia. Most significant scars are likely primarily developmental, not secondary or acquired.[26,27] Thus, routine use of VCUG has been increasingly criticized of late. Although some physicians regularly incorporate VCUG as part of follow-up after a first fUTI, the prevailing opinion is that this is not appropriate.[10–12] The UK National Institute for Health and Clinical Excellence (NICE) guidelines recommend that VCUG only be performed after the second fUTI or after the first fUTI if 1 or more of the following conditions is present: abnormal sonogram, unusual bacteria, poor urine flow, or renal insufficiency (see **Table 2**).[11] Although not as specific, the AAP and AUA guidelines include similar recommendations, particularly regarding the routine use of VCUG.[10,12]

The AAP recommends performing VCUG after a second UTI or if renal-bladder ultrasound reveals hydronephrosis, scarring, or other findings that suggest high-grade VUR, obstructive uropathy, or other atypical or complex clinical circumstances. The recommendation that VCUG not be routinely performed after fUTI, as Thomas Newman[28] pointed out in a Commentary in *Pediatrics*, greatly from the earlier 1999 AAP guideline. Based on evidence accumulated during the 12 years since the earlier guideline, the AAP concluded that the use of VCUG is difficult to justify, given the risks, costs, and discomfort of the procedure and lack of benefit derived from having VUR diagnosed. However, this recommendation for minimal radiographic evaluation is controversial, because many physicians think that a significant number of children will have complications of UTI that otherwise could have been avoided.

Box 3
AAP imaging guidelines

- Febrile infants with UTIs should undergo renal and bladder ultrasonography

- VCUG should not be performed routinely after the first fUTI; VCUG is indicated if renal-bladder ultrasound reveals hydronephrosis, scarring, or other findings that suggest either high-grade VUR or obstructive uropathy, as well as in other atypical or complex clinical circumstances

- Further evaluation should be conducted if there is a recurrence of fUTI

Data from Roberts KB and the Subcommittee on Urinary Tract Infection, Steering Committee on Quality Improvement and Management. Clinical practice guideline. Urinary tract infection: clinical practice guideline for the diagnosis and management of the initial UTI in Febrile infants and children 2 to 24 months. Pediatrics 2011;128(3):602, 603.

> **Box 4**
> **AUA imaging guidelines**
>
> - Ultrasonography is recommended every 12 months to monitor renal growth and any parenchymal scarring.
>
> - Voiding cystography (radionuclide cystogram or low-dose fluoroscopy, when available) is recommended every 12 to 24 months with longer intervals between follow-up studies in patients in whom evidence supports lower rates of spontaneous resolution (ie, those with higher grades of VUR [grades III–V], BBD, and older age).
>
> - Option: follow-up cystography may be done after 1 year of age in patients with VUR grade I to II; these patients tend to have a high rate of spontaneous resolution and boys have a low risk of recurrent UTI.
>
> - Option: a single normal voiding cystogram (ie, no evidence of VUR) may establish resolution. The clinical significance of grade I VUR and the need for ongoing evaluation is undefined.
>
> *Data from* Peters CA, Skoog SJ, Arant BS Jr, et al. Summary of the AUA guideline on management of primary vesicoureteral reflux in children. J Urol 2010;184(3):1134–44.

DMSA renal scanning is a nuclear imaging procedure that enables visualization of the kidneys and assessment of their function, and identifies areas of decreased perfusion. DMSA can be used acutely to confirm pyelonephritis during the acute phase, although persistence of hypoperfusion on a follow-up scan performed months later (eg, 4–5 months after acute infection) represents scarring.[11] The concept of a top-down approach incorporates a DMSA scan to identify upper tract involvement or APN during fUTI. As noted earlier, only 60% of patients with fUTI have confirmatory scans for APN. Only in cases with confirmed positive scans during the acute phase of a fUTI would a VCUG be performed in centers where the top-down approach is advocated.

Thus, in the conventional bottom-up approach, the initial diagnostic focus is the bladder, and primarily involves detection of urinary tract abnormalities and VUR, which is accomplished using VCUG. Detection of VUR on initial imaging leads to appropriate follow-up imaging and management, whereas normal imaging results indicate that no further work-up, at least for VUR, is required.[29] This approach has the potential to produce a high yield of VUR cases. The criticism is that patients will be diagnosed with VUR, especially low grades, even if they have little risk of acquiring renal scars. The argument may be countered by the potential of identifying all VUR in patients who ultimately may suffer the morbidity of recurrent fUTI.

The top-down approach focuses initially on the kidney and confirming the renal involvement in the setting of fUTI, APN. This confirmation is accomplished through DMSA renal scanning, or, in some cases, magnetic resonance imaging (MRI) or computed tomography (CT) have served as a substitute. Patients with cortical defects that indicate pyelonephritis go on to VCUG, whereas those with central photopenia that suggests hydronephrosis undergo RUS. Patients with normal DMSA results require no further work-up, with the exception of those with recurrent fUTI, who then undergo VCUG.[29] The top-down approach has been praised for being more selective in determining acute renal involvement at the time of infection. Criticisms include the necessity of sedation, or even general anesthesia, in some younger children (not required with the bottom-up approach), a higher radiation dose compared with VCUG, and the requirement for repeat scanning if acute infection is identified **(Fig. 1)**.[30]

Table 2
NICE guidelines: recommended imaging schedule

Test	Responds Well to Treatment Within 48 h	Atypical UTI[a]	Recurrent UTI
Infants <6 mo old			
Ultrasound during the acute infection	No	Yes[b]	Yes
Ultrasound within 6 wk	Yes[c]	No	No
DMSA 4–6 mo following the acute infection	No	Yes	Yes
VCUG	No	Yes	Yes
Infants and children 6 mo to <3 y old			
Ultrasound during the acute infection	No	Yes[b]	No
Ultrasound within 6 wk	No	No	Yes
DMSA 4–6 mo following the acute infection	No	Yes	Yes
VCUG	No	No[d]	No[d]
Children ≥3 y old			
Ultrasound during the acute infection	No	Yes[b,e]	No
Ultrasound within 6 wk	No	No	Yes[e]
DMSA 4–6 mo following the acute infection	No	No	Yes
VCUG	No	No	No

[a] Atypical UTI includes patients with 1 or more of the following: seriously ill, poor urine flow, abdominal or bladder mass, raised creatinine, septicemia, failure to respond to treatment with suitable antibiotics within 48 hours, or infection with non–*Escherichia coli* organisms. Recurrent UTI includes patients with 1 of the following: 2 or more episodes of UTI with APN/upper UTI, 1 episode of UTI with APN/upper UTI plus 1 or more episodes of UTI with cystitis/lower UTI, or 3 or more episodes of UTI with cystitis/lower UTI.
[b] In an infant or child with a non–*E coli* UTI, responding well to antibiotics and with no other features of atypical infection, the ultrasound can be requested on a nonurgent basis to take place within 6 weeks.
[c] If abnormal, consider VCUG.
[d] Although VCUG should not be performed routinely, it should be considered if the following features are present: dilatation on ultrasound, poor urine flow, non–*E coli* infection, or family history of VUR.
[e] Ultrasound in toilet-trained children should be performed with a full bladder with an estimate of bladder volume before and after micturition.
Data from National Institute for Health and Clinical Excellence (NICE). Urinary tract infection in children: diagnosis, treatment and long-term management. Clinical guideline 57. 2007. Available at: http://guidance.nice.org.uk/CG54. Accessed December 19, 2011.

ISSUES IN PEDIATRIC UTI: RENAL SCARRING

The impact of renal scarring in pediatric patients with UTI has been the subject of much discussion in recent years. As mentioned elsewhere in this issue, the natural history of VUR is resolution with time (and patience). However, the presence of renal scarring in patients with VUR, and especially in those patients experiencing recurrent fUTI, becomes a challenge. The issue of protecting renal reserve becomes paramount in this select group of patients. In the patient with normal kidneys before an fUTI, the presence of a new scar, or a hypoperfused area on scan, likely has little long-term

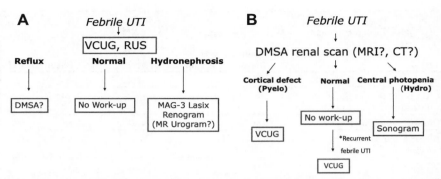

Fig. 1. Bottom-up versus top-down approaches for imaging follow-up in pediatric UTI. (A) The bottom-up, North American standard approach, and (B) the top-down approach to imaging evaluation of the child presenting with a UTI. Hydro, hydronephrosis; MAG-3, mercaptoacetyl-triglycine; MR, magnetic resonance; Pyelo, pyelonephritis. (From Koyle MA, Elder JS, Skoog SJ, et al. Febrile urinary tract infection, vesicoureteral reflux, and renal scarring: current controversies in approach to evaluation. Pediatr Surg Int 2011;27(4):337–46; with permission from Springer Science and Business Media.)

impact on renal reserve. However, that does not mean that an fUTI does not lead to other traumatic sequelae and expense. Furthermore, although the short-term effects of renal scarring, including hypertension in up to 30% of patients, are known, the long-term consequences are less well understood.[9] In one study comparing children with and without scars at 16 to 26 years after their initial diagnosis of UTI, patients with non-scarred kidneys had equivalent blood pressure measurements to those with unilateral or bilateral scars, whereas the glomerular filtration rate was only negatively affected in those with bilateral scars compared with those with unilateral scars or no scars.[31] In addition, increased use of antenatal ultrasonography has revealed that many of the scars attributed to VUR reflect a developmental abnormality and not acquired APN-associated damage; this has been confirmed by prenatal ultrasonographic studies.[26] Thus, the necessity of routinely screening the kidneys for reflux-related renal scarring in patients with VUR remains unclarified and has become an area of uncertainty that is beyond the scope of this article.[10,32,33]

ISSUES IN PEDIATRIC UTI: BBD

BBD describes any abnormalities of storage as well as emptying, and also includes constipation.[34] BBD has become a more common source of pediatric urology referrals in the past 2 decades. It constitutes a spectrum. Because BBD has been shown to negatively affect VUR spontaneous resolution rates and even surgical outcomes, the AUA guidelines state, "Symptoms indicative of BBD should be sought in the initial evaluation (including urinary frequency and urgency, prolonged voiding intervals, daytime wetting, perineal/penile pain, holding maneuvers [posturing to prevent wetting] and constipation/encopresis)."[10]

The rationale for addressing BBD in management of VUR is based on several factors. The risk of fUTI in children with VUR on CAP is greater in patients with BBD compared with those without BBD. In addition, children with BBD experience lower rates of reflux resolution within 24 months after diagnosis, lower cure rates following endoscopic therapy, and a higher rate of postoperative UTI compared with children without BBD.[10] Treatment of BBD is therefore urged before addressing VUR. However, no standardized treatment algorithm for BBD exists, and the impact of treating BBD on VUR outcomes has not been established. It is also important to recognize that the presence of VUR and BBD in the same patient may indicate a genetic component; this warrants further investigation.[7]

In the author's experience, many children referred with UTI for management have never had a UTI confirmed by urinalysis and culture. Many have dysuria or abdominal pain, but are often labeled as UTI or as needing reflux to be ruled out. Such misdiagnosis may occur in 50% or more referred for UTI. Furthermore, many parents are unaware that their child has constipation, as long they are not encopretic. When these families are counseled, we stress the mantra: "A happy bladder is an empty bladder. An even happier bladder is an empty rectum."

ISSUES IN PEDIATRIC UTI: RISK OF CHRONIC KIDNEY DISEASE

A perceived risk of chronic kidney disease (CKD) in patients with fUTI has existed for decades.[35] However, the contribution of UTI and VUR to the development of end-stage renal disease (ESRD; ie, stage 5 CKD) is difficult to ascertain and likely has been exaggerated. The risk of a child with a UTI developing ESRD is estimated to be 1 in 10,000 based on the incidence of UTI and the incidence of ESRD resulting from VUR, which is, at worst, a weak association.[27]

In the most recent study to evaluate the correlation between childhood UTI and ESRD, a Finnish group performed a systematic literature search as well as a retrospective single-center case series.[36] Together, the data indicated recurrent childhood UTI as a main cause of ESRD in 0.3% of patients. The study investigators thus concluded that a child with normal kidneys is not at significant risk of developing ESRD because of UTIs. Although this study has been cited for methodological concerns, such as a small data set, a lack of details about eligible study types and extraction steps, and no assessment of potential bias, the results add to the growing body of evidence that UTI in childhood does not cause CKD.

ISSUES IN PEDIATRIC UTI: CIRCUMCISION

The risk of UTI is higher in uncircumcised versus circumcised boys before the age of 1 year, and circumcision has been associated with a reduced risk of UTI.[37–39] However, this difference is diminished in older boys, because the overall frequency of UTI tends to decrease with increased age.[40] Whether or not circumcision should be performed to reduce the likelihood of UTI has been the subject of debate for many years. The results of a meta-analysis published in 2005 indicated that, to prevent 1 UTI, 111 circumcisions would need to be performed.[39] The study investigators concluded that, based on these results, circumcision as a means to prevent UTI may only be warranted in boys at high risk of UTI, such as those with high-grade VUR. Of the recently published pediatric UTI guidelines, only the AUA guidelines directly address circumcision in male infants.[10] The guidelines state that circumcision of the male infant with VUR may be considered based on an increased risk of UTI in boys who are not circumcised.

ISSUES IN PEDIATRIC UTI: WHEN TO REFER

Despite the current controversies and issues in pediatric UTI and VUR management, it is likely that some children will benefit from further evaluation by a pediatric urologist or nephrologist. The role of the pediatric urologist is to identify any contributory underlying conditions or issues, such as BBD, that may be promoting recurrent infections. Many centers have elimination dysfunction centers, using the skills of midlevel providers and even physical therapists and psychologists to assess and manage.

these children, because they are time consuming, and the care may require long-term follow-up. BBD is rarely 1-stop shopping and can be frustrating for the clinician and parents alike. Common elements of BBD treatment programs include bladder training with timed voiding, behavior therapy, relaxation measures, biofeedback anticholinergic medications, α-blockers, and treatment of constipation.[10,41]

In particular, referral should be considered for complex cases or patients at high risk of recurrent UTIs or renal damage. Such patients include infants less than 3 months old; infants and children 3 months or older with APN or upper UTI; children with congenital abnormalities; patients with symptoms that are nonspecific to UTI; and infants and children with a high risk of serious illness.[11]

SUMMARY

There is no single algorithm that fits every patient with fUTI. Although guidelines provide some help, they should serve only as learned opinions that are based on data scrutinized by a committed panel of experts. They should not serve as rigid rules requiring emphatic adherence. The understanding of fUTI and VUR and how they are evaluated and managed is in evolution. This evolution mandates a cooperative, open approach between the primary care provider, pediatric urologist/nephrologist, and the patient/parents to tailor a thoughtful, agreed-on therapeutic option for each individual patient.

REFERENCES

1. Hellstrom A, Hanson E, Hansson S, et al. Association between urinary symptoms at 7 years old and previous urinary tract infection. Arch Dis Child 1991;66:232–4.
2. Marild S, Jodal U. Incidence rate of first-time symptomatic urinary tract infection in children under 6 years of age. Acta Paediatr 1998;87:549–52.
3. Chesney RW, Carpenter MA, Moxey-Mims M, et al. Randomized intervention for children with vesicoureteral reflux (RIVUR): background commentary of RIVUR investigators. Pediatrics 2008;122(Suppl 5):S233–9.
4. Rajimwale A, Williams A, Shenoy M, et al. Critical analysis of the NICE guidelines on UTI in children: a perspective from the UK. Dialogues in Pediatric Urology 2011;32:7–9.
5. Pecile P, Miorin E, Romanello C, et al. Age-related renal parenchymal lesions in children with first febrile urinary tract infections. Pediatrics 2009;124:23–9.
6. Shaikh N, Ewing AL, Bhatnagar S, et al. Risk of renal scarring in children with a first urinary tract infection: a systematic review. Pediatrics 2010;126:1084–91.
7. Hudson RG. Lessons from the guidelines: understanding evidence-based vesicoureteral reflux treatment in 2010. Dialogues in Pediatric Urology 2011;32:5–6.
8. Jodal U, Smellie JM, Lax H, et al. Ten-year results of randomized treatment of children with severe vesicoureteral reflux. Final report of the International Reflux Study in Children. Pediatr Nephrol 2006;21:785–92.
9. Faust WC, Diaz M, Pohl HG. Incidence of post-pyelonephritic renal scarring: a meta-analysis of the dimercapto-succinic acid literature. J Urol 2009;181: 290–7.
10. Peters CA, Skoog SJ, Arant BS Jr, et al. Summary of the AUA guideline on management of primary vesicoureteral reflux in children. J Urol 2010;184: 1134–44.
11. National Institute for Health and Clinical Excellence (NICE). Urinary tract infection in children: diagnosis, treatment and long-term management. Clinical guideline 54. Available at: http://guidance.nice.org.uk/CG054. Accessed January 30, 2012.

12. Roberts KB, Subcommittee on urinary tract infection, Steering Committee on quality improvement and management. Urinary tract infection: clinical practice guideline for the diagnosis and management of the initial UTI in febrile infants and children 2 to 24 months. Pediatrics 2011;128:595–610.
13. Baraff LJ, Bass JW, Fleisher GR, et al. Practice guideline for the management of infants and children 0 to 36 months of age with fever without source. Agency for Health Care Policy and Research. Ann Emerg Med 1993;22:1198–210.
14. McCaig LF, Burt CW. National Hospital Ambulatory Medical Care Survey: 2002 emergency department summary. Adv Data 2004;(340):1–34.
15. Medical versus surgical treatment of primary vesicoureteral reflux: report of the International Reflux Study Committee. Pediatrics 1981;67:392–400.
16. Peters C, Rushton HG. Vesicoureteral reflux associated renal damage: congenital reflux nephropathy and acquired renal scarring. J Urol 2010;184:265–73.
17. Garin EH, Olavarria F, Garcia N, et al. Clinical significance of primary vesicoureteral reflux and urinary antibiotic prophylaxis after acute pyelonephritis: a multicenter, randomized, controlled study. Pediatrics 2006;117:626–32.
18. Pennesi M, Travan L, Peratoner L, et al. Is antibiotic prophylaxis in children with vesicoureteral reflux effective in preventing pyelonephritis and renal scars? A randomized, controlled trial. Pediatrics 2008;121:e1489–94.
19. Roussey-Kesler G, Gadjos V, Idres N, et al. Antibiotic prophylaxis for the prevention of recurrent urinary tract infection in children with low grade vesicoureteral reflux: results from a prospective randomized study. J Urol 2008;179:674–9.
20. Montini G, Rigon L, Zucchetta P, et al. Prophylaxis after first febrile urinary tract infection in children? A multicenter, randomized, controlled, noninferiority trial. Pediatrics 2008;122:1064–71.
21. Craig JC, Simpson JM, Williams GJ, et al. Antibiotic prophylaxis and recurrent urinary tract infection in children. N Engl J Med 2009;361:1748–59.
22. Brandstrom P, Esbjorner E, Herthelius M, et al. The Swedish Reflux Trial in children: I. Study design and study population characteristics. J Urol 2010;184:274–9.
23. Brandstrom P, Esbjorner E, Herthelius M, et al. The Swedish Reflux Trial in children: III. Urinary tract infection pattern. J Urol 2010;184:286–91.
24. Peters CA. Antibiotic prophylaxis for reflux: why and when I won't use it. Dialogues in Pediatric Urology 2011;32:3–4.
25. Keren R, Carpenter MA, Hoberman A, et al. Rationale and design issues of the Randomized Intervention for Children With Vesicoureteral Reflux (RIVUR) study. Pediatrics 2008;122(Suppl 5):S240–50.
26. Montini G, Tullus K, Hewitt I. Febrile urinary tract infections in children. N Engl J Med 2011;365:239–50.
27. Craig JC, Williams GJ. Denominators do matter: it's a myth–urinary tract infection does not cause chronic kidney disease. Pediatrics 2011;128:984–5.
28. Newman TB. The New American Academy of Pediatrics Urinary Tract Infection Guideline. Pediatrics 2011;128:572–5.
29. Koyle MA, Elder JS, Skoog SJ, et al. Febrile urinary tract infection, vesicoureteral reflux, and renal scarring: current controversies in approach to evaluation. Pediatr Surg Int 2011;27:337–46.
30. Routh JC, Lee RS, Chow JS. Radiation dose and screening for vesicoureteral reflux. AJR Am J Roentgenol 2010;194:W243.
31. Wennerstrom M, Hansson S, Jodal U, et al. Renal function 16 to 26 years after the first urinary tract infection in childhood. Arch Pediatr Adolesc Med 2000;154:339–45.

32. Rushton HG, Majd M, Jantausch B, et al. Renal scarring following reflux and non-reflux pyelonephritis in children: evaluation with 99mtechnetium-dimercaptosuccinic acid scintigraphy. J Urol 1992;147:1327–32.

33. Majd M, Rushton HG, Jantausch B, et al. Relationship among vesicoureteral reflux, P-fimbriated *Escherichia coli*, and acute pyelonephritis in children with febrile urinary tract infection. J Pediatr 1991;119:578–85.

34. Neveus T, von Gontard A, Hoebeke P, et al. The standardization of terminology of lower urinary tract function in children and adolescents: report from the Standardisation Committee of the International Children's Continence Society. J Urol 2006; 176:314–24.

35. Margileth AM, Pedreira FA, Hirschman GH, et al. Urinary tract bacterial infections: office diagnosis and management. Pediatr Clin North Am 1976;23:721–34.

36. Salo J, Ikaheimo R, Tapiainen T, et al. Childhood urinary tract infections as a cause of chronic kidney disease. Pediatrics 2011;128:840–7.

37. Wiswell TE, Smith FR, Bass JW. Decreased incidence of urinary tract infections in circumcised male infants. Pediatrics 1985;75:901–3.

38. Shaw KN, Gorelick M, McGowan KL, et al. Prevalence of urinary tract infection in febrile young children in the emergency department. Pediatrics 1998;102:e16.

39. Singh-Grewal D, Macdessi J, Craig J. Circumcision for the prevention of urinary tract infection in boys: a systematic review of randomised trials and observational studies. Arch Dis Child 2005;90:853–8.

40. Coulthard MG, Lambert HJ, Keir MJ. Occurrence of renal scars in children after their first referral for urinary tract infection. BMJ 1997;315:918–9.

41. Glassberg KI, Combs AJ. Nonneurogenic voiding disorders: what's new? Curr Opin Urol 2009;19:412–8.

Evidence Basis for Individualized Evaluation and Less Imaging in Febrile Urinary Tract Infection
An Editorial Commentary

Thomas B. Newman, MD, MPH[a],*

KEYWORDS

- Urinary tract infection • Vesicoureteral reflux • Voiding cystourethrogram
- Urine testing

KEY POINTS

- The past decade has seen a remarkable retreat from previous dogma regarding urinary tract infections (UTIs).
- The lack of evidence that treatment affects long term outcomes suggests urine testing decisions should be based primarily on patient preferences and estimated short-term benefits.
- Short-term benefits of diagnosing UTIs are limited in children with mild illness, because most UTIs resolve without treatment.
- An individualized approach to urine testing that is less aggressive than previous recommendations is warranted.

In this issue Drs Koyle and Shifrin[1] provided a thoughtful review on febrile urinary tract infections (UTIs) in children, acknowledging the uncertainty around many of the questions we used to think we knew the answers to. They concluded that there is not a single algorithm that fits all patients and that clinicians and parents should have an open and cooperative approach. I would like to expand on that conclusion in this commentary and focus on febrile infants younger than 2 years, for whom decisions are most difficult because the children cannot reliably report UTI symptoms, and obtaining the urine sample from this age group is often time consuming and unpleasant.

This editorial commentary was written in response to the article by Drs Martin Koyle and Donald Shifrin, entitled "Issues in Febrile Urinary Tract Infection Management" in *Pediatric Clinics of North America* (59:4), August 2012.

[a] Department of Epidemiology and Biostatistics, School of Medicine, University of California, San Francisco, CA 94143, USA
* Department of Epidemiology & Biostatistics, UCSF Box 0560, San Francisco, CA 94143.
E-mail address: newman@epi.ucsf.edu

It is clear from recent studies highlighted in Koyle and Shifrin's review that the past decade has seen a remarkable retreat from previous dogmas regarding UTIs. There are no good data demonstrating a relationship between febrile UTIs and subsequent renal diseases, and if there is such a relationship, it must be weak.[2,3] Although we know that vesicoureteral reflux (VUR) is frequently found in children with a history of febrile UTIs, we admit that most VUR resolves spontaneously and that we do not have evidence as to whether treatment of the rest improves outcome.[4]

These changes in the outlook toward UTIs are reflected in new, more conservative imaging recommendations, but their implications have not yet been sufficiently appreciated for the decisions pediatricians face most often when evaluating a young child with a fever: whether to obtain a urine sample, and if so, how to do so.

The decision to obtain a urine sample for testing should be based on both the probability of UTI and the projected health benefit of diagnosing it at the current visit. The former can be estimated by considering clinical and demographic risk factors, including absence of another likely source for the fever, fever duration, race, sex, and circumcision status.[4,5] The health benefit of early diagnosis of UTI is the improvement in health outcomes that can be accomplished by treatment. Now that we acknowledge that we do not know the extent to which imaging or treatment of UTI actually prevents late adverse outcomes, we can focus on short-term outcomes, such as reduction of symptoms and prevention of immediate complications, such as sepsis or meningitis.

Because febrile UTIs are easily treated, the benefit of reducing symptoms is directly related to symptom severity. Patients who present with high temperature, flank pain, and longer duration of illness (suggesting that their UTI is not resolving spontaneously) have the most to gain from having their UTIs diagnosed and treated sooner. Serious complications of UTI, such as bacteremia and meningitis, are rare and largely seen in infants younger than 6 months, especially those younger than 2 months.[6–8] It makes sense to test more aggressively for UTI in these infants.

What happens to children in whom a UTI is initially missed? In a prospective study of 15,781 episodes of febrile illness in children younger than 5 years, even those children whose bacterial infections were not initially diagnosed and treated did well.[9] Data from the Pediatric Research in Office Settings ("PROS") Febrile Infant Study suggest that even in the highest risk 0- to 3-month age group (in whom I recommend urine testing), the outcome is generally benign.[6] In this study, there were 807 infants aged 0 to 3 months with a temperature greater than or equal to 38°C, whose practitioners did not initially order for any urine tests, who were not initially treated with antibiotics, and were followed up until resolution of their illness. Based on the demographic and clinical risk factors for UTI recorded at their initial visit, about 61 patients (7.6%) would have had a UTI diagnosed if a urine test had been ordered. However, only 2 patients were diagnosed with UTI; both were treated and did well. The other approximately 59 infants (97%) recovered uneventfully, without ever having their UTIs diagnosed. Given this benign outcome in a group at highest risk of complications, it seems that the short-term risk of failing to diagnose UTI at the initial clinic visit is extremely low. Hence, the benefit of early diagnosis of UTI is primarily the opportunity to reduce symptoms sooner and prevent a small number of return visits for persistent fever.

An open question is at what risk of UTI these modest benefits justify the cost, discomfort, and inconvenience of urine testing, as well as the accompanying risk of false-positive results. The American Academy of Pediatrics practice guideline suggests that this point is 1% to 2%, implying that it is worth performing urine tests on 50 to 100 children to identify a UTI (sooner) in 1 child. This seems like a very low threshold (and high number needed to test) to me.[10] However, this threshold varies with the treatment and risk preferences of the family and clinician, as suggested by Drs Koyle and Shifrin.

Families and clinicians will also have a range of preferences regarding the relative value of a more accurate urine culture result obtainable by urethral catheterization weighed against the invasiveness of the procedure[11] and the risk of introducing a UTI.[12,13] Greater certainty is required if the consequence of a positive culture is to be imaging, particularly with a voiding cystourethrogram (VCUG). On the other hand, if the main decision made as a result of the urine culture is whether to discontinue antibiotics (already started because of a positive urinalysis result), it may not be worth doing about 20 urethral catheterizations to avoid administering antibiotics for an additional 8 days in 1 child.[14]

SUMMARY

There is growing consensus that most infants and children with UTI do not need invasive imaging, at least initially.[15–19] The importance of ultrasonography and VCUG after recurrence of UTI is uncertain.[10,17] The weak and uncertain relationship between diagnosing and treating UTI and the prevention of future renal diseases suggests that decisions about whether and how to obtain urine samples should depend on estimated short-term benefits[3] and patient values. As stated by Koyle and Shifrin, while guidelines can be helpful, "they should not serve as rigid rules requiring emphatic adherence."

REFERENCES

1. Craig JC, Irwig LM, Knight JF, et al. Does treatment of vesicoureteric reflux in childhood prevent end-stage renal disease attributable to reflux nephropathy? Pediatrics 2000;105:1236–41.
2. Salo J, Ikaheimo R, Tapiainen T, et al. Childhood urinary tract infections as a cause of chronic kidney disease. Pediatrics 2011;128:840–7.
3. Craig JC, Williams GJ. Denominators do matter: it's a myth—urinary tract infection does not cause chronic kidney disease. Pediatrics 2011;128:984–5.
4. Finnell S, Downs S, Carroll A. Technical report: the diagnosis and management of the initial urinary tract infection in febrile infants and young children. Pediatrics 2011;128:e749–70.
5. Shaikh N, Morone NE, Lopez J, et al. Does this child have a urinary tract infection? JAMA 2007;298:2895–904.
6. Newman TB, Bernzweig JA, Takayama JI, et al. Urine testing and urinary tract infections in febrile infants seen in office settings: the Pediatric Research in Office Settings' Febrile Infant Study. Arch Pediatr Adolesc Med 2002;156:44–54.
7. Schnadower D, Kuppermann N, Macias CG, et al. Febrile infants with urinary tract infections at very low risk for adverse events and bacteremia. Pediatrics 2010;126:1074–83.
8. Herz AM, Greenhow TL, Alcantara J, et al. Changing epidemiology of outpatient bacteremia in 3- to 36-month-old children after the introduction of the heptavalent-conjugated pneumococcal vaccine. Pediatr Infect Dis J 2006;25:293–300.
9. Craig JC, Williams GJ, Jones M, et al. The accuracy of clinical symptoms and signs for the diagnosis of serious bacterial infection in young febrile children: prospective cohort study of 15 781 febrile illnesses. BMJ 2010;340:c1594.
10. Newman TB. The new American Academy of Pediatrics urinary tract infection guideline. Pediatrics 2011;128(3):572–5.

11. Merritt KA, Ornstein PA, Spicker B. Children's memory for a salient medical procedure: implications for testimony. Pediatrics 1994;94:17–23.
12. Lohr JA, Downs SM, Dudley S, et al. Hospital-acquired urinary tract infections in the pediatric patient: a prospective study. Pediatr Infect Dis J 1994;13:8–12.
13. Lohr JA, Portilla MG, Geuder TG, et al. Making a presumptive diagnosis of urinary tract infection by using a urinalysis performed in an on-site laboratory. J Pediatr 1993;122:22–5.
14. Schroeder AR, Newman TB, Wasserman RC, et al. Choice of urine collection methods for the diagnosis of urinary tract infection in young, febrile infants. Arch Pediatr Adolesc Med 2005;159:915–22.
15. Newman TB. Evidence does not support American Academy of Pediatrics recommendation for routine imaging after a first urinary tract infection. Pediatrics 2005;116:1613–4.
16. Newman TB. Much pain, little gain from voiding cystourethrograms after urinary tract infection. Pediatrics 2006;118:2251.
17. National Collaborating Centre for Women's and Children's Health. Urinary tract infection in children: diagnosis, treatment and long-term management. National Institute for Health and Clinical Excellence Clinical Guideline. London: RCOG Press; 2007.
18. Schroeder AR, Abidari JM, Kirpekar R, et al. Impact of a more restrictive approach to urinary tract imaging after febrile urinary tract infection. Arch Pediatr Adolesc Med 2011;165:1027–32.
19. Schroeder AR, Harris SJ, Newman TB. Safely doing less: a missing component of the patient safety dialogue. Pediatrics 2011;128:e1596–7.

Advances in the Surgical Pediatric Urologic Armamentarium

Robert M. Turner II, MD*, Janelle A. Fox, MD, Michael C. Ost, MD

KEYWORDS

- Minimally invasive • Child • Laparoscopy • Robot • Single-site • Percutaneous
- Ureteroscopy

KEY POINTS

- Due to recent technological advancements and careful adaptations in the pediatric patient, minimally invasive approaches now have routine applications in pediatric urology.
- Robotic surgery has the potential to make some minimally invasive techniques more accessible to pediatric urologists by simplifying complex reconstructive procedures.
- Miniaturization of endoscopic equipment has expanded the indications of endourologic surgery in the pediatric stone patient.
- Challenges for the foreseeable future include cost-containment and further improvement in patient comfort and cosmesis.

INTRODUCTION

The last 2 decades have seen great changes in the surgical management of urologic disease in children. Following the emergence of minimally invasive approaches in the adult population, urologists have successfully applied these techniques in pediatric patients. The most notable advancements have occurred in laparoscopy, robotics, and endourology. Improvements in imagery and miniaturization of laparoscopic equipment have expanded the indications of laparoscopy in children from simple orchiopexy and pyeloplasty to ureteral reimplantation. Even more complex urologic surgery such as bladder reconstruction is being performed more readily with the aid of robotics. The treatment of stone disease in children has also changed for the better because of the availability of smaller and more flexible endourologic equipment.

The technical difficulty and steep learning curve of conventional laparoscopy led to the application of robotic assistance, namely with the da Vinci Surgical System

Disclosure statement: no competing financial interests exist. Additional disclosure: the views expressed in this presentation are those of the authors and do not necessarily reflect the official policy or position of the Department of the Navy, Department of Defense, or the US government.
Division of Pediatric Urology, Children's Hospital of Pittsburgh of UPMC, University of Pittsburgh, Pittsburgh, PA, USA
* Corresponding author. 3471 Fifth Avenue, Suite 700, Pittsburgh, PA 15213.
E-mail address: turnerrm@upmc.edu

Pediatr Clin N Am 59 (2012) 927–941
doi:10.1016/j.pcl.2012.05.011
0031-3955/12/$ – see front matter © 2012 Elsevier Inc. All rights reserved.

(Intuitive Surgical, Sunnyvale, CA, USA). Robotic assistance has the potential to make laparoscopic surgery more accessible to pediatric urologists by simplifying complex reconstructive procedures. Although still in its infancy, laparoendoscopic single-site surgery (LESS) is making the laparoscopic approach even less invasive.

ADAPTATIONS OF LAPAROSCOPY FOR THE PEDIATRIC PATIENT

The foundation of laparoscopy in urology has its origins in the use of the cystoscope to inspect the peritoneal cavity of children with nonpalpable undescended testes.[1,2] Despite this early use in the pediatric population, most of the equipment was developed for adults. Specific challenges of laparoscopy in children include a smaller working space, limited area for trocar insertion, delicacy of tissues, and manual dexterity required when working with smaller instruments and suture. This article first discusses recent technological advancements and considerations when applying them in children.

Insufflation

Abdominal insufflation is accomplished with carbon dioxide (CO_2) gas, which is noncombustible and highly soluble. Automated insufflation machines allow manual settings to regulate intra-abdominal pressure and CO_2 flow rates. Children are particularly sensitive to increases in intra-abdominal pressure, with potentially severe respiratory and hemodynamic changes, with greater risk of subcutaneous emphysema from dissection of insufflation gas.[3,4] Subcutaneous emphysema is disturbing on examination, but not a clinical problem provided it is not associated with pneumothorax. Peritoneal insufflation has cardiovascular, pulmonary, vascular, neurologic, and somatic effects. A common complaint during recovery is shoulder pain, a referred pain from diaphragmatic distension. Hypercapnia from CO_2 insufflation causes hypertension, tachycardia, and increased cardiac output; however, the reduced venous return from compression of the inferior vena cava during pneumoperitoneum often negates this sympathetic effect. Ventilatory difficulty should prompt reduced abdominal insufflation, return to supine position, and a check of the endotracheal tube, which can migrate during surgery. Perhaps the most feared, but very rare, complication of laparoscopy is venous gas embolism; a mill-wheel cardiac murmur is diagnostic but rarely encountered. Gas embolism is immediately treated with desufflation of the abdomen; positioning in a left lateral, decubitus, head-down position (which moves the gas bubble to the apex of the right ventricle); 100% oxygen supplementation; and hyperventilation to help reabsorb the carbon dioxide gas bubble.[5]

The current norms used for working pressure in infants (0–2 years), children (2–10 years), and adolescents (>10 years) are 8 to 10 mm Hg, 10 to 12 mm Hg, and 15 mm Hg, respectively.[6] Increasing the pressure beyond these levels does little to increase the working space in pediatric patients. Reduced abdominal wall laxity may require higher intra-abdominal insufflation pressures but directly increases risk of cardiopulmonary, vascular, or neurohumoral complications.

Trocars

Trocars enable the laparoscopic surgeon to introduce working instruments into the insufflated abdomen and provide a conduit for the carbon dioxide gas to maintain pneumoperitoneum. The typical trocar consists of an outer sheath (or port) that contains an inner obturator, which is removed following trocar insertion. In both infants and children, it is preferable to limit the trocar size because of the shorter body wall and limited working space. The authors have had success with a latex-free, radially dilated trocar system (Step system, Covidien, Mansfield, MA, USA) that incorporates an expandable sheath that accommodates 3-mm, 5-mm, and 10-mm ports.[7] An advantage to the Step system is elimination of the need for fascial closure after removal of the port. Fascia is closed to prevent bowel or omental herniation through the abdominal wall; however, in practice, a child's abdominal wall is so thin that fascia is easy to close regardless of trocar size. All nonradially dilating trocar sizes 10 mm and greater deserve proper fascial closure. Direct intra-abdominal visualization of port sites on trocar removal helps identify injury to abdominal wall vessels, typically the inferior epigastric artery or its superficial branches.

Laparoscopes and Camera Systems

Laparoscopes are typically rigid, contain a 0° or 30° lens, and range in size from 5 mm to 10 mm. Most pediatric urologic procedures can be completed with the use of a 30° lens, which allows the surgeon to see behind intra-abdominal structures. Aside from the camera, patient positioning is critical to successful laparoscopy. Renal surgery is performed in a lateral or flank position, allowing bowel to fall away. Bladder and ureteral surgery are often performed in dorsal lithotomy; Trendelenburg positioning lessens the need for bowel retraction. Diagnostic laparoscopy and orchiopexy are straightforward with children positioned supine. Careful padding of pressure points, securing of the endotracheal tube, and taping the patient to the bed are important, because patients can slide during frequent bed rotation or tilting during surgery (**Fig. 1**).

Optics are not uniform between laparoscopes and the quality of visualization is directly proportional to scope diameter. For example, a 3-mm telescope has fused bundle fiberoptics that produce pixilated images with reduced resolution. Many 3-mm and current 5-mm and 10-mm telescopes contain rod lens systems that provide excellent quality and brightness. The authors think that 5-mm optics offer acceptable light transmission and visualization in almost all pediatric applications.

The quality of the laparoscopic camera systems have markedly improved with time.[8] Digital equipment, as opposed to analog, offers high-fidelity imagery and picture recording, with better color, sharpness, contrast, and field depth. High-definition video towers with widescreen displays improve visualization. Two-dimensional (2D) images lack spatial depth information and require the laparoscopist to recognize this limitation and compensate.[9] This disadvantage has led to recent advances in 3-dimensional (3D) video technology, which uses 2 optic channels in a single metallic sheath to mimic the binocular function of a surgeon's eyes. Markedly improved images, digital input, and video recording capability have allowed surgeons to perfect and teach minimally invasive techniques, which is an asset not widely available in open surgery.

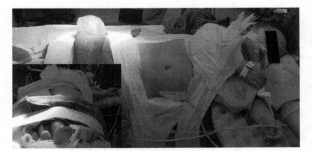

Fig. 1. A 12-month-old girl is placed in flank position for a right laparoscopic pyeloplasty with arms extended 90° from her body and pressure points carefully padded to prevent decubitus ulceration or rhabdomyolysis. The patient will receive a paralytic agent for laparoscopy to maximize abdominal wall compliance; therefore, an endotracheal tube is chosen rather than other airways.

Laparoscopic Instruments

Although instrumentation for open surgery has seen little change in the last several decades, laparoscopic instrumentation is constantly adapting to meet the demands of expanded applications of minimally invasive surgery. The use of laparoscopy in pediatric urology has required miniaturization of standard adult laparoscopic instruments. The decreased diameter of these instruments affects their rigidity. Although 5-mm and 10-mm instruments are effectively rigid rods, 3-mm instruments flex to varying degrees based on manufacturer, length, and instrument type. However, 3-mm instruments are sufficiently rigid to prove immediately functional to most surgeons.[6] One compromise in the use of smaller instruments is that the 3-mm arsenal is more limited than the 5-mm arsenal.

Manual dexterity and finesse are required when working with laparoscopic needle drivers, especially in the infant or child. A fine needle driver (ie, 3 mm or 5 mm) is required when working with the fine 5-0 or 6-0 suture that is commonly used for laparoscopic pyeloplasty in children.[6] Needles can get caught within the sheath of a 5-mm trocar, and, at that small size, are not easily visualized on radiograph. Therefore, carefully watching needles as they enter the abdomen or placing them through a larger 8-mm to 10-mm trocar minimizes this risk. A lost needle means removal of the trocar to cut open its sheath, and, if still not found, then open surgical conversion. The EndoStitch suturing device (Covidien, Mansfield, MA, USA) is a disposable, 1-handed, 10-mm suturing instrument that shuttles its needle from one jaw through tissue, then to the other jaw; Although it makes tissue closure easier, its application in children is limited because of large instrument size.[10]

Electrosurgical Instruments

Electrosurgical devices combine laparoscopic instruments with an energy source, providing a means to cauterize vessels during dissection. Monopolar energy can be added to most laparoscopic dissectors and scissors and is useful in the cauterization of small vessels. The monopolar hook electrode is particularly useful for dissection around tubular structures.[11] Monopolar cautery must be used with great caution because of the pattern of current spread across tissue as well as the risk of current arcing through a gap in the instrument's insulation. These risks are increased in the limited working space of pediatric laparoscopy. Monopolar coagulation runs the highest risk of electrosurgical injury outside the surgeon's visual field via the mechanisms of insulation failure, direct coupling (conduction of current from direct touching of an energized instrument and other metal device), and capacitative coupling (induction of current in nearby conductors despite normal insulation).

Bipolar electrocautery involves flow of radiofrequency-based current from one jaw to the other, which reduces thermal spread and capacitive coupling. Simple bipolar instruments do not cut tissue and are generally powered by the standard electrosurgical unit (Bovie). One example of a more advanced so-called smart bipolar device is the LigaSure vessel sealing system (Valleylab, Boulder, CO, USA), which generates more current with only a percentage of the voltage required by a simple bipolar instrument.[11] The LigaSure actively monitors changes in tissue impedance, provides real-time adjustment of the energy output, and can coagulate vessels of up to 7 mm. A 5-mm diameter device is available for pediatric applications.

The Harmonic scalpel (Ethicon Endosurgery, Cincinnati, OH, USA) is a disposable ultrasonic cutting and coagulating surgical device. The handpiece of the device transforms electrical energy into mechanical energy by the use of a piezoelectric crystal system. The rapid mechanical vibrations significantly increase the temperature of the active blade, denaturing proteins by breaking hydrogen bonds and creating a coagulum that seals vessels of up to 5 mm. The intracorporeal portion of the instrument dissipates heat (and steam), so care must be taken to avoid inadvertent thermal injury to adjacent structures. In comparison, the Harmonic scalpel coagulates and cuts tissues at lower temperatures (50–150°C) than its radiofrequency-based counterparts (150–400°C) and may therefore be safer in tight spaces or near important structures.[12]

da Vinci Surgical System

The da Vinci Surgical System consists of a surgeon console, patient-side cart with interactive robotic arms, and a vision cart. It was approved for clinical use by the United States Food and Drug Administration in 2000. Although the system allows for the use of 4 working arms, the fourth arm is seldom used in the pediatric population because of the limited working space. The camera arm contains 2 optic channels in a single metallic sheath, which mimics the surgeon's binocular vision, and transmits a high-definition 3D image at the surgeon console (**Fig. 2**). Although smaller cameras are available in 8.5 mm (3D) and 5 mm (2D), the best image is achieved through the 12-mm camera, giving the surgeon a 10× magnified, 3D picture. The surgeon sits comfortably at the surgeon console, from where the robotic controls including arm position, focus, zoom, camera position, and instrument movement can be manipulated. Among the principal advantages for the use of robotic-assisted surgery are tremor filtration and motion scaling.[13] Tremor filtration results in steadier and smoother movements even with longer laparoscopic instruments that would otherwise magnify unintentional movement.[14] Computerized motion scaling allows large movements by the surgeon to be translated into delicate manipulations in the surgical field.

Robotic Instrumentation

The robotic instruments have proprietary EndoWrist technology (Intuitive Surgical, Sunnyvale, CA, USA) that allows the surgeon to move the instrument with the 7 degrees of freedom present in the human wrist. The instrument's movement is more

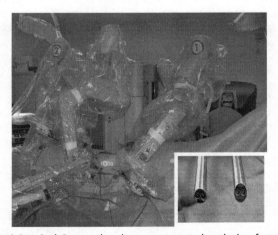

Fig. 2. The da Vinci Surgical System has become a popular choice for minimally invasive surgery involving extensive suturing, such as a pyeloplasty. Improved 3D imagery with binocular lenses is achieved with the 8.5-Fr robotic laparoscope; 0° and 30° lenses are shown (inset). The surgeon sits several feet from the patient's side at the console. The patient cart contains the robotic arms that are docked at the patient's side, and a vision cart with high-definition monitor and insufflation device is in easy view of a scrubbed surgical assistant.

similar to the surgeon's hand and wrist motion than conventional laparoscopy in which the surgeon's movements are opposite to those of the internal instruments.

Most EndoWrist instruments, which require special 8-mm robotic trocars, were created for use in adults. Five-millimeter instruments have been created for use in children and infants and rely on a 3-joint wrist. However, the arsenal of 5-mm robotic instruments is limited. Notably absent are the Hot Shears (Intuitive Surgical, Sunnyvale, CA, USA), curved scissors that are electrocautery capable and one of the more common instruments used in robotic surgery; for these reasons, most surgeons still use 8-mm instruments in pediatric urologic surgery. Bipolar electrocautery can be used through 8-mm Maryland bipolar forceps, which function as a dissector, grasper, and retractor. PK Dissecting Forceps (Intuitive Surgical, Sunnyvale, CA, USA) require a proprietary generator that provides audio feedback that signifies adequate coagulation of tissue. Although robotic instrumentation is still limited, all 5-mm laparoscopic instruments, including the suction/irrigator, can be used through a separate port or 8-mm robotic port by a skilled bedside assistant.

APPLICATIONS OF CONVENTIONAL AND ROBOTIC-ASSISTED LAPAROSCOPY

Laparoscopic approaches have proved beneficial, with reports of less postoperative pain, less blood loss, and shorter hospital stays after pediatric urologic surgery. Although not every application is addressed in this article, the following procedures represent key minimally invasive techniques now accepted into the surgical armamentarium.

Orchiopexy

Laparoscopy remains the central diagnostic tool for evaluation of a nonpalpable testis, although classic open approaches like the Jones technique are still used by some. Differential diagnosis includes a viable or hypotrophic intra-abdominal testis, nubbin, intracanalicular testis (within the inguinal canal), or absent testis (testicular agenesis or vanishing testis). Laparoscopy allows both diagnostic and therapeutic modalities, and laparoscopic orchiopexy has become the therapeutic procedure of choice in boys with an intra-abdominal testis (**Fig. 3**). If primary orchiopexy is not feasible because of short gonadal vessels, a staged Fowler-Stephens orchiopexy can be performed, initially ligating the gonadal vessels to allow collateral blood flow to develop from the deferential artery (artery of the vas) to the testis. Second-stage laparoscopic orchiopexy then involves tunneling of the testis lateral to the bladder, medial to the epigastric vessels over the pubic tubercle, and into the scrotum. Overall outcomes are excellent; one of the largest series by Chang and colleagues[15] reported an overall success rate of 85% and a 96% success rate with testes that had no previous surgery.

Nephrectomy

The safety and efficacy of laparoscopic nephrectomy in children has been firmly established.[16–19] This procedure can be performed using transperitoneal or retroperitoneal approaches and is used for removal of a poorly functioning kidney secondary to ureteropelvic junction (UPJ) obstruction, reflux nephropathy, calculi, malignancy, cystic degeneration, dysplasia, and pediatric renal transplant recipients (**Fig. 4**).[6] Surgical outcomes and success rates for laparoscopic nephrectomy have been compared with the open approach; although operative times are longer, postoperative hospital stay was significantly shorter than for open surgery.[20] The use of robotic assistance is feasible, but cost-effectiveness and any improvement in outcomes have yet to be shown.[4]

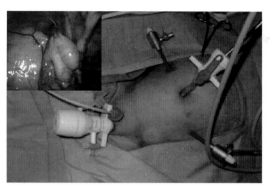

Fig. 3. Laparoscopic trocar placement (for camera and 2 working instruments) with light transilluminating the abdominal wall in the area of a left intra-abdominal testis. The intra-abdominal testis is clearly viable on laparoscopy (inset). A 10-mm trocar placed through the scrotum, over the pubic symphysis, is used to retrieve the mobilized testis.

Partial Nephrectomy

The most common indication for laparoscopic partial nephrectomy in children is a nonfunctioning renal moiety in a duplicated system secondary to obstruction or vesicoureteral reflux. This procedure may also be performed transperitoneally or retroperitoneally in a manner similar to nephrectomy. Acceptable outcomes have been achieved with both conventional and robotic-assisted laparoscopic approaches. Lee and colleagues[21] successfully completed robotic-assisted partial nephrectomy in 9 patients with a mean age of 7.2 years. Overall, patients had a mean hospitalization of 2.9 days. The only complication was an asymptomatic urinoma that resolved following percutaneous drainage.

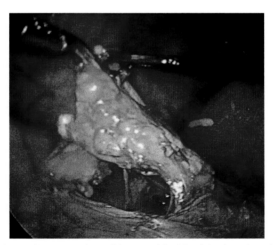

Fig. 4. Laparoscopic nephrectomy in a 14-year-old girl with chronic urinary incontinence secondary to an ectopic ureter inserting in the vagina. The renal moiety may be significantly atrophied, but still capable of filtering urine, as seen here.

Pyeloplasty

Laparoscopic pyeloplasty for the surgical management of UPJ obstruction was first reported in 1995.[22] Surgical outcomes and success rates have been found to be equivalent with the open procedure, with benefits including less incisional discomfort, quicker convalescence, and excellent surgical cosmesis.[23] Despite these benefits, laparoscopic pyeloplasty has not been widely adopted by all pediatric urologists because of its steep learning curve and the difficulty of intracorporeal suturing with laparoscopic instruments. Robotic-assisted pyeloplasty has subsequently emerged with the distinct advantage of easier suturing, and thus has a more rapid learning curve with potential for superior results (**Fig. 5**).[24] A systematic review and meta-analysis comparing conventional laparoscopic pyeloplasty with the robotic-assisted approach suggested benefits of a decreased operative time and shorter hospital stay, with no difference in success rates or complications.[25] At present, no cost analyses have been published to determine whether robotic pyeloplasty is efficient enough to replace conventional laparoscopy. The only limitation of the robot in pediatric renal or pelvic surgery seems to be size of the child, although experienced robotic surgeons have determined feasibility for children of 5 kg and heavier. The reported success rates among multiple series are 94% to 100%.[24]

Ureteral Reimplantation

The management of vesicoureteral reflux (VUR) has changed greatly in the last 25 years. Until further data become available, suppressive antibiotic use is recommended after discussion of risks and benefits with a child's caregivers, to reduce the risk for pyelonephritis and subsequent renal scarring, while awaiting spontaneous resolution. Current recommendations for VUR management by the pediatric urologist are summarized in the American Urological Association's (AUA) Clinical Guidelines from 2010: *Management and Screening of Primary Vesicoureteral Reflux in Children*. Surgical correction is considered appropriate for recurrent pyelonephritis despite prophylactic antibiotics or because of parental preference[25]; failure of VUR to resolve and medication noncompliance have recently become relative indications for surgery, because the true long-term risk of VUR and clear benefit of prophylactic antibiotics have been brought into question. Similar to pyeloplasty, minimally invasive approaches to ureteral reimplantation have not been widely adopted by pediatric urologists because of the high success rates of open surgery and the requirement of advanced laparoscopic skills to perform the procedure successfully.[26]

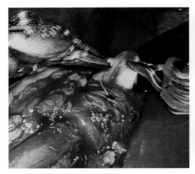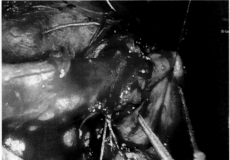

Fig. 5. Laparoscopic pyeloplasty can be accomplished with conventional or robotic assistance. Robotic pyeloplasty eases suturing of the new anastomosis after transecting the UPJ. The reconstructed UPJ (*right*) is transposed anterior to the obstructing crossing vessel (*left*).

Laparoscopic ureteral reimplantation can be performed using extravesical or transvesical (vesicoscopic) approaches. Early reports of laparoscopic extravesical reimplantation were met with skepticism because of high operative times and lack of obvious benefit. However, robotic-assisted extravesical reimplantation has reported success rates as high as 97.6% without significant urinary retention, an uncommon but feared risk of the open bilateral extravesical (Lich-Gregoir) ureteroneocystostomy. Reports of transvesical laparoscopy are slowly emerging.[27–29]

Bladder Reconstruction and Continence Surgery

Increasingly complex pelvic surgeries are being attempted in children with robotic assistance, given the advantage of smaller steady movements in a pediatric pelvis and ease of suturing. Bladder neck reconstruction, bladder neck slings, bladder augmentation, and creation of a continent channel that can be catheterized (Mitrofanoff) to treat a neurogenic bladder are now feasible with robotic assistance.[30,31] Intraabdominal laparoscopy and robotic surgery do not seem to adversely affect modern ventriculoperitoneal shunts with respect to infection or intracranial pressure.[32,33] Although the following are theoretic benefits, outcomes data are lacking for shortened hospital stay, improved pain management, reduced adhesions translating to fewer bowel obstructions, and equivalent outcomes when compared with open surgery. The next decade should provide such data.

LESS

Although in its infancy, LESS surgery has the potential to further minimize the invasiveness of laparoscopic surgery. The theoretic advantage of LESS surgery is that a procedure can be performed through a single umbilical incision; however, the advantages of this approach compared with conventional laparoscopy have yet to be shown. This technique is made possible by a multichannel, single-port access device for the camera and up to 3 working instruments; 2 examples are the Covidien SILS port (Covidien, Mansfield, MA, USA) and the Olympus TriPort (Olympus, New York, NY, USA and Advanced Surgical Concept, Wicklow, Ireland). Depending on the company, laparoscopic instruments with an outward curve at the tip prevent each instrument from crossing each other and allow, for example, the right arm to have control of the right instrument. In addition, flexible laparoscopes help to maintain good visualization of the surgical site while deflecting out of the path of the working instruments.

Successful use of LESS nephrectomy and LESS pyeloplasty have been reported in small retrospective series, with similar perioperative parameters and short-term outcomes to those of historical cohorts. Koh and colleagues[34] recently reported the largest series of pediatric LESS nephrectomy to date, with 11 patients having only 2 minor complications and a mean operative time of 139 minutes. LESS pyeloplasty has similar feasibility reports, with a series of 11 patients having 2 minor, common complications and a respectable mean operative time of 182.5 minutes.[35] Additional applications of single-site surgery in pediatric urology have included nephroureterectomy, partial nephrectomy, gonadectomy, orchiopexy, and varicocelectomy.[36] Further clinical evaluation of LESS surgery including larger series, performance in multiple centers, and, ideally, randomized trials comparing standard laparoscopic techniques are required before its widespread use is adopted.

ADVANCES IN ENDOUROLOGY

Surgical management of urolithiasis in children has evolved greatly in the past 2 decades under the influence of improvements in lithotripsy and endourologic techniques, and reports of the rising incidence of pediatric urolithiasis. After successful use of extracorporeal shock wave lithotripsy (SWL) was initially reported in children in 1986,[37] management shifted from open surgical lithotomy to minimally invasive techniques. With success rates varying from 68% to 86% according to stone burden (size and number), composition, and location,[38–43] SWL became the primary treatment modality for renal and proximal ureteral calculi of 15 mm or less.[38] Historically, the surgical management of large stone burden relied on open approach. During the past decade, both the miniaturization of endoscopic equipment and refinements in technique have led to the adoption of percutaneous techniques that previously had been only applied to the adult population. The adaptations of endoscopic equipment have also permitted safe use of ureteroscopy in the treatment of both renal and ureteral stones in children.

Percutaneous Nephrolithotomy

After its initial description in 1976,[44] percutaneous nephrolithotomy (PCNL) quickly became accepted for management of large stone burden in adults. However, reluctance to perform PCNL in children persisted because of concerns regarding the use of large instruments in small pediatric kidneys, resultant parenchymal damage, radiation exposure, and the risk of major complications including hemorrhage and sepsis. The earliest PCNL series were performed using standard, adult-sized instruments through an access tract dilated as much as 30 French (30 Fr).[45,46] Despite these initial successes, PCNL was still largely avoided in children younger than 5 years of age. In 1998, Jackman and colleagues[47] described a novel miniperc technique using an 11-Fr peel-away vascular access sheath that significantly reduced the size of the access tract (**Fig. 6**). Additional advances include smaller nephroscopes (15–18 Fr) or use of pediatric cystoscopes, in combination with better energy sources for intracorporeal lithotripsy, namely the holmium yttrium aluminum garnet (holmium:YAG) laser.[38] Pneumatic and ultrasonic probes have smaller versions that fit through miniaturized access, but any combination with simultaneous suction of fragmented stones still requires larger access tracts of more than 24 Fr. As a result, PCNL has now replaced open

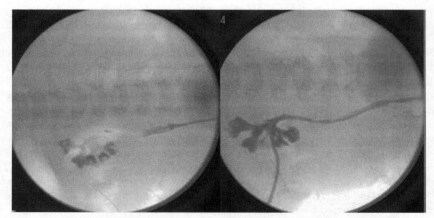

Fig. 6. A retrograde pyelogram nephrostogram, with a ureteral orifice draining into it. The 2 hemiscrotal halves before stone treatment show a large filling defect within the renal pelvis, representing stone (*left*). Antegrade nephrostogram after PCNL, using the miniperc technique, shows complete clearance of stone burden (*right*). This technique minimizes blood loss, pain, and hospital stay, and is practical for the smaller kidneys of pre–school aged children.

pelviolithotomy or nephrolithotomy as the standard of care in the management of large stone burden in children of all ages.

PCNL is currently being used both as monotherapy and in combination with SWL (sandwich therapy) in the pediatric population. It may be the only option for renal or ureteral stone treatment in children who have undergone ureteral reimplantation or bladder neck reconstruction. Recent retrospective series of PCNL monotherapy report stone-free rates that approach 90%.[48–50] Guven and colleagues[51] recently reported a multicenter retrospective review of 140 PCNLs performed in 130 children stratified by age (mean age 10.7 years). Stone-free rates for those patients 3 years or younger, 4 to 7 years, and 8 to 16 years were 87%, 76%, and 83.6%, respectively. Although techniques varied among the institutions, mean postoperative hemoglobin reduction and blood transfusion rates were higher in those patients in whom adult-sized instruments were used. Bilen and coworkers[50] reported an 88% stone-free rate using intracorporeal electrohydraulic lithotripsy, ultrasound, and holmium laser. When stratified by tract size (14 Fr, 20 Fr, and 24 Fr), efficacy rates were similar in all groups, but there no complications or transfusions in the 14-Fr tract group. These reports and others suggest that every effort should be made to use appropriately sized equipment in the pediatric population. In an effort to reduce morbidity of multiple tracts and/or repeat percutaneous procedures, some centers have had success with adjunctive SWL following primary PCNL (sandwich therapy).[52,53] Others prefer to perform second-look nephroscopy through the original tract during the same hospitalization when further stone fragments are suspected. There is no acceptable small size at which pediatric urologists are comfortable observing fragments after lithotripsy, so every attempt is made to clear the initial stone. Potential complications of PCNL include retained fragments causing renal colic, bleeding, renal pseudoaneurysm, sepsis, renal pelvic perforation, ureteral injury, pneumothorax, hemothorax, urothorax, and colonic or nearby bowel injury.

Ureteroscopy

Adoption of ureteroscopy (URS) in the management of pediatric stone disease also lagged behind that of the adult population because of a concern that the use of large instruments in small-caliber ureters would result in high rates of ureteral perforation, stricture formation, and development of vesicoureteral reflux.[38] With the acceptance of SWL as primary therapy for upper tract stones smaller than 1.5 cm, URS was historically reserved for calculi below the iliac crests and for upper tract calculi following SWL failure.[54,55] The early success and safety of distal URS in addition to the miniaturization of flexible endoscopes led several centers to expand their use of URS to the treatment of upper tract calculi.

A wide variety of semirigid and flexible ureteroscopes are available, and use is based on surgeon preference, anatomy, and stone location. The semirigid ureteroscopes range in size from 4.5 Fr to 8 Fr with working channels of 2.4 Fr to 3.5 Fr. Flexible ureteroscopes have been enhanced with 270° deflection capabilities and are available in sizes as small as 6.9 Fr, with working channels of 1.8 Fr to 3.5 Fr. Flexible ureteroscopes are generally placed through ureteroscopic sheaths for repeated, safe access to the kidney, as well as maintaining safe intrarenal pressures with pressurized irrigation (**Fig. 7**). Most commonly used, the holmium:YAG laser, with its 2100-nm wavelength and short, 0.4-mm depth of tissue penetration, has the greatest safety margin of any of the intracorporeal lithotripters.[56] The decision to place a ureteral stent is made at the conclusion of the procedure and is typically based on surgeon preferences and anticipation of significant ureteral edema. A string tether can be left on the

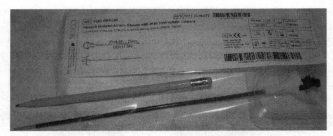

Fig. 7. The smallest ureteroscopic sheath available for renal or proximal ureteral stone treatment has an inner diameter of 9.5 Fr and outer diameter of 11.5 Fr, which is roughly half the width of a pencil and feasible for passage in most children. Younger children may require passive ureteral dilation with a stent before successful ureteroscopy. Ureteral access is safe in children, without significant risk of inducing vesicoureteral reflux and with low rates of ureteral stricture.

stent to allow removal in the home or clinic and avoid a second anesthetic for operative stent removal.

Ureteroscopy is a highly effective endourologic technique to treat stone disease in the pediatric population, with recent series reporting initial stone-free rates of 88% to 98%.[56–60] Smaldone and colleagues[58] retrospectively reviewed a series of 100 children treated with ureteroscopy for kidney and ureteral stones and reported a 91% stone-free rate with 9% requiring staged procedures. De Dominicis and colleagues[55] randomized children with distal ureteral calculi to either SWL or URS. Stone-free rates were significantly higher after 1 treatment (93% vs 43%) for children treated with URS. Factors affecting the success of URS in the management of ureteral stones are stone size and location; large proximal stones are most difficult to treat.[61] URS is successful in the management of lower pole calculi. Bozkurt and coworkers[62] recently reviewed their series of lower pole renal stones with a diameter of 15 to 20 mm treated with either PCNL or URS. In those patients who underwent primary URS, 89.2% were stone free following a single treatment.

With an experienced operator, ureteroscopy can be safely performed with minimal morbidity. Careful manipulation avoids complications of ureteral perforation, avulsion, ischemia, and stricture. Risk factors for ureteral stricture formation, which occurred in only 1% of patients in 1 large series,[58] are impacted stone, ureteral perforation, and mucosal damage secondary to oversized instrumentation.[63]

SUMMARY

Robotic surgery for pediatric urologic indications is becoming routine. Technological advancements in digital imagery and recorders are helping to safely train a new generation of minimally invasive pediatric urologists. Challenges for the foreseeable future of robotic surgery may include improvements in cost and even cosmesis, through the use of smaller instruments, single-site ports, or creatively placed incisions. In addition, as the pediatric urologic stone problem worsens, there will continue to be see advances in lithotripsy techniques, energy sources, and endourologic equipment. It is hoped that techniques that enhance stone clearance will also be adapted to improve patient comfort.

REFERENCES

1. Timchenko AD. Methods of laparoscopy in children. Klinicheskaia Khirurgiia 1969;5:10–4.

2. Cortesi N, Ferrari P, Zambarda E, et al. Diagnosis of bilateral abdominal cryptorchidism by laparoscopy. Endoscopy 1976;8:33–4.
3. Halachmi S, El-Ghoneimi A, Bissonnette B, et al. Hemodynamic and respiratory effect of pediatric urological laparoscopic surgery: a retrospective study. J Urol 2003;170:1651–4 [discussion: 4].
4. Casale P. Laparoscopic and robotic approach to genitourinary anomalies in children. Urol Clin North Am 2010;37:279–86.
5. Diehl K. Complications of laparoscopic surgery. In: Mullholland M, Doherty G, editors. Complications in surgery. Philadelphia: Lippincott Williams & Wilkins; 2006.
6. Tomaszewski JJ, Casella DP, Turner RM, et al. Pediatric laparoscopic and robot-assisted laparoscopic surgery: technical considerations. J Endourol 2012;26(6): 602–13.
7. Docimo SG. Re: Experience with the Bailez technique for laparoscopic access in children. J Urol 2004;171:806.
8. Kourambas J, Preminger GM. Advances in camera, video, and imaging technologies in laparoscopy. Urol Clin North Am 2001;28:5–14.
9. Storz P, Buess GF, Kunert W, et al. 3D HD versus 2D HD: surgical task efficiency in standardised phantom tasks. Surg Endosc 2012;26(5):1454–60.
10. Chen RN, Moore RG, Kavoussi LR. Laparoscopic pyeloplasty. Indications, technique, and long-term outcome. Urol Clin North Am 1998;25:323–30.
11. Borin JF. Laparoscopic and robotic instrumentation for urologic reconstructive surgery in adults. In: Ost MC, editor. Robotic and laparoscopic reconstructive surgery in children and adults. New York: Humana; 2011. p. 3–15.
12. Greenberg JA. The harmonic ACE pistol grip. Rev Obstet Gynecol 2008;1:198–9.
13. Cassilly R, Diodato MD, Bottros M, et al. Optimizing motion scaling and magnification in robotic surgery. Surgery 2004;136:291–4.
14. Prasad SM, Maniar HS, Soper NJ, et al. The effect of robotic assistance on learning curves for basic laparoscopic skills. Am J Surg 2002;183:702–7.
15. Chang B, Palmer LS, Franco I. Laparoscopic orchidopexy: a review of a large clinical series. BJU international 2001;87:490–3.
16. Yao D, Poppas DP. A clinical series of laparoscopic nephrectomy, nephroureterectomy and heminephroureterectomy in the pediatric population. J Urol 2000; 163:1531–5.
17. Borzi PA. A comparison of the lateral and posterior retroperitoneoscopic approach for complete and partial nephroureterectomy in children. BJU Int 2001;87:517–20.
18. Gundeti MS, Patel Y, Duffy PG, et al. An initial experience of 100 paediatric laparoscopic nephrectomies with transperitoneal or posterior prone retroperitoneoscopic approach. Pediatr Surg Int 2007;23:795–9.
19. Baez JJ, Luna CM, Mesples GF, et al. Laparoscopic transperitoneal and retroperitoneal nephrectomies in children: a change of practice. J Laparoendosc Adv Surg Tech A 2010;20:81–5.
20. Hamilton BD, Gatti JM, Cartwright PC, et al. Comparison of laparoscopic versus open nephrectomy in the pediatric population. J Urol 2000;163:937–9.
21. Lee RS, Sethi AS, Passerotti CC, et al. Robot assisted laparoscopic partial nephrectomy: a viable and safe option in children. J Urol 2009;181:823–8 [discussion 8–9].
22. Peters CA, Schlussel RN, Retik AB. Pediatric laparoscopic dismembered pyeloplasty. J Urol 1995;153:1962–5.
23. Jarrett TW, Chan DY, Charambura TC, et al. Laparoscopic pyeloplasty: the first 100 cases. J Urol 2002;167:1253–6.

24. Peters CA. Pediatric robot-assisted pyeloplasty. J Endourol 2011;25:179–85.
25. Braga LH, Pace K, DeMaria J, et al. Systematic review and meta-analysis of robotic-assisted versus conventional laparoscopic pyeloplasty for patients with ureteropelvic junction obstruction: effect on operative time, length of hospital stay, postoperative complications, and success rate. Eur Urol 2009;56:848–57.
26. Capolicchio JP. Laparoscopic extravesical ureteral reimplantation: technique. Adv Urol 2008:567980.
27. Kutikov A, Guzzo TJ, Canter DJ, et al. Initial experience with laparoscopic transvesical ureteral reimplantation at the Children's Hospital of Philadelphia. J Urol 2006;176:2222–5 [discussion: 5–6].
28. Peters CA, Woo R. Intravesical robotically assisted bilateral ureteral reimplantation. J Endourol 2005;19:618–21 [discussion: 21–2].
29. Kawauchi A, Naitoh Y, Soh J, et al. Transvesical laparoscopic cross-trigonal ureteral reimplantation for correction of vesicoureteral reflux: initial experience and comparisons between adult and pediatric cases. J Endourol 2009;23:1875–8.
30. Bagrodia A, Gargollo P. Robot-assisted bladder neck reconstruction, bladder neck sling, and appendicovesicostomy in children: description of technique and initial results. J Endourol 2011;25:1299–305.
31. Gundeti MS, Acharya SS, Zagaja GP, et al. Paediatric robotic-assisted laparoscopic augmentation ileocystoplasty and Mitrofanoff appendicovesicostomy (RA-LIMA): feasibility of and initial experience with the University of Chicago technique. BJU international 2011;107:962–9.
32. Casperson KJ, Fronczak CM, Siparsky G, et al. Ventriculoperitoneal shunt infections after bladder surgery: is mechanical bowel preparation necessary? J Urol 2011;186:1571–5.
33. Fraser JD, Aguayo P, Sharp SW, et al. The safety of laparoscopy in pediatric patients with ventriculoperitoneal shunts. J Laparoendosc Adv Surg Tech A 2009;19:675–8.
34. Koh CJ, De Filippo RE, Chang AY, et al. Laparoendoscopic single-site nephrectomy in pediatric patients: initial clinical series of infants to adolescents. Urology 2010;76:1457–61.
35. Tugcu V, Ilbey YO, Polat H, et al. Early experience with laparoendoscopic single-site pyeloplasty in children. J Pediatr Urol 2011;7:187–91.
36. Kawauchi A, Naitoh Y, Miki T. Laparoendoscopic single-site surgery for pediatric patients in urology. Curr Opin Urol 2011;21:303–8.
37. Newman DM, Coury T, Lingeman JE, et al. Extracorporeal shock wave lithotripsy experience in children. J Urol 1986;136:238–40.
38. Smaldone MC, Docimo SG, Ost MC. Contemporary surgical management of pediatric urolithiasis. Urol Clin North Am 2010;37:253–67.
39. Myers DA, Mobley TB, Jenkins JM, et al. Pediatric low energy lithotripsy with the Lithostar. J Urol 1995;153:453–7.
40. Muslumanoglu AY, Tefekli A, Sarilar O, et al. Extracorporeal shock wave lithotripsy as first line treatment alternative for urinary tract stones in children: a large scale retrospective analysis. J Urol 2003;170:2405–8.
41. Landau EH, Shenfeld OZ, Pode D, et al. Extracorporeal shock wave lithotripsy in prepubertal children: 22-year experience at a single institution with a single lithotriptor. J Urol 2009;182:1835–9.
42. Elsobky E, Sheir KZ, Madbouly K, et al. Extracorporeal shock wave lithotripsy in children: experience using two second-generation lithotripters. BJU Int 2000;86:851–6.

43. Rizvi SA, Naqvi SA, Hussain Z, et al. Management of pediatric urolithiasis in Pakistan: experience with 1,440 children. J Urol 2003;169:634–7.
44. Fernstrom I, Johansson B. Percutaneous pyelolithotomy. A new extraction technique. Scand J Urol Nephrol 1976;10:257–9.
45. Woodside JR, Stevens GF, Stark GL, et al. Percutaneous stone removal in children. J Urol 1985;134:1166–7.
46. Mor Y, Elmasry YE, Kellett MJ, et al. The role of percutaneous nephrolithotomy in the management of pediatric renal calculi. J Urol 1997;158:1319–21.
47. Jackman SV, Docimo SG, Cadeddu JA, et al. The "mini-perc" technique: a less invasive alternative to percutaneous nephrolithotomy. World J Urol 1998;16:371–4.
48. Zeren S, Satar N, Bayazit Y, et al. Percutaneous nephrolithotomy in the management of pediatric renal calculi. J Endourol 2002;16:75–8.
49. Desai MR, Kukreja RA, Patel SH, et al. Percutaneous nephrolithotomy for complex pediatric renal calculus disease. J Endourol 2004;18:23–7.
50. Bilen CY, Kocak B, Kitirci G, et al. Percutaneous nephrolithotomy in children: lessons learned in 5 years at a single institution. J Urol 2007;177:1867–71.
51. Guven S, Istanbulluoglu O, Gul U, et al. Successful percutaneous nephrolithotomy in children: multicenter study on current status of its use, efficacy and complications using Clavien classification. J Urol 2011;185:1419–24.
52. Mahmud M, Zaidi Z. Percutaneous nephrolithotomy in children before school age: experience of a Pakistani centre. BJU Int 2004;94:1352–4.
53. Samad L, Aquil S, Zaidi Z. Paediatric percutaneous nephrolithotomy: setting new frontiers. BJU Int 2006;97:359–63.
54. Wu HY, Docimo SG. Surgical management of children with urolithiasis. Urol Clin North Am 2004;31:589–94, xi.
55. De Dominicis M, Matarazzo E, Capozza N, et al. Retrograde ureteroscopy for distal ureteric stone removal in children. BJU Int 2005;95:1049–52.
56. Tan AH, Al-Omar M, Denstedt JD, et al. Ureteroscopy for pediatric urolithiasis: an evolving first-line therapy. Urology 2005;65:153–6.
57. Kim SS, Kolon TF, Canter D, et al. Pediatric flexible ureteroscopic lithotripsy: the Children's Hospital of Philadelphia experience. J Urol 2008;180:2616–9 [discussion: 9].
58. Smaldone MC, Cannon GM Jr, Wu HY, et al. Is ureteroscopy first line treatment for pediatric stone disease? J Urol 2007;178:2128–31 [discussion: 31].
59. Thomas JC, DeMarco RT, Donohoe JM, et al. Pediatric ureteroscopic stone management. J Urol 2005;174:1072–4.
60. Nerli RB, Patil SM, Guntaka AK, et al. Flexible ureteroscopy for upper ureteral calculi in children. J Endourol 2011;25:579–82.
61. Turunc T, Kuzgunbay B, Gul U, et al. Factors affecting the success of ureteroscopy in management of ureteral stone diseases in children. J Endourol 2010;24:1273–7.
62. Bozkurt OF, Resorlu B, Yildiz Y, et al. Retrograde intrarenal surgery versus percutaneous nephrolithotomy in the management of lower-pole renal stones with a diameter of 15 to 20 mm. J Endourol 2011;25:1131–5.
63. Johnson DB, Pearle MS. Complications of ureteroscopy. Urol Clin North Am 2004;31:157–71.

Is Bladder Dysfunction in Children Science Fiction of Science Fact

Editorial Comment

Darius J. Bägli, MDCM, FRCSC[a,b,*]

KEYWORDS

- Bladder dysfunction management • Psychosocial stress • Bladder strategies
- Constipation • Brain and behavior

KEY POINTS

- A functional bladder problem in the child is in many ways the pediatric urologist's hypertension diagnosis. It is insidious. It is often ignored. It can be caused or aggravated by psychosocial stressors.
- Bladder retraining strategies must be maintained lifelong, even once overt symptoms are corrected, in order to ensure bladder health.
- Bladder dysfucntion can lead to bladder muscle hypertrophy, excessive intralumenal pressure, and bladder wall failure, and can permanently damage other systems. The condition may even likely affect the brain.
- Consider bladder and bowel sphicter proximity in addressing management. Always treat and correct constipation first.
- Modern considerations of bladder dysfunction reveal bi-directional neural trafficking and imprinting between the bladder and higher cerebral centres.

In 1957, legendary science fiction writer Isaac Asimov penned *Strikebreaker*.[1] In this short story, a small idiosyncratic human outer space colony has for generations relegated and ostracized a single family to care for its waste processing facility, for the colonists will have nothing to do with such matters. When the colony refuses to end his family's isolation, Igor goes on strike. With the ruling council intransigent, the

This editorial commentary was written in response to the article by Dr Franco I, "Functional Bladder Problems in Children: Pathophysiology, Diagnosis, and Treatment" in *Pediatric Clinics of North America* (59:4), August 2012.
a Divisions of Developmental & Stem Cell Biology, and Urology, The Hospital For Sick Children and Research Institute, Toronto, Ontario, Canada; b Institute of Medical Science, and Faculty of Medicine, University of Toronto, Toronto, Ontario, Canada
* 555 University Avenue, Toronto, Ontario, Canada M5G 1X8.
E-mail address: darius.bagli@sickkids.ca

Pediatr Clin N Am 59 (2012) 943–946
doi:10.1016/j.pcl.2012.05.002
0031-3955/12/$ – see front matter © 2012 Elsevier Inc. All rights reserved.

imminent breakdown of the waste processing machinery threatens to wipe out the colony. However, a volunteer reluctantly operates the facility and breaks the strike and Igor capitulates. Meanwhile, instead of gratitude, now that the volunteer has worked in the job, the colony shuns him as well and he may never return.

The present excellent review of "Functional Bladder Problems in Children" by Dr Franco has many metaphors in this story. It has been decades since Terry Allen's landmark description of nonneurogenic bladder dysfunction.[2] However, the medical community on this planet has largely relegated the critical attention this problem demands to specific dedicated practitioners and specialists. And if they were to strike, it could easily wipe out the health and welfare of the patient.

As the author indicates, if bladder dysfunction remains unidentified and uncorrected in childhood, it frequently manifests in life-long lower urinary tract problems in adulthood such as prostadynia/prostatitis or interstitial cystitis and urethral syndrome. Ask any adult urologist how impossibly common or unmanageable these conditions can be. Even more devastating is the notion that attendant kidney damage and loss of function are preventable consequences of failure to recognize and correct bladder dysfunction in childhood. There are reports of children progressing to total renal failure and kidney transplantation in the face of the most severe forms of elimination dysfunction.

In our institution, trainees are taught to think that virtually all children presenting to the pediatric urology service (indeed one could say all children) are suspect for some degree of constipation and/or bladder dysfunction until proven otherwise. Given its great prevalence, it is somewhat ironic, then, that the colony of practicing physicians perennially takes a cursory view of this problem or relegates it to superficial management strategies with little goal or conviction. And as with the volunteer in the story, there is often little sense of obligation or urgency for the importance of the role played by those few who do manage this problem effectively and thoroughly.

An appreciation of the protean manifestations and subtle diagnostic clues to bladder dysfunction, as outlined by the author, can be extremely useful in identifying patients at risk. When the primary inciting problem is addressed at the bladder level, the added and more obvious problems of urinary tract infection (UTI), or even ongoing vesicoureteral reflux then often become secondary management issues. Nevertheless, it is easy for recurrent UTI or reflux to become a distraction as these can be more objectively diagnosed. However, their resolution is most often inexorably tied to effectively treating bladder dysfunction; little progress will be made with the former without correcting the latter.

Of all the internal organs, only the colon and bladder can come under such rigid control of their owner. Moreover, the term dysfunctional elimination syndrome (DES), coined by Koff and colleagues[3] is more apropos when one considers the intimate proximity of the anal and bladder outlet muscle sphincter complexes. It is difficult for the young child who is just beginning to appreciate their ability to voluntarily control these muscle groups, to contract or relax them independently of each other. Thus, when children experience the dysuria of UTI or pain from voiding through a meatal stenosis, they will engage in the most primitive of responses and stop the pain by stopping voiding (permanently, if they could). In contracting the bladder outlet complex, the anal sphincter also contracts, ostensibly unnecessarily. Thus begins the vicious cycle of secondary constipation brought on by the primary bladder problem. Conversely, an anal fissure, hard stool, or even repeated avoidance of undesirable or unfamiliar bathroom conditions can lead to anal sphincter contraction, bowel movement avoidance, and sympathetic (and here I refer not to autonomic function) contracting of the bladder outlet, with the same outcome. Despite the eventual resolution of the painful stimulus, during such a formative period, this bladder/bowel behavior becomes locked in and learned.

The learned sympathy of the 2 sphincters for each other leads to the brain and to behavior. In perhaps one of the more important considerations in this field to date, the author lays out what is undoubtedly the tip of the iceberg in the complex interplay between higher brain centers and lower urinary tract (and gastrointestinal tract) control. It comes as no surprise, therefore, that when outward psychosocial pressures perturb the intense developmental stages of functional brain development in the child, this creates the neurobiological potential to modulate lower urinary tract function.

One of the most profound and well-known examples of psychosocial stress in this context (but unfortunately not always inquired about because social moirés continue to inhibit even the health professional) is the ability of child abuse or sexual abuse to alter the voiding behavior of the victim. Therapy for such assaults on the psyche, even in adults, can have a positive and corrective effect on even longstanding bladder dysfunction.[4] Recently, Zderic and Valentino and their research teams, using animal models of social stressing, have begun to show that social stress leads to acquired (and measurable) bladder dysfunction and tissue remodeling.[5] Even more intriguing are the emerging associations between the ability of the brain and the bladder to affect each other, such that the dysfunctional bladder (or colon or other pelvic organs) can neuroanatomically project to specific neuronal regions in the brain to incite neurobehavioral consequences, and vice versa.[6] It should come as no surprise then that corticotropin releasing factor, a stress hormone, has been identified as a principle neurotransmitter projecting to and emanating from the Barrington nucleus in the pons, the Grand Central Station for micturition.[6] This raises the intriguing possibility of targeting cerebral centers in the management of distinct lower urinary tract pathology.

Presaging this association on a more clinical basis, although somewhat arbitrarily at the time, we specifically included additional scoring points for the presence of psychosocial pressures or events (positive or negative) when we established the first bladder dysfunction scoring system for children in 2000.[7] Using this or one of the modified voiding scoring systems that followed can help to provide a somewhat more objective measure of bladder functional status before and after institution of bladder management programs and strategies such as those outlined by the author.

A functional bladder problem in the child is in many ways the pediatric urologist's hypertension diagnosis. It is insidious. It is often ignored. It can be caused or aggravated by psychosocial stressors. It can lead to muscle hypertrophy, excessive intralumenal pressure, and bladder wall failure. Untreated, it can permanently damage other systems, and may even likely affect the brain. Unsupported by their family and health professional, the patient is often noncompliant with therapy. Like antihypertensive therapy, retraining bladder strategies and good bladder habits must be adhered to for life. The author treats many of these issues in depth and from familiar personal experience derived from many years of dedicated consideration of these problems. As Asimov suggests, we need to pay more attention to Igor and his family.

REFERENCES

1. Asimov I. The Best Science Fiction of Isaac Asimov. New York: Roc; 1986. p. 384.
2. Allen TD. The non-neurogenic neurogenic bladder. J Urol 1977;117:232–8.
3. Koff SA, Wagner TT, Jayanthi VR. The relationship among dysfunctional elimination syndromes, primary vesicoureteral reflux and urinary tract infections in children. J Urol 1998;160:1019–22.
4. Ellsworth PI, Merguerian PA, Copening ME. Sexual abuse: another causative factor in dysfunctional voiding. J Urol 1995;153:773–6.

5. Chang A, Butler S, Sliwoski J, et al. Social stress in mice induces voiding dysfunction and bladder wall remodeling. Am J Physiol Renal Physiol 2009;297:F1101–8.
6. Valentino RJ, Wood SK, Wein AJ, et al. The bladder-brain connection: putative role of corticotropin-releasing factor. Nat Rev Urol 2011;8:19–28.
7. Farhat W, Bägli DJ, Capolicchio G, et al. The dysfunctional voiding scoring system: quantitative standardization of dysfunctional voiding symptoms in children. J Urol 2000;164:1011–5.

Pediatric Urologic Oncology

Gwen M. Grimsby, MD, Michael L. Ritchey, MD*

KEYWORDS

- Rhabdomyosarcoma • Wilms tumor • Nephroblastoma • Yolk sac tumor • Teratoma

KEY POINTS

- Patients with disorders of sexual development are at increased risk for gonadal tumors. Children with a history of undescended testis have a slight increased risk of testis cancer after puberty.
- Benign lesions, such as mature teratomas and epidermoid cysts, should be managed with testis-sparing surgery.
- Yolk sac tumor should be managed with radical inguinal orchiectomy. Greater than 90% are stage I at diagnosis; thus, chemotherapy and retroperitoneal lymph node dissection are rarely indicated.

GENITOURINARY RHABDOMYOSARCOMA
Epidemiology, Pathology, and Staging

Rhabdomyosarcoma (RMS) is the most common soft tissue sarcoma in infants and children, with 15% to 20% arising from genitourinary sites, including prostate, bladder, paratesticular, vagina, and uterus.[1] There is a bimodal age distribution with a peak incidence in the first 2 years of life and again at adolescence. A genetic predisposition is found in the Li-Fraumeni syndrome and neurofibromatosis.[2] Embryonal RMS is the most common subtype that includes sarcoma botryoides, a polypoid variety that occurs in the bladder or vagina.[1] Alveolar RMS, the second most common form, has a worse prognosis with a higher rate of local recurrence.[1] As with most solid tumors, tumor stage is most predictive of clinical outcome. Preoperative studies to determine the extent of disease include chest CT, CT or MRI of the primary site, bone scan, and bone marrow biopsy. The most common site of metastatic spread of RMS is the lung. Unfavorable prognostic factors include unfavorable sites (eg, bladder or prostate, presence of distant metastases at diagnosis, involved regional lymph nodes, primary tumors greater than 5 cm, and age less than 1 or greater than 10 years old).[3,4]

An editorial commentary by Dr Armando Lorenzo, "Genitourinary Malignancies in Children: Editorial Commentary" is based on this article and found in *Pediatric Clinics of North America* (59:4), August 2012.

Phoenix Children's Hospital, 1919 East Thomas Road, Phoenix, AZ 85016, USA
* Corresponding author. 1920 East Cambridge Avenue, Suite 302, Phoenix, AZ 85006.
E-mail address: Michael.ritchey@gmail.com

Treatment

The treatment of RMS has evolved from radical surgical excision. Several advances have been made by cooperative group studies, including identification of prognostic factors (histology, site, biology, and extent of disease)[3–5]; reduction or elimination of radiation therapy for special groups or sites[6]; reduced need for radical surgery leading to increased bladder salvage[7]; and elimination of routine lymphadenectomy for some patients with localized paratesticular RMS.[1,8]

Bladder and prostate rhabdomyosarcoma

RMS of the bladder or prostate often presents with symptoms of urinary obstruction, including urinary frequency, stranguria, acute urinary retention, and hematuria. Tumors of the bladder usually occur as a botryoid form and grow intraluminally (**Fig. 1**), whereas prostatic RMS tends to present as a solid mass and often has a poorer prognosis.[1,7] On physical examination, an abdominal mass may be present. CT/MRI can delineate the extent of tumor and evaluate pelvic and retroperitoneal nodes. Cystoscopy can confirm the diagnosis and facilitates transurethral biopsy.

The treatment of bladder/prostate RMS is focused on preserving an intact bladder. Unfortunately, many of these tumors are not amenable to partial resection. Most centers recommend chemotherapy and radiation before surgery, with the exception of those children amenable to partial cystectomy at diagnosis, to allow for bladder sparing after multimodal treatment. Pooled data from multiple cooperative groups have demonstrated 5-year overall survival rate of 84% for patients with nonmetastatic embryonal bladder/prostate RMS.[9] In the International Rhabdomyosarcoma Study (IRS)-IV, the bladder was able to be retained in 55 patients. At last follow-up of the IRS-IV patients, however, only 36 patients (40%) had no relapse and a normally functioning intact bladder. Thus, although radiation is important to prevent local treatment failure, radiation may affect bladder function in children. Urodynamic evaluation of bladder function after radiation has shown a reduced bladder capacity and abnormal voiding patterns.[10]

The concern regarding bladder function has led some groups to explore treatment of bladder/prostate RMS without routine radiation therapy. These include risk-based approaches that use response to chemotherapy to stratify patients and determine the need for radiation therapy.[11] There are reports of high relapse rates after complete remission by imaging and biopsy, however.[12] Thus, close follow-up of patients with apparent complete remission is indicated.

Paratesticular rhabdomyosarcoma

Paratesticular RMS accounts for 7% to 10% of genitourinary RMS tumors with the peak age of presentation between 1 and 5 years old.[13] Presentation is often a unilateral

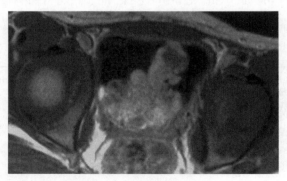

Fig. 1. MRI of botryoid type sarcoma of the bladder.

Key Points: Rhabdomyosarcoma

- Embryonal rhabdomyosacroma is the most common subtype and may exist as the sarcoma botryoides forms, which grows in hollow organs, such as the bladder or vagina.

- Sixty percent to 80% of paratesticular RMSs are stage I at presentation. Patients older than 10 years, however, are at higher risk for retroperitoneal relapse and thus should undergo staging with ipsilateral retroperitoneal lymph node dissection before chemotherapy.

- Goals of treatment include organ preservation; thus, initial neoadjuvant chemotherapy and/ or radiation are performed to improve rates of organ sparing after urgical resection.

---

painless mass or scrotal swelling that is distinct from the testis. At diagnosis, 60% to 80% of paratesticular tumors are stage I compared with 13% of RMS overall.[13] More than 90% of paratesticular RMS are embryonal in histology and have a good prognosis. Abdominal CT is needed to rule out extension to retroperitoneal lymph nodes that occurs in up to 20% of patients.

Initial treatment is radical inguinal orchiectomy. The current Children's Oncology Group (COG) protocols recommend that children 10 years and older have an ipsilateral retroperitoneal lymph node dissection as part of routine staging before chemotherapy. Patients with positive lymph nodes require intensified chemotherapy and nodal irradiation.[13] With current multimodal treatment, survival rates of 90% are expected.[8,13,14]

Vaginal and uterine rhabdomyosarcoma

Vaginal RMS generally presents in the first few years of life with vaginal bleeding, discharge, or a vaginal mass. Uterine RMS may present as a tumor originating from the cervix with vaginal bleeding or mass or as a tumor originating in the uterine body presenting as an abdominal mass. Vaginal and uterine lesions generally have embryonal or botryoid histology and have an excellent prognosis.[15–17]

In the past, patients were frequently treated with anterior pelvic exenteration. With the development of effective chemotherapy, attempts to preserve the vagina and uterus have become a priority and definitive surgery is delayed until after an initial course of chemotherapy.[16,17] Once an adequate response is demonstrated, repeat biopsies are performed. If there is persistence of disease, delayed tumor resection is performed with partial vaginectomy or vaginectomy with hysterectomy. Unfortunately, treatment of pelvic RMS in female patients may result in significant late complications secondary to multimodal therapy, including vaginal stenosis, ureteral obstruction, intestinal stricture or fistula, and ovarian failure.[18]

WILMS TUMOR
Epidemiology and Biology

Wilms tumor is the most common renal tumor of childhood, accounting for 6% to 7% of all childhood cancers. The annual incidence is approximately 7 to 10 cases per million with greater than 80% of cases diagnosed before age 5.[19] Approximately 10% of children with Wilms tumor have congenital anomalies and syndromes, 5% to 10% of tumors are bilateral/multicentric, and 1% to 2% are familial. **Table 1** lists syndromes that are associated with development of Wilms tumor. The genetics of Wilms tumor has been intensely studied. *WT1*, located on chromosome 11 p, was the first Wilms tumor gene identified. The *WT1* gene is important for normal kidney and gonadal development. Deletions or mutations of *WT1* are associated with aniridia, Wilms tumor, Aniridia, Genitourinary anomalies and mental Retardation (WAGR) syndrome, and Denys-Drash syndrome.[20] Wilms tumor develops in approximately 40% to 70% of

Table 1
Syndromes associated with development of Wilms tumor

Syndrome	Genes	Wilms Tumor Risk
WAGR	*WT1*	50%
Denys-Drash	*WT1*	50%
Frasier	*WT1*	5%–10%
Beckwith-Wiedemann	*WT2*	5%–10%
Familial Wilms tumor	*FWT1/FWT2*	30%
Perlman	Unknown	>20%
Simpson-Golabi-Behmel	*GPC3*	10% (in males)
Li-Fraumeni	*p53*	Low
Neurofibromatosis	*NF1*	Low
Sotos	*NSD1*	Low
Trisomy 18	Unknown	Low
Bloom	*BLM*	Low

aniridia patients with deletions of *WT1*.[21] Overgrowth syndromes, including hemihypertrophy alone or as part of the Beckwith-Wiedemann syndrome (BWS), are associated with an increased risk for the development of Wilms tumor. A second Wilms tumor gene, *WT2*, identified at the 11p15 locus, has been linked to BWS.[22] The risk of nephroblastoma in children with BWS and hemihypertrophy is estimated to be 4% to 10%.[23] Another Wilms tumor gene on the X chromosome, or *WTX* at Xq11.1, has been found inactivated in up to one-third of Wilms tumors.[24]

Screening with serial renal ultrasounds every 3 to 4 months is recommended for children at high risk for development of Wilms tumor. Tumors detected by screening generally are a lower stage but no studies have demonstrated that early detection improves patient survival.[25] Screening may detect smaller tumors, making them more amenable to renal-sparing surgery (**Fig. 2**). The Wilms Tumor Surveillance Working Group recommends screening when a condition has a Wilms tumor incidence of greater than 5% (see **Table 1**).[26] Screening of the contralateral kidney after nephrectomy for unilateral Wilms tumor is also recommended to monitor for metachronous tumor development.

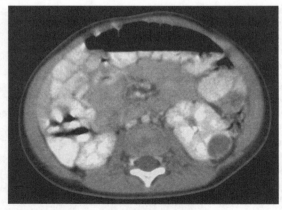

Fig. 2. CT scan of small renal tumor initially found on serial screening by ultrasound. The small lesion was amenable to renal-sparing surgery.

Preoperative Evaluation and Staging

The most common presentation of Wilms tumor is the finding of an abdominal mass by a caregiver. Abdominal pain, gross hematuria, and fever are less-frequent presentations. Rupture of the tumor with hemorrhage into the peritoneal cavity may result in the presentation of an acute abdomen. During physical examination, it is important to assess for signs of associated Wilms tumor syndromes, including aniridia, hemihypertrophy, and genitourinary anomalies.

Ultrasound demonstrates the solid nature of the lesion and Doppler ultrasound is particularly helpful to exclude intracaval tumor extension.[27] CT of the chest and abdomen is recommended in all children suspected of having a solid renal tumor. These studies are important to assess for evidence of metastatic spread. Another important role of imaging is to evaluate the contralateral kidney before surgery. If the kidney is normal on imaging, exploration is not needed at the time of surgery.[28] Alternatively, evidence of bilateral tumors leads to attempts at renal-sparing surgery (discussed later). Preoperative imaging studies of all solid renal tumors of childhood have some common radiographic features, and a precise diagnosis is not always possible before surgery.[29]

The most important determinants of outcome in children with Wilms tumor are tumor stage and histopathology. The majority of patients with Wilms tumor have favorable histology associated with a good prognosis. A small percentage of patients have anaplastic tumors associated with resistance to chemotherapy and a poor prognosis even when the tumor is confined to the kidney.[30] More than one-third of kidneys resected for Wilms tumor contain precursor lesions, known as nephrogenic rests.[31] Presence of nephrogenic rests may indicate an increased risk of developing contralateral disease in children under 1 year of age.[32] The current staging system used by the COG is based primarily on the surgical and histopathological findings (**Box 1**). Examination for extension through the capsule, residual disease, and vascular and lymph node involvement are essential to properly assess the extent of the tumor at presentation. Any tumor spill is now a criterion for stage III designation due to the increased risk for local tumor recurrence.[33,34]

Treatment

The majority of children with Wilms tumor are enrolled in randomized clinical trials that evaluate the appropriate role for the different therapeutic modalities (chemotherapy, radiation, or surgery) available. The duration of these trials are now longer because the survival for patients with all stages of favorable histology Wilms tumor exceeds 90%. The ability of traditional staging factors to predict outcomes is diminished.

Box 1
Wilms tumor staging system of the Children's Oncology Group

Tumor is confined to the kidney and completely resected.

Extracapuslar penetration completely resected. The tumor may extend into the renal sinus or extrarenal vessels may contain tumor thrombus or be infiltrated by tumor.

Residual nonhematogenous tumor is confined to the abdomen: lymph node involvement, any tumor spillage, tumor beyond surgical margin either grossly or microscopically, or residual tumor.

Hematogenous metastases are present.

Bilateral renal involvement is present.

Clinical cancer trials are now evaluating biologic factors that may predict tumor behavior. In the National Wilms Tumor Study (NWTS)-5, loss of heterozygosity of a portion of chromosome 16q and/or 1p was evaluated prospectively and found associated with an increased risk for relapse, independent of histology and stage.[35] Ongoing COG studies are using this biologic marker to stratify patients for treatment.

Current management now emphasizes reducing the morbidity of treatment of low-risk patients, reserving more-intensive treatment for those high-risk patients for whom survival remains poor.[36–38] Over the years, the number of children who receive postoperative radiation therapy has decreased and the duration of chemotherapy has been reduced. Surgery is an integral part of treatment of Wilms tumor. In the COG trials conducted primarily in North America, the majority of patients undergo nephrectomy at diagnosis. The exceptions are those patients with either inoperable disease or bilateral renal tumors. The latter patients are given chemotherapy in an attempt to reduce the tumor burden to allow renal-sparing surgical procedures. Although there has been a great effort to reduce the morbidity of treatment from radiation and chemotherapy, surgical morbidity cannot be overlooked.[39,40]

In the randomized clinical trials conducted by the Société Internationale D'oncologie Pédiatrique [International Society of Pediatric Oncology] (SIOP), preoperative therapy is given before surgery. There is usually a marked reduction in the size of the tumor. This facilitates tumor removal, reducing the risk of intraoperative spill.[40] SIOP investigators have reported a lower rate of complications when nephrectomy is performed after preoperative chemotherapy.[40] Another finding after preoperative therapy is that more patients have lower-stage tumors due to disappearance of micrometastases after neoadjuvant therapy. This was thought a significant advantage in terms of decreasing morbidity of treatment, in particular the late effects of radiotherapy. There have been some concerns regarding the ability of postchemotherapy stage, however, to predict the risk of abdominal relapse.[37]

The United Kingdom Children's Cancer Study Group trials also use prenephrectomy chemotherapy but, unlike SIOP, they perform biopsy before treatment to avoid giving chemotherapy to benign conditions and to non-Wilms tumors.[41] The Wilms' Tumour Study 9101 (UKW3) trial randomly assigned patients to either immediate surgery or 6 weeks of preoperative chemotherapy with delayed surgery and reported that event-free and overall survival at 5 years similar in the 2 groups.[41] They concluded, like the SIOP group, that all children with nonmetastatic Wilms tumor should receive chemotherapy before tumor resection.

The SIOP studies have yielded important information on tumor response after preoperative chemotherapy in terms of tumor volume and histology. Stromal and epithelial predominant tumors are found more often after chemotherapy. These histologic subtypes may demonstrate a poor clinical response to therapy but have an excellent prognosis if the tumor is completely excised.[42] Patients with blastemal predominant tumors after chemotherapy have a high relapse rate.[43] SIOP stratifies patients for treatment based on these histologic patterns after treatment. Tumors with diffuse anaplasia and blastemal predominance after chemotherapy are classified as high risk and are treated with an intensified postoperative chemotherapy regimen. Patients with stage I tumors with complete tumor necrosis after preoperative chemotherapy are considered low risk and receive no further chemotherapy.[44]

The COG has also identified a select group of children in whom postoperative chemotherapy can be avoided. Children less than 2 years of age with stage I favorable histology tumors weighing less than 550 g do not receive chemotherapy after nephrectomy. A prior NWTS Group study reported that 5-year overall survival was the same as for similar patients treated with postoperative dactinomycin and vincristine.[45] There is a trade-off between more-intensive therapy and its potential long-term sequelae required for the 16% of children who relapse versus the avoidance of any postoperative chemotherapy in the majority.

Bilateral Wilms Tumors and Renal-Sparing Surgery

On the COG renal tumor protocols, preoperative chemotherapy is only recommended for children in whom renal-sparing surgery is planned, whose tumors are inoperable, or in whom surgery is associated with increased morbidity.[27,39,46,47]

Synchronous bilateral Wilms tumors occur in 5% to 7% of children with Wilms tumor and preservation of renal tissue is important to decrease the incidence of renal failure, which approaches 15% at 15 years post-treatment in patients with bilateral Wilms tumor.[48,49] The current COG protocol for patients with bilateral Wilms tumor recommends 6 weeks of chemotherapy after which tumor response is assessed with CT or MRI to determine the reduction in tumor volume and feasibility of partial resection. Patients with tumors amenable to renal-sparing procedures can proceed with surgery. Tumors not responding to therapy require bilateral open biopsy to determine histology. Open biopsies are recommended because they are more accurate than percutaneous needle biopsies when assessing for anaplasia.[47] Failure to achieve a reduction in volume is often due to tumor differentiation.[50] Differentiated tumors may show a poor clinical response to therapy but have an excellent prognosis if the tumor is completely excised. Patients with progressive disease have a poor prognosis and require treatment with a different chemotherapeutic regimen.[46,50,51]

Renal-sparing surgery has been explored in children with unilateral Wilms tumors.[52,53] The incidence of renal failure after nephrectomy for most children with unilateral Wilms tumor, however, is low, 0.6% at 20 years post-treatment.[48,49] The COG has a renal-sparing protocol for select patients with unilateral Wilms tumors known to be at risk for bilateral disease and those at increased risk for renal failure.

Late Effects of Treatment

Several organ systems are subject to the late sequelae of anticancer therapy. Clinicians must be aware of the spectrum of problems that face children as they grow into adulthood. Chemotherapy and gonadal radiation may produce ovarian failure and pregnancy related complications.[54] An increased incidence of second malignant neoplasms has also been noted in children treated for Wilms tumor, with a 1% cumulative incidence at 10 years post-diagnosis and with prior irradiation one of the greatest risk factors.[55] As discussed previously, renal failure is noted with increased frequency in children with bilateral Wilms tumors. Children with *WT1* mutations, such as those with aniridia, however, also have an increased risk of renal failure if they survive into puberty.[48]

Key Points: Wilms tumor

- Deletions of *WT1* are associated with aniridia, WAGR syndrome, and Denys-Drash syndrome, and Wilms tumor. Deletions of *WT2* are associated with hemihypertrophy and BWS.

- Contralateral renal exploration is no longer necessary at the time of radical nephrectomy if imaging of the contralateral kidney is normal on preoperative staging CT or MRI.

- Bilateral Wilms tumor should be treated initially with chemotherapy with the goal of umor shrinkage and renal-sparing surgery.

TESTICULAR TUMORS

Testicular tumors account for 2% of all pediatric solid tumors, with an annual incidence of 5.9:100,000 for boys less than 15 years of age.[56] Recent reports have shown that the benign lesions represent 74% of primary testis tumors in prepubertal children. The incidence of childhood testicular tumors peaks at age 2, tapers after age 4, and begins to rise again at puberty.[57] Several etiologic factors have been investigated. Patients with disorders of sexual development have an increased incidence of gonadal tumors and those with hypovirilization and gonadal dysgenesis are at the highest risk. The risk of tumor formation in gonadal dysgenesis is increased if there is a Y chromosome present, with the incidence of tumor development approximately 10% by 20 years old. Patients with a prior history of undescended testis have an increased risk of testicular malignancy. The relative risk of cancer increases with age at orchidopexy with the greatest risk after puberty.[58]

Diagnosis and Staging

The most common presentation is a painless testicular mass. Disorders that must be excluded are epididymitis, hydrocele, hernia, and spermatic cord torsion. The latter can present as a painless mass in the neonate with little scrotal wall inflammation if the event occurred prenatally. Color Doppler testicular ultrasound is useful for evaluating testicular problems and can identify both solid and cystic testicular neoplasms. There are no sonographic features, however, that can reliably distinguish benign and malignant tumors. Prepubertal teratomas typically appear cystic on ultrasound and epidermoid cysts of the testis also have a fairly characteristic appearance (**Fig. 3**). When these are identified preoperatively, the surgeon can plan for a testicular-sparing procedure.[59,60]

The COG staging for testis tumors is based on imaging finding, serum tumor markers, and pathologic findings. CTs of the retroperitoneum and chest are obtained to evaluate the retroperitoneal lymph nodes and to exclude other metastatic lesions. Serum α-fetoprotein (AFP) and β–human chorionic gonadotropin (β-hCG) are obtained at diagnosis and monitored after orchiectomy to determine if there is an appropriate half-life decline. β-hCG is rarely elevated in preadolescent tumors. Yolk sac tumors invariably produce AFP, which makes it a useful marker to distinguish benign from malignant prepubertal testis tumors. AFP has a half-life of approximately 5 days and

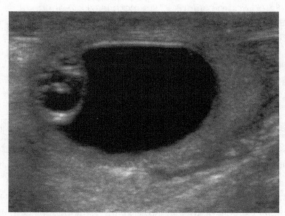

Fig. 3. Testicular ultrasound demonstrating cystic lesion that proved to be a teratoma of the testicle. The patient underwent a testis-sparing procedure.

AFP levels may be elevated in infant boys and this does not always represent persistent disease after orchiectomy because normal adult levels (<10 mg/mL) are not reached until 8 months of age.[61]

Mature Teratoma

Teratoma accounts for more than 40% of testis tumors in prepubertal children.[59,60] Prepubertal mature teratomas have a benign clinical course that contrasts the metastatic nature of adult teratomas.[62] As discussed previously, the presumptive diagnosis of teratoma can often be made on ultrasound and these tumors are currently managed with a testicular-sparing approach, with no recurrences reported to date.[59,60] Ultrasound can underestimate the amount of normal parenchyma due to compression by the tumor against the capsule.[63]

Epidermoid Cyst

Epidermoid cysts account for 15% of pediatric testicular tumors.[59,60,64] They occur within the testicular parenchyma and are filled with keratinous debris leading to the characteristic ultrasound finding of concentric rings of alternating hypoechoic and hyperechoic layers that give rise to an onion-skin appearance.[65] Epidermoid cysts represent a monodermal teratoma and follow a benign clinical course, and testis-sparing surgery has been advocated both in children and adults.[56,59,60]

Yolk Sac Tumor

Yolk sac tumor is the second most common prepubertal testicular tumor of germ cell origin and occurs primarily in children younger than 2 years old.[57] More than 90% of prepubertal children present with stage I disease.[66] The most common site of distant metastases is the lung and metastasis to the retroperitoneal lymph nodes occurs in only 4% to 6% of children.[66] Initial treatment is radical inguinal orchiectomy and is curative in most children. Thus, routine retroperitoneal lymph node dissection and/or adjuvant chemotherapy are not indicated.[66] Staging of patients with tumor markers and imaging studies is performed (discussed previously). Clinical stage I patients do not receive additional adjuvant treatment after radical orchiectomy. Patients who have persistent elevation of AFP and retroperitoneal adenopathy are presumed to have metastatic disease and can be treated as stage III.

Combination chemotherapy with platinum-based therapies (cisplatin, etoposide, and bleomycin) has been used in pediatric patients with advanced GCTs.[66,67] The 6-year overall survival of children with stage II and III testicular tumors approaches 100%.[67,68] Several patients, however, experienced significant ototoxicity and nephrotoxicity with the cisplatin-based chemotherapy regimens.

REFERENCES

1. Crist WM, Anderson JR, Meza JL, et al. IRS-IV: results for patients with nonmetastatic disease. J Clin Oncol 2001;19(12):3091–102.
2. Malkin D, Li FP, Strong LC, et al. Germ line p53 mutations in a familial syndrome of breast cancer, sarcomas, and other neoplasms. Science 1990;250:1233–8.
3. Meza JL, Anderson J, Pappo AS, et al. Analysis of prognostic factors in patients with nonmetastatic rhabdomyosarcoma treated on IRS III and IV: the COG. J Clin Oncol 2006;24:3844–51.
4. Malempati S, Rodeberg DA, Donaldson SS, et al. Rhabdomyosarcoma in infants younger than 1 year: a report from the Children's Oncology Group. Cancer 2011; 117:3493–501.

5. Rodary C, Gehan EA, Flamant F, et al. Prognostic factors in 951 nonmetastatic rhabdomyosarcoma in children: report from the International Rhabdomyosarcoma Workshop. Med Pediatr Oncol 1991;19:89–95.

6. Flamant F, Rodary C, Rey A, et al. Treatment of non-metastatic rhabdomyosarcomas in childhood and adolescence. Results of the second study of the International Society of Paediatric Oncology: MMT84. Eur J Cancer 1998;34:1050–62.

7. Arndt C, Rodeberg D, Breitfeld PP, et al. Does bladder preservation (as a surgical principle) lead to retaining bladder function in bladder/prostate rhabdomyosarcoma? Results from the IRSG-IV. J Urol 2004;171:2396–403.

8. Ferrari A, Bisogno G, Casanova M, et al. Paratesticular rhabdomyosarcoma: report from the Italian and German cooperative group. J Clin Oncol 2002;29:449–55.

9. Rodeberg DA, Anderson JR, Arndt CA, et al. Comparison of outcomes based on treatment algorithms for rhabdomyosarcoma of the bladder/prostate; combined results from the Children's Oncology Group, German Cooperative Soft Tissue Sarcoma Study, Italian Cooperative Group, and International Society of Pediatric Oncology Malignant Mesenchymal Tumors Committee. Int J Cancer 2011;128:1232–9.

10. Yeung CK, Ward HC, Ransley PG, et al. Bladder and kidney function after cure of pelvic rhabdomyosarcoma in childhood. Br J Cancer 1994;70:1000–3.

11. Seitz G, Dantonello TM, Int-Veen C, et al. Treatment efficiency, outcome and surgical treatment problems in patients suffering from localized embryonal/prostate rhabdomyosarcoma: a report from the Cooperative Soft Tissue Sarcoma trial CWS-96. Pediatr Blood Cancer 2011;56:718–24.

12. Godzinski J, Flamant F, Rey A, et al. Value of postchemotherapy bioptical verification of complete clinical remission in previously incompletely resected (stage I and II pT3) malignant mesenchymal tumors in children: International Society of Pediatric Oncology 1984 Malignant Mesenchymal Tumors Study. Med Pediatr Oncol 1994;22:22–6.

13. Wiener ES, Anderson JR, Ojimba JI, et al. Controversies in the management of paratesticular rhabdomyosarcoma: is staging retroperitoneal lymph node dissection necessary for adolescents with resected paratesticular rhabdomyosarcoma? Semin Pediatr Surg 2001;10:146–52.

14. Stewart RJ, Martelli H, Oberlin, et al. Treatment of children with nonmetastatic paratesticular rhabdomyosarcoma: results of the Malignant Mesenchymal Tumors studies of the International Society of Pediatric Oncology. J Clin Oncol 2003;21:793–8.

15. Waterhouse DO, Meza JL, Breneman JC, et al. Local control and outcome in children with localized vaginal rhabdomyosarcoma: a report from the Soft Tissue Sarcoma committee of the Children's Oncology Group. Pediatr Blood Cancer 2011;15:76–83.

16. Martelli H, Oberlin O, Rey A, et al. Conservative treatment for girls with nonmetastatic rhabdomyosarcoma of the genital tract: a report from the study committee of the International Society of Pediatric Oncology. J Clin Oncol 1999;17:2117–22.

17. Arndt CA, Donaldson SS, Anderson JR, et al. What constitutes optimal therapy for patients with rhabdomyosarcoma of the female genital tract? Cancer 2001;91:2454–68.

18. Spunt SL, Sweeney TA, Judson MM, et al. Late effects of pelvic rhabdomyosarcoma and its treatment in female survivors. J Clin Oncol 2005;23:7143–51.

19. Breslow N, Olshan A, Beckwith JB, et al. Epidemiology of Wilms' Tumor. Med Pediatr Oncol 1993;21:172–81.

20. Coppes MJ, Huff V, Pelletier J. Denys-Drash syndrome: relating a clinical disorder to genetic alterations in the tumor suppressor gene WT1. J Pediatr 1993;123: 673–8.
21. Van Heyningen V, Hoovers JM, de Kraker J, et al. Raised risk of Wilms tumour in patients with aniridia and submicroscopic WT1 deletion. J Med Genet 2007;44:787–90.
22. Koufos A, Grundy P, Morgan K, et al. Familial Wiedemann-Beckwith syndrome and a second Wilms tumor locus both map to 11p15.5. Am J Hum Genet 1989;44:711–9.
23. Debaun MR, Tucker MA. Risk of cancer during the first four years of life in children from the Beckwith- Wiedemann syndrome registry. J Pediatr 1998;132:377–9.
24. Ruteshouser EC, Robinson SM, Huff V. Wilms tumor genetics: mutations in WT1, WTX and CTNNB1 account for only about one-third of tumors. Genes Chromosomes Cancer 2008;47:461–70.
25. Green DM, Breslow NE, Beckwith JB, et al. Screening of children with hemihypertrophy, aniridia, and Beckwith-Wiedemann syndrome in patients with Wilms' tumor: a report from the NWTSG. Med Pediatr Oncol 1993;21:188–92.
26. Scott RH, Walker L, Olsen OE, et al. Surveillance for Wilms tumour in at-risk children: pragmatic recommendations for best practice. Arch Dis Child 2006;91: 995–9.
27. Shamberger RC, Ritchey ML, Haase GM, et al. Intravascular extension of Wilms tumor. Ann Surg 2001;234:116–21.
28. Ritchey ML, Shamberger RC, Hamilton T, et al. Fate of bilateral lesions missed on preoperative imaging: a report of the NWTSG. J Urol 2005;174:1519–21.
29. Miniati D, Gay AN, Parks KV, et al. Imaging accuracy and incidence of Wilms' and non-Wilms' tumors in children. J Pediatr Surg 2008;43:1301–7.
30. Dome JS, Cotton CA, Perlman EJ, et al. Treatment of anaplastic histology Wilms tumor: results from the fifth National Wilms Tumor Study. J Clin Oncol 2006;24: 2352–8.
31. Beckwith JB. Precursor lesions of Wilms tumor: clinical and biological implications. Med Pediatr Oncol 1993;21:158–68.
32. Coppes MJ, Arnold M, Beckwith JB, et al. Factors affecting the risk of contralateral Wilms tumor development. Cancer 1999;85:1616–25.
33. Shamberger RC, Guthrie KA, Ritchey ML, et al. Surgery-related factors and local recurrence of Wilms tumor in National Wilms Tumor Study 4. Ann Surg 1999;229: 292–7.
34. Kalapurakal JA, Li SM, Breslow NE, et al. Intraoperative spillage of favorable histology Wilms tumor cells: influence of irradiation and chemotherapy regimens on abdominal recurrence: a report from the NWTSG. Int J Radiat Oncol Biol Phys 2010;76:201–6.
35. Grundy PE, Breslow NE, Li S, et al. Loss of heterozygosity for chromosomes 1p and 16q is an adverse prognostic factor in favorable histology wilms tumor. a report from the NWTSG. J Clin Oncol 2005;23:7312–21.
36. Green DM, Breslow NE, Beckwith JBB, et al. Effect of duration of treatment on treatment outcomes and cost of treatment for Wilms' tumor: a report from the NWTSG. J Clin Oncol 1998;16:3744–51.
37. Tournade MF, Com-Nougue C, Voute PA, et al. Results of the sixth International Society of Pediatric Oncology Wilms' tumor trial and study: a risk-adapted therapeutic approach in Wilms' tumor. J Clin Oncol 1993;11:1014–23.
38. DeKraker J, Graf N, van Tinteren H, et al. Reduction of postoperative chemotherapy in children with stage I intermediate-risk and anaplastic Wilms' tumour (SIOP 93-01 trial): a randomized controlled trial. Lancet 2004;364:1229–35.

39. Ritchey ML, Shamberger RC, Haase G, et al. Surgical complications after nephrectomy for Wilms tumor: report from the National Wilms Tumor Study Group. J Am Coll Surg 2001;192:63–8.
40. Godzinski J, Tournade MF, deKraker J, et al. Rarity of surgical complications after post-chemotherapy nephrectomy for nephroblastoma. Experience of the International Society of Paediatric Oncology-Trial and study "SIOP-9". International Society of Paediatric Oncology Nephroblastoma Trial and Study committee. Eur J Pediatr Surg 1998;8:83–6.
41. Mitchell C, Pritchard-Jones K, Shannon R, et al. Immediate nephrectomy versus preoperative chemotherapy in the management of non-metastatic Wilms' tumour: results of a randomised trial (UKW3) by the UK Children's Cancer Study Group. Eur J Cancer 2006;42:2554–62.
42. Verschuur AC, Vujanic GM, Tinteren HV, et al. Stromal and epithelial predominant tumours have an excellent outcome: the SIOP 93 experience. Pediatr Blood Cancer 2010;55:233–8.
43. Reinhard H, Semler O, Burger D, et al. Results of the SIOP 93-01/GPOH trial and study for the treatment of patients with unilateral nonmetastatic Wilms Tumor. Klin Padiatr 2004;216:132–40.
44. Boccon-Gibod L, Rey A, Sandstedt B, et al. Complete necrosis induced by preoperative chemotherapy in Wilms tumor as an indicator of low risk: report of the international society of paediatric oncology (siop) nephroblastoma trial and study 9. Med Pediatr Oncol 2000;34:183–90.
45. Shamberger RC, Anderson JR, Breslow NE, et al. Long-term outcomes of infants with very low risk Wilms tumor treated with surgery alone on National Wilms Tumor Study-5. Ann Surg 2010;251:555–8.
46. Ritchey ML, Pringle K, Breslow N, et al. Management and outcome of inoperable Wilms tumor. A report of National Wilms' Tumor Study. Ann Surg 1994;220:683–90.
47. Hamilton TE, Ritchey ML, Haase GM, et al. The management of synchronous bilateral Wilms tumor: a report from the National Wilms Tumor Study Group. Ann Surg 2011;253:1004–10.
48. Breslow NE, Collins AJ, Ritchey ML, et al. End stage renal disease in patients with Wilms tumor: results from the NWTSG and the United States Renal Data System. J Urol 2005;174:1972–5.
49. Lange J, Peterson SM, Takashima JR, et al. Risk factors for end stage renal disease in non-WT1-syndromic Wilms tumor. J Urol 2011;186:378–86.
50. Shamberger RC, Haase GM, Argani P, et al. Bilateral Wilms' tumors with progressive or nonresponsive disease. J Pediatr Surg 2006;41:652–7.
51. Ora I, van Tinteren H, Bergeron C, et al. Progression of localized Wilms' tumour during preoperative chemotherapy is an independent prognostic factor: a report from the SIOP 93-01 nephroblastoma trial and study. Eur J Cancer 2007;43:131–6.
52. Haecker FM, vonSchweinitz D, Harms D, et al. Partial nephrectomy for unilateral Wilms tumor: result of study SIOP 93-01/GPOH. J Urol 2003;170:939–44.
53. Zani A, Schiavetti A, Gambino M, et al. Long-term outcome of nephron sparing surgery and simple nephrectomy for unilateral localized Wilms tumor. J Urol 2005;173:946–8.
54. Green DM, Peabody EM, Nan B, et al. Pregnancy outcome after treatment for Wilms tumor: a report from the NWTSG. J Clin Oncol 2002;20:2506–13.
55. Taylor AJ, Winter DL, Pritchard-Jones K, et al. Second primary neoplasms in survivors of Wilms' tumour—a population-based cohort study from the British Childhood Cancer Survivor Study. Int J Cancer 2008;122:2085–93.

56. Pohl HG, Shukla AR, Metcalf PD, et al. Prepubertal testis tumors: actual prevalence rate of histological types. J Urol 2004;172:2370–2.

57. Walsh TJ, Grady RW, Porter MJ, et al. Incidence of testicular germ cell cancers in U.S. children: SEER program experience 1973 to 2000. Urology 2008;68:402–5.

58. Petersson A, Richiardi L, Nordenskjold A, et al. Age at surgery for undescended testis and risk of testicular cancer. N Engl J Med 2007;356:1835–41.

59. Metcalfe PD, Farivar-Mohseni J, Farhat W, et al. Pediatric testicular tumors: contemporary incidence and efficacy of testicular preserving surgery. J Urol 2003;170:2412–6.

60. Shukla AR, Woodard C, Carr MC, et al. Experience with testis sparing surgery for testicular teratoma. J Urol 2004;171:161–3.

61. Huddart SN, Mann JR, Gornall P, et al. The UK Children's Cancer Study Group: testicular malignant germ cell tumours 1979-1988. J Pediatr Surg 1990;25:406–10.

62. Grady RW, Ross JH, Kay R. Epidemiological features of testicular teratoma in a prepubertal population. J Urol 1997;158:1191–2.

63. Patel AS, Coley BD, Jayanthi VR. Ultrasonography underestimates the volume of normal parenchyma in benign testicular masses. J Urol 2007;178:1730–2.

64. Rushton G, Belman AB, Sesterhenn I, et al. Testicular sparing surgery for prepubertal teratoma of the testis: a clinical and pathological study. J Urol 1990;144:726–30.

65. Ulbright TM. Germ cell tumors of the gonads: a selective review emphasizing problems in differential diagnosis, newly appreciated, and controversial issues. Mod Pathol 2005;18(Suppl 2):S61–79.

66. Mann JR, Pearson D, Barrett A, et al. Results of the United Kingdom Children's Cancer Study Group's malignant germ cell tumor studies. Cancer 1989;63:1657–67.

67. Rogers PC, Olson TA, Cullen JW, et al. Treatment of children and adolescents with stage II testicular and stages I and II ovarian malignant germ cell tumors: a Pediatric Intergroup Study–Pediatric Oncology Group 9048 and Children's Cancer Group 8891. J Clin Oncol 2004;22:3563–9.

68. Cushing B, Giller R, Cullen JW, et al. Randomized comparison of combination chemotherapy with etoposide, bleomycin, and either high-dose or standard-dose cisplatin in children and adolescents with high-risk malignant germ cell tumors: a pediatric intergroup study—Pediatric Oncology Group 9049 and Children's Cancer Group 8882. J Clin Oncol 2004;22:2691–700.

Geintourinary Malignancies in Children: Editorial Comment

Armando J. Lorenzo, MD, MSc, FRCSC

KEYWORDS

- Pediatric genitourinary malignancies • Wilms' tumor • Rhabdomyosarcoma
- Testicular tumors • Tissue-sparing surgery • Long-term outcomes

KEY POINTS

- Many pediatric genitourinary malignant conditions have experienced favorable improvements in survival.
- As children affected by these conditions live longer and become young adults, long-term consequences of the malignant process and its treatment become more prominent.
- Balancing under and over-treatment is likely to become an important future goal, with the judicious introduction more selective strategies along with minimally invasive and tissue-sparing procedures.

Genitourinary malignancies in children, not unlike many other cancers, comprise heterogeneous tumors grouped together under the realm of pediatric urologic oncology, loosely bound by anatomic proximity, related embryologic origins, and functional ties or similarities in the organs they arise from. This artificial and rather rudimentary classification system serves as a framework for specialization, better understanding, protocol development, and treatment. Looking ahead, as understanding about them—as well as of cancer in general—increases, the broad categories created by histology and staging will likely begin to break down, making way for more sophisticated diagnostic tools based on differences and unique characteristics at the molecular level.

The current state of the art, a culmination of collaborative efforts by many scientists, health care providers, patients, and families, has been clearly and masterfully summarized in this issue of the *Pediatric Clinics of North America*. Years of clinical and basic science innovation have translated into better prognosis, albeit often achieved with aggressive therapeutic strategies that have important side effects and long-term consequences that are yet to be fully characterized.[1] In many circumstances, improved survival has come at a cost, and we are becoming increasingly aware of the impact on survivors of childhood neoplasms. Thus, it is important to pick up on new trends and

Pediatric Urology, Hospital for Sick Children, University of Toronto, 555 University Avenue, Toronto, Ontario M5G 1X8, Canada
E-mail address: armando.lorenzo@sickkids.ca

Pediatr Clin N Am 59 (2012) 961–964
doi:10.1016/j.pcl.2012.05.017
0031-3955/12/$ – see front matter © 2012 Elsevier Inc. All rights reserved.

common denominators in the recent advances described by Drs Grimsby and Ritchey, in the article elsewhere in this issue: a movement toward tissue-sparing procedures, tailored chemotherapy, selective and more accurately delivered radiation therapy, protocols generated by collaborative study groups, and extended long-term monitoring. These advances should allow for the shared goal of decreasing morbidity from the condition itself as well as the treatment, function preservation, and better quality and quantity of life.

From a surgical point of view, the preservation of grossly normal-appearing or unaffected parts of the organ during resection has become increasingly appealing. In some situations, such as renal neoplasms or prepubertal testicular teratomas, experience has shown that some tumors tend to splay out the surrounding parenchyma, creating an optical illusion on imaging studies and intraoperative evaluation that there is little tissue to be saved by performing a selective versus radical resection (**Fig. 1**).[2,3] For chemosensitive neoplasms, the introduction of neoadjuvant therapy for the purpose of decreasing the size of the primary tumor and allowing less radical resection has also gained momentum based on experience with bilateral renal involvement or inoperable tumors (notably Wilms tumors[4]). Regardless of the tissue of origin, we should ask ourselves if it is fair to remove the whole organ to embrace the concept of radical resection, so often the default when it comes to solid tumors. Selective surgical resection of the tumor from the whole organ has already gained acceptance (even becoming standard of care) in the treatment of many other conditions, such as breast, kidney, penile, and urothelial cancers. Although more technically challenging, the investment may pay off down the road, particularly for patients who are at risk for further functional decline with age or from acute events related to metachronous neoplasms[5] or injury to the

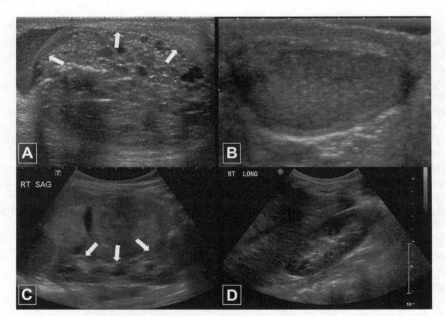

Fig. 1. Examples of imaging studies before and after tissue-sparing procedures. Prepubertal testicular teratoma before (*A*) and after (*B*) resection; renal neoplasm in a teenager before (*C*) and after (*D*) partial nephrectomy. Notice normal parenchyma displaced and distorted by the neoplastic process (*white arrows*), followed by almost-normal sonographic appearance of the organ during postoperative monitoring.

contralateral organ. If this rationale is acceptable for older patients with multiple comorbidities and shorter overall life expectancy, it stands to reason that an even stronger case can be made for children and adolescents. Particularly for this patient population, who should be offered hope for life expectancies in the order of decades, slight early increases in morbidity trends can translate into exponential worsening over time, with a detrimental impact on quantity and quality of life. Ultimately, the careful balance between the potential benefits of organ preservation compared with the risk of local recurrence and subsequent need for intensified multimodal treatment protocols need to be frequently assessed. These are some of the fundamental questions likely to be addressed in future trials as survival outlooks aim way past the traditional 5-year and 10-year curve cutoffs.

Moving forward, the definition of "preserved function" should be critically evaluated, particularly when insults occur early in life or before all demands are placed on the affected system. We now realize that long-term deterioration can occur even in the face of seemingly normal or near-normal measures during early monitoring, and many functional handicaps may not become manifest until appropriate developmental milestones have been reached (notably puberty). Examples of how this can have a huge impact on quality of life and morbidity include the possibility of early-raising trends in renal insufficiency for selected patients who have previously undergone resection of renal malignancies (beyond what would be expected for a cohort of patients of the same age without prior kidney surgery), the issue of bladder function deterioration after aggressive radiation therapy for local control of pelvic rhabdomyosarcomas,[6] the likely adverse impact on future fertility by various neoplastic processes or treatments,[7] and the possibility of erectile dysfunction after aggressive pelvic surgery and/or radiation.[8]

Last but not least, it is not uncommon that there is an impact on body image and cosmesis, particularly by surgical procedures. Although it is hard to defend less than optimal outcomes in favor of less-invasive interventions, successfully introduced minimally invasive techniques for the management of neoplasms in adults are slowly being brought to the pediatric arena. A highly critical yet open mind in this process may translate into smaller, well-concealed scars and quicker recovery from attempts at surgical resection.

We are living in rapidly changing and exciting times. Although it is important to temper overtly enthusiastic embracement of new approaches, it is always nice to dream of better, less-invasive, more-effective treatment paradigms. Defeating cancer is more than just achieving short-term or medium-term remission. As more is learned about childhood malignancies and the impact of treatment, this should be kept in mind. Our patients are entitled to hope for a long and close to "normal" life. It is our job to help them achieve that. With judicious innovation and restless research efforts, soon enough many of the ideas presented in the Review Article elsewhere in this issue and my Editorial Comment will be outdated, making way for revolutionary changes that are bound to make cancer a less-frightening and far more curable condition.

If you can dream it, you can do it.
—Walt Disney

Let us dream...

REFERENCES

1. Rebholz CE, Reulen RC, Toogood AA, et al. Health care use of long-term survivors of childhood cancer: the British Childhood Cancer Survivor Study. J Clin Oncol 2011;29(31):4181–8.

2. Davidoff AM, Giel DW, Jones DP, et al. The feasibility and outcome of nephron-sparing surgery for children with bilateral Wilms tumor. The St Jude Children's Research Hospital experience: 1999-2006. Cancer 2008;112(9):2060–70.
3. Patel AS, Coley BD, Jayanthi VR. Ultrasonography underestimates the volume of normal parenchyma in benign testicular masses. J Urol 2007;178(4 Pt 2):1730–2.
4. Ritchey ML. Nephron sparing surgery for Wilms tumor—where is the future? J Urol 2011;186(4):1179–80.
5. Rich BS, McEvoy MP, La Quaglia MP. A case of renal cell carcinoma after successful treatment of Wilms tumor. J Pediatr Surg 2010;45(9):1883–6.
6. Ferrer FA. Re: Does bladder preservation (as a surgical principle) lead to retaining bladder function in bladder/prostate rhabdomyosarcoma? Results from Intergroup Rhabdomyosarcoma Study IV. J Urol 2004;172(5 Pt 1):2084.
7. Winther JF, Olsen JH. Adverse reproductive effects of treatment for cancer in childhood and adolescence. Eur J Cancer 2011;47(Suppl 3):S230–8.
8. Macedo A, Ferreira PV, Barroso U, et al. Sexual function in teenagers after multimodal treatment of pelvic rhabdomyosarcoma: a preliminary report. J Pediatr Urol 2010;6(6):605–8.

Pediatric Urological Emergencies

Sarah M. Lambert, MD

KEYWORDS

- Abdominal pain • Scrotal mass • Testicular torsion • Renal trauma
- Urologic emergencies

KEY POINTS

- Children with acute abdominal pain should be evaluated immediately. In addition to a thorough abdominal examination to rule out surgical disease, these children should be evaluated for urinary tract infection, constipation, and spermatic cord torsion.
- A child with acute scrotal pain must be presumed to have spermatic cord torsion regardless of age until proven otherwise; however, in some cases, an accurate evaluation may prevent an unnecessary surgical exploration.
- The differential diagnosis of a vaginal mass includes benign periurethral cysts, skin tags, urethral prolapse, imperforate hymen, prolapsed ureterocele, or rarely, malignancies such as a rhabdomyosarcoma.
- Blunt force renal trauma requires immediate evaluation but does not necessarily require operative intervention. The conservative treatment of high-grade blunt renal injuries has been successfully described in children. Children with high-grade injuries at risk for failure of conservative management include those with vascular avulsion or extensive urinary extravasation, especially in the setting of ureteropelvic junction disruptions.
- Infants with ambiguous genitalia require immediate evaluation because congenital adrenal hyperplasia may result in salt wasting, which can be life-threatening.

Urological emergencies represent a small percentage of office and emergency department visits, but the rapid assessment and management of these conditions are essential to preservation of urological health. In many cases, the initial contact with the child and family will be through a phone call to the office or an urgent office visit. A thorough understanding of the chief compliant, history of the present illness, and past medical history is vital to appropriate management of all pediatric urologic patients. In addition, the physical examination will identify abnormalities and narrow the differential diagnosis; however, because other acute processes, such as appendicitis, may mimic genitourinary disease, the clinician must be alert for evidence of disease in other organ systems.

Department of Urology, Columbia University, The Morgan Stanley Children's Hospital of New York, 3959 Broadway, CHN-1117, New York, NY 10032, USA
E-mail address: lamberts@email.chop.edu

Pediatr Clin N Am 59 (2012) 965–976
doi:10.1016/j.pcl.2012.05.014
0031-3955/12/$ – see front matter © 2012 Published by Elsevier Inc.

pediatric.theclinics.com

The initial assessment must accurately determine the degree of acuity and the level of care required. Although few children are severely ill when evaluated in the pediatric office, developing the skills to recognize an infant or child who requires hospitalization is critical. Some children will require treatment in an emergency department or direct admission to an inpatient facility, whereas other children can be managed as outpatients. Determining when an infant requires an inpatient admission is particularly important because the metabolic reserve is less abundant in the newborn.[1] Patients with hemodynamic instability must be emergently addressed. This article outlines the most common urgent and emergent pediatric urological conditions with the goal to direct initial evaluation and treatment.

ACUTE ABDOMINAL CONDITIONS

Children with acute abdominal pain should be evaluated immediately. An accurate history of the nature of the pain may be the best indicator of the source of the pain. Details about the character of the pain, including timing, acuity of onset, radiation, and migration are important and should, if possible, be elicited directly from the child. Associated loss of appetite, nausea, vomiting, or a change in bowel pattern may help to distinguish gastrointestinal from genitourinary sources. Causes of abdominal pain in children vary widely and are often unique to the pediatric population. Pyelonephritis, renal colic, or cystitis are potential etiologies within the differential diagnosis. Renal colic can result from obstructing nephrolithiasis, ureteropelvic junction obstruction, ureterovesical junction obstruction, or clot obstruction. Nonurological intra-abdominal etiologies in children include gastroenteritis, constipation, mesenteric adenitis, pyloric stenosis, midgut volvulus, appendicitis, and intussuception. Nonabdominal sources, such as sickle cell crisis, streptococcal pharyngitis, or pneumonia, should also be considered. In addition to a thorough abdominal examination designed to rule out surgical abdominal disease, these children should be evaluated for urinary tract infection (UTI), constipation, and spermatic cord torsion. Usually an acute abdominal series is ordered, which will demonstrate considerable amounts of stool throughout the colon if constipation is the cause. Occasionally, some children with spermatic cord torsion complain of abdominal pain and have minimal scrotal complaints. Therefore, a scrotal examination must always accompany an abdominal examination. Most abdominal masses originate in genitourinary organs and should be evaluated immediately.[2] In neonates, transillumination of the abdomen may assist in distinguishing between solid and cystic lesions. The most common malignant abdominal tumor in infants is neuroblastoma, followed by Wilms tumor.[3] Children with neuroblastoma typically relate a history of more constitutional symptoms than children with Wilms tumor.

If an abdominal mass is suspected, an abdominal ultrasound evaluation should be ordered. If the mass is solid, computed tomography (CT) is almost always required. Renal pathology is the source of up to two-thirds of neonatal abdominal masses.[4] Cystic abdominal masses include hydronephrosis, multicystic dysplastic kidneys, adrenal hemorrhage, hydrometrocolpos, intestinal duplication, and choledochal ovarian omental or pancreatic cysts. Solid masses include neuroblastoma, congenital mesoblastic nephroma, hepatoblastoma, and teratoma. A solid flank mass may be caused by renal venous thrombosis, which becomes apparent with signs of hematuria, hypertension, and thrombocytopenia. Renal venous thrombosis in infants is associated with polycythemia, dehydration, diabetic mothers, asphyxia, sepsis, and coagulopathies, such as antithrombin-3 or protein C deficiencies.

NEPHROLITHIASIS

The incidence of nephrolithiasis in children is increasing in the United States: 1000 to 7500 hospital admissions in the United States result from pediatric nephrolithiasis.[5,6]

Nephrolithiasis can be associated with significant metabolic disturbances and underlying medical conditions. The presence of nephrolithiasis does not represent an emergent situation but does require urology and nephrology evaluation. Certain clinical signs and patient characteristics must be assessed to determine the acuity of the patient. Children with renal calculi often present with renal colic. Patients often complain of abdominal pain, flank pain, lower quadrant pain, and or scrotal pain. In young children, abdominal symptoms can often be vague and more difficult to localize. Although nephrolithiasis is more common in adolescents, 20% of pediatric nephrolithiasis occurs in newborns and infants.[7] Children with renal ectopia, such as pelvic kidneys, also present with atypical symptoms. Nausea, emesis, and gross hematuria often accompany the abdominal pain.

Children with obstruction of a solitary system, urinary tract infection, renal insufficiency, immunosuppression, uncontrollable pain, and/or the inability to tolerate oral intake should be evaluated emergently. These children should be assessed in the emergency department with a complete blood count, metabolic panel, urine analysis, urine culture, and abdominal imaging. A renal and bladder ultrasound often provides adequate diagnostic information, but a CT scan of the abdomen and pelvis is warranted in some cases. The sensitivity of ultrasound is significantly lower than CT imaging but the risk of malignancy associated with irradiation must be considered.[8] An infected obstructing ureteral calculus can result in urosepsis and death; therefore, these children should be stabilized, administered broad-spectrum intravenous (IV) antibiotics, and the obstructed renal unit decompressed. In an unstable patient, percutaneous nephrostomy tube placement is the safest and most efficient management.

ACUTE SCROTAL CONDITIONS
Testicular Torsion

The annual incidence of testicular torsion in boys younger than 18 years is 3.8 per 100,000.[9] A child with acute scrotal pain must be presumed to have spermatic cord torsion regardless of age until proven otherwise; however, in some cases, an accurate evaluation may save the child an unnecessary surgical exploration. The differential diagnosis of the acute scrotum includes testicular torsion, torsion of the appendix testis or epididymis, epididymitis/orchitis, hernia/hydrocele, trauma, sexual abuse, tumor, idiopathic scrotal edema, dermatitis, cellulitis, and vasculitis, such as Henoch-Schonlein purpura.[10] Gradual onset of the pain is more consistent with epididymitis, whereas abrupt pain suggests spermatic cord torsion or torsion of one of the testicular appendices. The classical presentation of testicular torsion is the sudden onset of severe, unilateral pain that is often associated with nausea and emesis. Pain is present with palpation and at rest. A history of similar intermittent episodes may suggest intermittent testicular torsion.

The acute scrotum should be examined carefully to determine the true etiology. Observation of the child's general appearance and level of distress should be recognized. Scrotal erythema, edema, or ecchymoses should be readily identifiable. To begin the scrotal examination, the inguinal canal should be inspected on each side for signs of asymmetry or mass. The inguinal canal is then palpated to identify a fullness or mass suggestive of a hernia or hydrocele of the spermatic cord. Testicular torsion may present with varied clinical findings, but the involved testis often demonstrates signs such as higher riding in the hemiscrotum, a transverse orientation, an anterior epididymis, absent cremasteric reflex, and tenderness of the testis and epididymis. Associated scrotal wall swelling or erythema is suggestive of spermatic cord torsion if presentation is delayed. The absence of edema or erythema or the presence of a cremasteric reflex does not rule out the possibility of acute testicular torsion, especially if the onset of pain was recent.

In contrast, torsion of the appendix testis or epididymis often results in localized tenderness at the superior pole of the testis or caput epididymis and is often associated with a reactive hydrocele. Additionally, in boys with thin scrotal skin, the "blue dot" sign can be seen reflective of a necrotic appendix. Epididymitis classically has a gradual onset and is not associated with nausea or emesis but can have similar clinical signs, including a firm, tender, enlarged testis with an erythematous and edematous scrotum.[10]

The normal newborn scrotum is relatively large. Its size may be increased with the trauma of breech delivery or by a newborn hydrocele. A hydrocele can be distinguished from hernia by palpation and transillumination, as well as from the absence of a mass in the inguinal canal. In the absence of volume changes within the hydrocele, the processus vaginalis is usually not patent and the newborn hydrocele resolves by 1 year of age without surgery. Neonatal extravaginal testicular torsion can also occur prenatally resulting in a firm, enlarged, nontender mass in the hemiscrotum that is usually associated with dark discoloration of the overlying skin. A normal scrotal examination at birth and subsequent development of erythematous, tender, edematous hemiscrotum suggests postnatal extravaginal testicular torsion and should be addressed immediately with surgical intervention if the neonate is clinically stable.

Traditionally significant ischemic damage is believed to occur after 4 to 8 hours. Therefore, testicular torsion represents a true surgical emergency. If there is a concern for testicular torsion, the patient should be sent to the emergency department for immediate evaluation. Patients presenting after 8 hours are usually still explored because the viability of the testis is difficult to predict.[11,12] Despite emergent scrotal exploration and detorsion, 32% of testes are nonviable and result in orchiectomy based on a review of the Pediatric Health Information System database.[13] Intraoperatively, the ipsilateral hemiscrotum will be explored and the testis will be identified and the spermatic cord torsion is released. At that time, the affected testis is observed for return of blood flow and wrapped in moist gauze. The contralateral hemiscrotum is then explored and a contralateral scrotal orchidopexy or septopexy is performed. The objective of exploring the contralateral testis and performing a septopexy is to prevent metachronous testicular torsion. If the ipsilateral testis appears healthy, a septopexy is performed. If the affected testis is unable to be salvaged, an orchiectomy is performed.

Hernia/Hydrocele

Infants and children with an inguinal hernia or a hydrocele that changes in volume should be seen within 24 hours and sooner if there is history of inguinal or scrotal pain. Most of these children will need surgical intervention, but a few will require emergent surgery. If there is a history of scrotal or inguinal pain, the child's parents should be taught to recognize the signs of an incarcerated inguinal hernia and instructed to go to the emergency department if symptoms occur before the planned surgical correction. Infants with asymptomatic hydrocele rarely require surgery initially. In most cases, the hydrocele will resolve in the first year of life. An exception should be made if the hydrocele is particularly large or palpable in the inguinal region. A large hydrocele with a palpable inguinal component or one that is enlarging may indicate the presence of an abdominoscrotal hydrocele. These do not spontaneously resolve and usually enlarge. These should be corrected, usually at 6 to 12 months through an initial scrotal incision that will decompress the hydrocele.[14]

Testicular Masses

Testicular masses should be evaluated immediately. Prepubertal testicular and paratesticular tumors should be considered in the differential diagnosis of a scrotal mass.

Although much less common than epididymal cysts or spermatoceles, a complaint of a painless testicular or paratesticular mass should be addressed urgently. A physical examination and scrotal ultrasound should determine if the mass is concerning for neoplasia. Scrotal masses can be transilluminated to determine if the component is primarily fluid, such as a tense hydrocele or solid, such as a testicular tumor. If a firm intratesticular mass is palpated, a thorough examination of the lymph nodes should be performed to evaluate for lymphoma, leukemia, or metastatic disease. Patients with a nontender testicular mass and signs of precocious puberty should be evaluated for a Leydig cell tumor or, less commonly, a Sertoli cell tumor.[15] Epididymal cysts and spermatoceles can present as extratesticular masses but are characteristically smooth, round, and located within the epididymis. A scrotal ultrasound can further differentiate these physical examination findings. Boys with a complaints of a scrotal mass should be assessed by a pediatric urologist urgently due to the rapid growth and malignant potential of many lesions. If the ultrasound or examination are suggestive of a intratesticular or paratesticular mass, tumor markers including beta human chorionic gonadotropin, alpha fetoprotein, and lactate dehydrogenase must be obtained. Additionally, in most instances a CT scan of the abdomen and pelvis with oral and IV contrast is indicated.

In a contemporary series from a tertiary center, the most common prepubertal testis tumor was a teratoma followed by rhabdomyosarcoma, epidermoid cyst, yolk sac tumor, and germ cell tumor, respectively.[16] This histologic distribution was corroborated by a multicenter review including 4 tertiary pediatric hospitals demonstrating that 74% of tumors were benign with 48% teratoma.[17] Testicular tumors occur in the newborn and in early childhood as well as after adolescence. The peak incidence of testicular tumors in young children and infants occurs at age 2. In this population, yolk sac tumors are most common and approximately 75% of tumors are malignant.[18,19] Tumors of nontesticular origin, such as leukemia and lymphoma, must also be considered in the pediatric population.

Varicocele

Varicoceles are uncommon in prepubertal boys and increase in incidence to around 15% by 15 years of age.[20] A physical examination and scrotal ultrasound confirm the diagnosis. From the 3-dimensional measurements on ultrasound, the relative testicular volumes may be calculated and used to guide further treatment.[21] Varicoceles are 90% left-sided and 10% right-sided.[22] Although a left-sided varicocele is not a urological emergency, a right-sided varicocele in the absence of a left-sided varicocele should prompt an evaluation for a retroperitoneal process. If only the right side is involved, there exists a possibility that a retroperitoneal tumor is present and compressing the vein.

MALE PENILE OR URETHRAL SYMPTOMS

Boys with painful priapism must be evaluated immediately. Pain may suggest ischemia of the corporeal bodies, which may progress to corporeal fibrosis if untreated. Children with sickle cell anemia are especially at risk for priapism, with 75% of patients experiencing their first episode by the age of 20 years.[23] Outpatient treatment with penile aspiration and epinephrine irrigation has successfully been used in the treatment of this condition.[24] Patients receiving epinephrine should be observed in a monitored setting because of the risk of cardiac effects.

Paraphimosis also requires immediate attention and manual reduction. In children, this procedure may require some level of sedation. Conversely, phimosis is physiologic in young infants and attempts to manually retract the foreskin in boys less than 2 years of age should be avoided. Phimosis in older children is typically treated with 1 or 2 courses of low-dose steroid cream and circumcision if necessary.[25]

FEMALE GENITAL SYMPTOMS

Infant girls with introital masses commonly present to the pediatric outpatient office. Vaginal masses may be palpable or may protrude from the introitus. The differential diagnosis of these masses includes benign periurethral cysts, skin tags, urethral prolapse, imperforate hymen, prolapsed ureterocele, or rarely, malignancies such as a rhabdomyosarcoma. Bladder outlet obstruction may result from a prolapsed ureterocele. Most of these lesions are differentiated by physical examination, but historical information, such as pain, bleeding, or voiding difficulties help solidify the diagnosis.

Urethral prolapse is relatively common, particularly in young African American females. The prolapse is through the meatus, forming a hemorrhagic, often sensitive mass that bleeds with palpation or when in contact with the underwear. Girls may have difficulty with urination depending on the size of the prolapse and whether it compromises the urethral meatus.

Benign and malignant tumors of the vagina should be considered when vaginal bleeding occurs in young girls. A broad spectrum of entities ranging from capillary hemangioma, rhabdomyosarcoma, or carcinoma may be associated with vaginal bleeding. Labial masses may be associated with hernia or hydrocele of the canal of Nuck.[26]

We evaluate adolescent girls who have not menstruated and in whom there is concern about ureteral or vaginal anomaly. Many of these girls have an imperforate hymen or uterine anomaly that results in poor uterine drainage that may be uncomfortable. If left untreated, retrograde drainage of the uterus may place these patients at risk of endometriosis and infertility.[27] Patients with complete androgen insensitivity can also present with primary amenorrhea. A pelvic ultrasound or magnetic resonance imaging can further delineate the anatomy and guide intervention if necessary.

URINARY TRACT INFECTION

Febrile UTIs in the newborn are treated emergently because newborns are particularly susceptible to significant renal damage if the infection is not treated promptly. A urine culture should be obtained, and these infants require IV antibiotics as early as possible after the urine culture is obtained because they have a higher prevalence of concomitant bacteremia (10%–22%).[28] Appropriate antibiotic therapy administered without delay has been shown to reduce the incidence of renal scarring.[29]

Febrile UTIs in children older than newborns should be treated acutely. Children of all ages with a severe UTI may be subject to renal scarring and should be seen within 24 hours or sooner.[30] Children older than newborns with nonfebrile UTI should be seen semi-urgently. Nearly all children with culture-proven UTI should be evaluated with ultrasound and, if indicated, voiding cystourethrogram (VCUG). Some groups are reevaluating the role of renal nuclear scans in these children.

GROSS HEMATURIA

Gross hematuria in children is less common than microscopic hematuria, with an estimated prevalence of 1.3 per 1000.[31] The most common diagnoses are UTI (26%), perineal irritation (11%), trauma (7%), meatal stenosis with ulceration (7%), coagulation abnormalities (3%), and urinary tract stones (2%). Children with gross hematuria associated with trauma, nephrolithiasis, flank pain, fever, or bladder outlet obstruction should be assessed emergently with abdominal imaging. The most common glomerular causes of gross hematuria in children are poststreptococcal glomerulonephritis and immunoglobulin A (IgA) nephropathy. An antecedent sore throat, pyoderma, edema, or red blood cell casts suggest glomerulonephritis. IgA nephropathy can cause recurrent gross hematuria with flank or abdominal pain and may be preceded by an upper respiratory tract infection.[32] Adenoviral infection, hypercalciuria, and hyperuricosuria are other sources to consider. In the setting of asymptomatic gross hematuria, an ultrasound of the kidneys, ureters, and bladder should be performed, although the yield is low.[33] Contrary to the adult patient, cystoscopic examination in children rarely reveals a cause for hematuria but should be performed when bladder pathology is a consideration.

Gross hematuria in the newborn is an emergency because it may indicate renal venous thrombosis or renal arterial thrombosis. Both may be life-threatening. Renal venous thrombosis affects boys twice as often as girls, with a left-sided predominance. These infants require resuscitation and, occasionally, anticoagulant or operative therapy.[34] Gross hematuria outside the newborn period, although not life-threatening, should be evaluated without delay. Many children have an easy-to-recognize source, such as UTI, urethral prolapse, trauma, and meatal stenosis with ulceration, coagulation abnormalities, or urinary tract stones. Less obvious sources include acute nephritis, ureteropelvic junction obstruction, cystitis cystica, epididymitis, or tumor.[32,35] As with adult patients, a thorough history including a specific description of the color of the urine, the presence of clots, and timing of hematuria, such as terminal hematuria or hematuria on initiation of micturation, should facilitate the diagnostic process. A directed history should include medications, exercise habits, propensity for bleeding diathesis, and a travel history to rule out exposure to infectious diseases such as schistosomiasis or tuberculosis.

RENAL TRAUMA

The pediatric trauma patient usually presents to the emergency department and is evaluated by the emergency medicine and trauma teams often with the assistance of the urology service. Blunt force trauma is the primary mechanism for major renal trauma.[36] The pediatric kidney is particularly susceptible to trauma because of the limited visceral adipose tissue, limited chest wall protection, relatively increased renal size, and increased mobility of the kidney.[37] The mechanism of injury should be determined and a thorough history obtained from the patient and caregivers or observers. Epidemiologic data demonstrate that most renal injuries result from motor vehicle accidents, falls, or high-velocity activities, such as sledding, skiing, all terrain vehicle accidents, and skateboarding.[38,39] Therefore, injuries of this nature should alert the clinician to potential renal damage. The history should include any congenital renal anomalies, such as an ureteropelvic junction obstruction, a solitary kidney, or renal ectopia. Finally, evaluation of associated injuries must be undertaken. Any abdominal injury in a toddler or young child without an antecedent history of blunt force trauma should be evaluated for physical abuse.[40]

Blunt force renal trauma represents a urologic emergency that requires immediate attention but does not necessarily require operative intervention. It is well accepted that low-grade blunt renal injuries are managed conservatively. More recently, the conservative treatment of high-grade blunt renal injuries have been successfully described in children. A consecutive series of 101 patients from The Children's Hospital of Philadelphia with blunt renal injury demonstrated that a nonoperative management strategy was advantageous and successful in 94.7% of pediatric blunt renal injuries.[41] The children with high-grade injuries at risk for failure of conservative management include those with major vascular avulsion or extensive urinary extravasation, especially in the setting of ureteropelvic junction disruptions.[42] These patients require close urological observation and repeated examinations. We recommend conservative management and recognize that a complete evaluation is necessary to accurately determine which patients require further intervention.

Many patients presenting with blunt force renal trauma will have associated extrarenal injuries, such as other solid organ injuries, a pneumothorax, pelvic fractures, and bladder or urethral injuries. Therefore, complete physical examination in trauma patients is essential.[36,38] During examination for renal trauma, the urine should be assessed for gross hematuria. A urethral catheter should be postponed in the setting of gross hematuria until the lower urinary tract is assessed by the urology team.

AMBIGUOUS GENITALIA

Infants with ambiguous genitalia also require immediate evaluation. In the newborn period, all patients require a karyotype and laboratory evaluation by serum electrolytes, 17-OH progesterone, testosterone, luteinizing hormone, and follicle stimulation hormone levels. Once the karyotype is determined, serum analysis will assist in narrowing the differential diagnosis. Noninvasive, quick, and inexpensive, an ultrasound should be the first radiologic examination obtained. Although only 50% accurate in detecting intra-abdominal testes, ultrasound can detect gonads in the inguinal region and can assess Müllerian structures.[43] Although more expensive, magnetic resonance imaging scan can further delineate the anatomy. Because congenital adrenal hyperplasia (CAH) may result in salt wasting, which can be life-threatening, infants with ambiguous genitalia must be evaluated quickly and stabilized.[44] If CAH is suspected, the infant should not be discharged home from the nursery before appropriate testing is complete. In some cases, a genotypic female neonate with CAH may be incorrectly identified as a male neonate. The correct diagnosis should be made as quickly as possible to establish the appropriate sex of rearing. A history of a discordant karyotype from an amniocentesis and infant phenotype should prompt an evaluation. The parents should be asked about a family history of infertility, amenorrhea, and infant mortality. The complete evaluation of infants with ambiguous genitalia should include urology, neonatology, endocrinology, genetics, and psychology.

ANTENATAL HYDRONEPHROSIS

In neonates with prenatally detected hydronephrosis and a normal bladder, the postnatal evaluation of the hydronephrosis should begin within the first few days of life. If the postnatal renal and bladder ultrasound demonstrates bilateral hydronephrosis, a solitary kidney, or a thickened bladder wall, the child should be evaluated in the newborn nursery. The infant must be thriving and have normal electrolytes and normal blood urea nitrogen and creatinine levels before discharge home.

The postnatal history should also include the sex of the infant, laterality of the hydronephrosis, the level of obstruction (ie, ureteropelvic junction [UPJ], ureterovesical junction [UVJ], urethra), the presence or absence of oligohydraminos, and any other associated anomalies. The additional tests to be scheduled include a repeat ultrasound, a renal scan, or a VCUG to evaluate the relative drainage and percentage of function of the kidneys, as well as to evaluate for vesicoureteral reflux. Until this postnatal evaluation is completed, most infants are maintained on amoxicillin prophylaxis. The differential diagnosis for antenatal hydronephrosis most commonly includes UPJ obstruction, vesicoureteral reflux, ectopic ureter, ureterocele, megaureter (UVJ obstruction), multicystic dysplastic kidney, posterior urethral valves, prune belly syndrome, and megacystis microcolon syndrome.

Certain conditions require more immediate intervention, especially when bladder outlet obstruction is present. If posterior urethral valves are considered, the bladder should be drained with a feeding tube and a VCUG performed at an appropriate interval. Conversely, if prune belly syndrome is considered, urethral catheterization should be avoided if possible to minimize the risk of UTI. Additionally, a ureterocele may obstruct the bladder outlet and result in bilateral upper tract dilation. This situation can be ameliorated by placement of a urinary catheter.

CONGENITAL ANOMALIES IN THE NEONATE

Patients with major abdominal defects, such as bladder or cloacal exstrophy, require direct admission to the neonatal nursery for stabilization and surgical planning. In many cases, a team is assembled and provides orthopedic, general surgical, and urologic care during the surgery.[45] Patients with imperforate anus and variants, such as a cloacal anomaly, require decompression of the intestinal tract, usually within the first 24 to 48 hours.[46] At the time of the colostomy, the urologist may evaluate the perineum and perform endoscopy to further assess the urinary anomalies. In bladder exstrophy, the posterior bladder wall is visible through a midline defect in the abdominal wall and a pubic diastasis is appreciated. In addition, a bifid clitoris or epispadias is present. In cloacal exstrophy, an omphalocele is superior to the cecal plate and lateral bladder halves with prolapsed ileum typically in the midline. Additionally, a bifid clitoris or penis, imperforate anus, and spinal abnormalities are present. Procedures to correct these major defects must be planned by surgeons who are familiar with the potential risks and complications associated with the reconstruction of the urethra, vagina, and colon. The anesthesia team must be skillful in the management of the complex metabolic changes that may occur in infants who are under anesthesia for long periods. The neonatologists must be expert in the management of infants who have undergone major surgical procedures.

Currently, most spinal dysraphisms in children are diagnosed antenatally.[47] These infants are referred by direct admission to the neonatal intensive care nursery. Most of these children are not in urinary retention initially, but many develop spinal shock after neurosurgery in the newborn period and have a transient period of overflow urinary drainage. As soon as possible after closure of the spinal defect, a baseline renal and bladder ultrasound is performed to evaluate for evidence of bladder or upper tract abnormalities. If the newborn is not voiding spontaneously or has elevated post-void residual volumes, clean intermittent catheterization should be initiated. Initial urodynamics investigation is performed after resolution of the spinal shock to ensure that bladder storage pressures are not excessive.[48,49] High-risk infants (those with a detrusor leak-point pressure greater than 40 cm H_2O or detrusor-sphincter dyssynergia) are started on anticholinergic therapy and intermittent catheterization.[50]

Emergent urological conditions occur in every age group and involve the entire genitourinary tract. Many acute signs and symptoms are not unique to genitourinary etiologies and a broad differential diagnosis should be considered. A thorough understanding of emergent urological conditions results in efficient assessment and management.

REFERENCES

1. Park JW. Fever without source in children: recommendations for outpatient care in those up to 3. Postgrad Med 2000;107:259–62, 265–6.
2. Chandler JC, Gauderer MW. The neonate with an abdominal mass. Pediatr Clin North Am 2004;51:979–97.

3. Golden CB, Feusner JH. Malignant abdominal masses in children: quick guide to evaluation and diagnosis. Pediatr Clin North Am 2002;49:1369–92.
4. Pinto E, Guignard JP. Renal masses in the neonate. Biol Neonate 1995;68: 175–84.
5. Walther PC, Lamm D, Kaplan GW. Pediatric urolithiases: a ten-year review. Pediatrics 1980;65:1068–72.
6. Milliner DS, Murphy ME. Urolithiasis in pediatric patients. Mayo Clin Proc 1993; 68:241–8.
7. Mohamed J, Riadh M, Abdellatif N. Urolithiasis in infants. Pediatr Surg Int 2007; 23:295–9.
8. Fowler KA, Locken JA, Duchesne JH, et al. US for detecting renal calculi with nonenhanced CT as a reference standard. Radiology 2002;222:109–13.
9. Zhao LC, Lautz TB, Meeks JJ, et al. Pediatric testicular torsion epidemiology using a national database: incidence, risk of orchiectomy and possible measures toward improving the quality of care. J Urol 2011;186(5):2009–13.
10. Gatti JM, Murphy JP. Current management of the acute scrotum. Semin Pediatr Surg 2007;16:58.
11. Bartsch G, Frank S, Marberger H, et al. Testicular torsion: late results with special regard to fertility and endocrine function. J Urol 1980;124(3):375.
12. Beard CM, Benson RC Jr, Kelalis PP, et al. The incidence and outcome of mumps orchitis in Rochester, Minnesota, 1935 to 1974. Mayo Clin Proc 1977;52(1):3.
13. Cost NG, Bush NC, Barber TD, et al. Pediatric testicular torsion: demographics of national orchiopexy versus orchiectomy rates. J Urol 2011;185(Suppl 6): 2459–63.
14. Belman AB. Abdominoscrotal hydrocele in infancy: a review and presentation of the scrotal approach for correction. J Urol 2001;165:225–7.
15. Agarwal PK, Palmer JS. Testicular and paratesticular neoplasms in prepubertal males. J Urol 2006;176:875.
16. Metcalfe PD, Farivar-Mohseni H, Farhat W, et al. Pediatric testicular tumors: contemporary incidence and efficacy of testicular preserving surgery. J Urol 2003;170:2412.
17. Pohl HG, Shukla AR, Metcalfe PD, et al. Prepubertal testis tumors: actual prevalence rate of histological types. J Urol 2004;172:2370.
18. Levy DA, Kay R, Elder JS. Neonatal testis tumors: a review of the Prepubertal Testis Tumor Registry. J Urol 1994;151:715–7.
19. Ciftci AO, Bingol-Kologlu M, Senocak ME, et al. Testicular tumors in children. J Pediatr Surg 2001;36:1796–801.
20. Schiff J, Kelly C, Goldstein M, et al. Managing varicoceles in children: results with microsurgical varicocelectomy. BJU Int 2005;95:399–402.
21. Diamond DA, Paltiel HJ, DiCanzio J, et al. Comparative assessment of pediatric testicular volume: orchidometer versus ultrasound. J Urol 2000;164:1111–4.
22. MacLellan DL, Diamond DA. Recent advances in external genitalia. Pediatr Clin North Am 2006;53:449.
23. Adeyoju AB, Olujohungbe AB, Yardumian A, et al. Priapism in sickle-cell disease: incidence, risk factors and complications—an international multicentre study. BJU Int 2002;90:898–902.
24. Mantadakis E, Canvender JD, Rogers ZR, et al. Prevalence of priapism in children and adolescents with sickle cell anemia. J Pediatr Hematol Oncol 1999; 21:518–22.
25. Ashfield JE, Nickel KR, Siemens DR, et al. Treatment of phimosis with topical steroids in 194 children. J Urol 2003;169(3):1106.

26. Kizer JR, Bellah RD, Schnaufer L, et al. Meconium hydrocele in a female newborn: an unusual cause of a labial mass. J Urol 1995;153:188–90.
27. Rock JA, Zacur HA, Dlugi AM, et al. Pregnancy success following surgical correction of imperforate hymen and complete transverse vaginal septum. Obstet Gynecol 1982;59:448–51.
28. Pitetti RD, Choi S. Utility of blood cultures in febrile children with UTI. Am J Emerg Med 2002;20:271–4.
29. Ransley PG, Risdon RA. Reflux nephropathy: effects of antimicrobial therapy on the evolution of the early pyelonephritic scar. Kidney Int 1981;20:733–42.
30. van der Voort J, Edwards A, Roberts R, et al. The struggle to diagnose UTI in children under two in primary care. Fam Pract 1997;14:44–8.
31. Ingelfinger JR, Davis AE, Grupe WE. Frequency and etiology of gross hematuria in a general pediatric setting. Pediatrics 1977;59:557–61.
32. Meyers KE. Evaluation of hematuria in children. Urol Clin North Am 2004;31: 559–73.
33. Fernbach SK. The dilated urinary tract in children. Urol Radiol 1992;14:34–42.
34. Kuhle S, Massicotte P, Chan A, et al. A case series of 72 neonates with renal vein thrombosis: data from the 1-800-NO-CLOTS Registry. Thromb Haemost 2004;92: 729–33.
35. Diven SC, Travis LB. A practical primary care approach to hematuria in children. Pediatr Nephrol 2000;14:65–72.
36. Mohamed AZ, Morsi HA, Ziada AM, et al. Management of major blunt pediatric renal trauma: single center experience. J Pediatr Urol 2010;6(3):301–5.
37. Brown SL, Elder JS, Spirnak JP. Are pediatric patients more susceptible to major renal injury from blunt trauma? A comparative study. J Urol 1998;160:138.
38. Margenthaler JA, Weber TR, Keller MS. Blunt renal trauma in children: experience with conservative management at a pediatric trauma center. J Trauma 2002; 52(5):928.
39. Rogers CG, Knight V, Macura KJ, et al. High-grade renal injuries in children: is conservative management possible? Urology 2004;64(3):574.
40. Barnes PM, Norton CM, Dunstan FD, et al. Abdominal injury due to child abuse. Lancet 2005;366:234.
41. Nance ML, Lutz N, Carr MC, et al. Blunt renal injuries in children can be managed nonoperatively: outcome in a consecutive series of patients. J Trauma 2004;57: 474.
42. Henderson CG, Sedberry-Ross S, Pickard R, et al. Management of high grade renal trauma: 20 year experience at a pediatric level I trauma center. J Urol 2007;178:246.
43. Kolon TF. Intersex. In: Schwartz MW, editor. The 5-minute pediatric consult. New York: Lippincott, Williams & Wilkins; 2003. p. 480–1.
44. Forest MG. Recent advances in the diagnosis and management of congenital adrenal hyperplasia due to 21-hydroxylase deficiency. Hum Reprod Update 2004;10:469–85.
45. Gearhart JP. Bladder exstrophy: staged reconstruction [review]. Curr Opin Urol 1999;9:499–506.
46. Chen CJ. The treatment of imperforate anus: experience with 108 patients. J Pediatr Surg 1999;34:1728–32.
47. Babcook CJ, Goldstein RB, Filly RA. Prenatally detected fetal myelomeningocele: is karyotype analysis warranted? Radiology 1995;194:491–4.
48. McGuire EJ, Diddel G, Wagner F. Balanced bladder function in spinal cord injury patients. J Urol 1977;118:626–8.

49. Bauer SB. The challenge of the expanding role of urodynamic studies in the treatment of children with neurological and functional disabilities [editorial; comment]. J Urol 1998;160:527–8.

50. Snodgrass WT, Adams R. Initial urologic management of myelomeningocele. Urol Clin North Am 2004;31:427–34.

Circumcision Controversies

Kirk Pinto, MD

KEYWORDS

- Circumcision • Informed consent • Phimosis • Neonatal

KEY POINTS

- The fate of neonatal circumcision is as obscure as its origin. Despite the exhaustive research on this subject, the lack of consensus calls for even more unbiased study.
- If medical research does not answer ongoing questions regarding neonatal circumcision, clinicians should be aware of the sobering reality that there are legal and socioeconomic forces marshaling, which are eager to answer these questions for us.
- The controversies surrounding neonatal circumcision behooves individual clinicians to be knowledgeable of the history of the procedure, to be aware of the details of the procedure, to keep abreast of new findings on the subject, and to decide for themselves a defensible opinion (pro, con, or neutral) so that they can provide honest, and most importantly, competent care of their patients.

INTRODUCTION

Circumcision, in the simplest terms, is "... the removal of the prepuce of a male."[1] Beyond this basic definition nearly every aspect of circumcision from its origin to its indications, and with whom the responsibility for consent for this operation truly lays, contains some aspect of controversy.

Most newborns in this country are circumcised and there is little disagreement about the technical aspects of this common procedure. There have been volumes written on the potential harms and benefits of circumcision. The American Academy of Pediatrics, to whom many look to for guidance in the treatment of children, have traditionally taken a noncommittal stance on this matter.[2] In the modern political environment in the United States, the newest controversies surrounding circumcision exist in the legal and socioeconomic arenas.

Although sober proponents and detractors of circumcision agree that there is no overwhelming medical evidence to support either side, there is considerable disagreement regarding parents consenting to a nonemergency prophylactic procedure in their minor children. Also, at a time when the cost of health care has become a national issue, many question the government funding for these procedures because there

Urology Associates of North Texas and Cook Children's Hospital, 1325 Pennsylvania Avenue #550, Fort Worth, TX 76104, USA
E-mail address: Kpinto@UANT.com

Pediatr Clin N Am 59 (2012) 977–986
doi:10.1016/j.pcl.2012.05.015
0031-3955/12/$ – see front matter © 2012 Elsevier Inc. All rights reserved.

pediatric.theclinics.com

is no overwhelming proof that they are beneficial, necessary, or the only method to achieve the desired goals.

Although there are accepted reasons for circumcision in adults, in the United States, most circumcisions are done on neonates, which is the most discussed and controversial procedure. This article examines neonatal circumcision and the difficult problems surrounding this seemingly simple procedure.

HISTORY

Adequate knowledge of all aspects of the procedure is essential for the health care providers who advise parents about their child's potential circumcision so they can provide comprehensive information to help with this important decision. Circumcision is one of the oldest and one of the most commonly performed operations, even in contemporary medicine. The origin of this procedure dates back millennia and there is some controversy, along with a fascination, as to where and how it actually began.

Although most are familiar with the Jewish and Muslim traditions, circumcision is practiced in many societies from all over the globe. Throughout history, men in societies in Africa, Australia, the Americas, and other parts of the world have been circumcised with no connection to a Muslim or Jewish faith. Much research has gone into the origins of these rituals and how they evolved, but in most cases no written history can pinpoint the origin or reason for these often elaborate rituals.

There are some historical records of circumcision. The first recorded history of circumcision is from ancient Egypt, where wall paintings in Egyptian tombs depict the operation. Also, studies of mummies from nearly 4000 years ago show that they were circumcised.[3,4] Researchers have surmised that circumcisions may have been performed to help break a young child's bond with his mother or, in older boys, to initiate the young men fully into the tribe. Circumcision has been used as a less lethal and morbid way for oppressors to mark and humiliate enslaved men. Also, from antiquity to the nineteenth century, circumcision was thought of as a way to stanch the emerging sexual desires of young men. The existence of so many rites in so many places proves that circumcision has no single origin.

The Jewish tradition of circumcision is the most familiar, iconic, and well documented. Although it is hypothesized that the practice may have originated with the mutilation of Jewish slaves to demonstrate the hegemony of their masters, the tradition begins with Abraham in the Old Testament (Genesis 17:23). Within Judaism, there has always been some minor controversy as to the necessity of circumcision; however, more recently, there have been external forces attempting to limit the Jewish practice.[5] For example, in San Francisco, there was a resolution entertained to ban circumcision, even for religious reasons, within the city limits.[6]

Muslims, too, have a long tradition of circumcision also dating from the same covenant between God and Abraham. Muhammad, the Muslim prophet, was circumcised. Unlike the Jewish tradition, which requires circumcision for inclusion in the faith, circumcision is not necessary to be a Muslim because it is never mentioned in the Qur'an. Although circumcision is considered a strong tradition (*sunnah*) for men, circumcision in women, practiced by Muslims in some parts of the world, is considered less of a tradition (*makrumah*) in the Muslim faith but has engendered great concern in the West. The United States government enacted The Female Genital Mutilation act to criminalize the practice.[4,7]

For Christians, who make up the majority of Americans, circumcision holds no particular religious significance. Christians were excused from the circumcision covenant in many New Testament verses; Romans (2: 28–29) and Galatians (5:6) among them. Despite this exclusion, more than 1.2 million circumcisions were performed in the United States in 2005, indicating that religious tradition is not the biggest driver in a family's decision.[8]

Beyond the religious history of circumcision, there is a transition, mostly in the late nineteenth and early twentieth century, of this religious practice into a medical procedure. The first serious medical discussions of circumcision were directed toward phimosis and other foreskin problems associated with sexually transmitted diseases. Medicine was a fledgling specialty at this time and medical knowledge was rapidly expanding, although not always in beneficial directions. In America, Dr Lewis Sayer, a nineteenth century orthopedic surgeon, became a strong champion of circumcision after he used either amputation or manipulation of the foreskin to cure young male patients with paralysis. Dr Sayer was an influential physician and his support of circumcision encouraged others to expand the indications for the procedure. On both sides of the Atlantic, circumcision soon became a treatment of impotence, masturbation, bedwetting, night terrors, and even homosexuality.[3,4,9,10]

As medical knowledge advanced, so did surgical technique. Beyond better techniques, 2 developments in the late nineteenth century made newborn circumcision possible. First, better anesthesia and analgesia made procedures on younger patients safer. Second, the acceptance of germ theory prompted physicians to suspect the moist environment under the foreskin as a breeding ground for future pathologic conditions. If the foreskin caused significant problems in adults, the reasoning went, then earlier circumcision would prevent those problems all together.[3,4] Modern advocates of circumcision continue to use this notion, the prevention of further problems, as their primary argument, although they wish to prevent different pathologies than prior proponents. The central controversy surrounding circumcision is the question as to whether this prevention is medically, financially, or morally justified.

INDICATIONS

Patients with true phimosis, balanitis, noniatrogenic paraphimosis, and localized pathologic conditions of the foreskin (warts for example) are accepted as candidates for circumcision, and it is also accepted that these conditions are not present in the newborn. Rickwood[11] says a generous estimate would be that less than 2.5% of newborns would require circumcision based on these criteria. Newborn circumcision is motivated by the prevention of these problems during a period when the operation is purportedly cheaper, safer, and easier. The counter-argument from a medical standpoint is that operating on many healthy boys to relieve potential problems is not preferable to operating on the few boys who might actually develop those problems when they are adults and have demonstrable improvement from surgery.

PHIMOSIS AND URINARY TRACT INFECTION

Phimosis is a pathologic condition in which the patient's foreskin is not retractable. This condition is painful and can cause the foreskin to balloon during urination, hurt during erection, and lead to urinary tract infection (UTI). In adults, this condition is effectively treated with circumcision. Men are born with a physiologic phimosis in that, in most, the foreskin does not easily retract at birth. This condition is usually asymptomatic and resolves as the boy ages, and most boys by puberty will have a retractable foreskin. If the foreskin does become symptomatic, boys are candidates for circumcision.[11] Topical steroids have also been used in the treatment of pathologic phimosis with success in most patients.[12]

Boys with foreskin, whether or not true phimosis is present, have an increased incidence of UTI, especially in the first months of life. Wiswell[13] followed up a large number of boys born at military hospitals and showed a dramatic difference in the rate of infection between boys who were circumcised and uncircumcised and in the morbidity and mortality between the groups. Wiswell found that the circumcised boys had few complications from the removal of their foreskin, whereas the uncircumcised group had UTI's, hospitalizations, as well as 2 deaths and concluded that routine circumcision seemed justified and medically prudent.[13] More recently, Spach and colleagues[14] showed that a foreskin may predispose young adults to infection.

Opponents of this approach, correctly point out that most problems Dr Wiswell found were easily treated with antibiotics that death was rare, and that 98 boys would have to undergo circumcision to prevent just 2 urinary infections.[15,16] They advocate treating only the boys who have demonstrable foreskin-related pathologic conditions.

COST

Medical cost has become an enormous concern in American society. The United States spends between $150 and $200 million per year to perform newborn circumcisions.[2] The true measures of costs are difficult to assess because the complications of having foreskin are a small but a life-long risk. Compared with other medical interventions, including circumcision under anesthesia, neonatal circumcision is relatively inexpensive. Schoen and colleagues[17] compared the costs of circumcising newborns and the life-long medical expenses associated with having foreskin, and concluded that circumcision was justified on financial and medical grounds.

The rate of newborn circumcision seems affected by a patient's insurance status.[18] Leibowitz and collesgues[18] found that newborns on Medicaid were significantly less likely to be circumcised in states where Medicaid no longer funded the procedure although other, more limited studies found no such link.[18,19] At present, 15 states have stopped the funding for newborn circumcision and 2 states have variable coverage.[20] As Medicaid currently covers about 40% of births in the United States, the financial aspects of circumcision may become more predictive of its future than the medical ones.[21]

Proponents of newborn circumcision state that the newborn procedure is less expensive in the long run. Newborn circumcision reduces expenditures on the up to 10% of patients who may require later circumcision. There is also mounting evidence that HIV, syphilis, and other sexually transmitted diseases, in both men and women, can be prevented or reduced by circumcision along with their attendant costs of treatment.[22,23] Advocates of circumcision maintain an unintended consequence of circumcision being culled from the government payment plans will be a disproportional risk and burden on the poor who will not be able to afford this valuable prophylaxis.[24]

Opponents of newborn circumcision would be correct to point out that most of these problems could be prevented with changes in life-style. They also propose that elective circumcision should only be done on men of an age to consent to the removal of their foreskin. Opponents are adamant that the monetary costs of this procedure are not fungible with the harm circumcision causes.[25]

PARENTAL CONCERNS

Although it is laudable to pursue the scientific and economic truths, most parents decide on the newborn circumcision without strong information about its benefits or risks. Bean and Egelhoff[26] found that most parents had decided the fate of their child's foreskin before the boy's birth. Most parents and physicians believe that the discussion they have with their physician about the circumcision after birth is unbiased.

The reasons parents cite to circumcise their child are their wish that the child look like his father, their wish that he be like other boys, cleanliness, or their fears of sexual rejection later in life as being more important than any medical indications. Despite parental concerns, most of these issues are not critically germane. There is evidence that young men are not always aware of their own circumcision status. Conflicting evidence exists as to the effects neonatal circumcision has on a man's psychological well-being as well as his personal and sexual relationships in adulthood.[26–30] Opponents of circumcision argue that, these concerns could be addressed later when a child's own wishes could be considered.

HEALTH CONCERNS

Another proffered reason to circumcise newborns is the prevention of penile cancer and other penile maladies. There has been renewed interest in circumcision in places where it has not traditionally been performed because of the research into this particular aspect of circumcision. Cancer of the penis is a rare but serious condition, and in 2011, there were 1360 new reported cases in the United States,[31] where most men affected are uncircumcised, and the majority die from the disease.[32,33] Although circumcision status is a risk factor for penile cancer, it is not the only factor. Some countries, without a tradition of circumcision, also have very low and falling rates of penile cancer. This decline may be associated with an increased socioeconomic status, better hygiene, marital status, and possibly other lifestyle issues that may or may not make circumcision the only method of prevention for this disease.[34]

As HIV continues to take its toll around the world, the medical community has searched desperately for ways to stanch the morbidity and mortality of this tragic epidemic. Circumcision, in adult men, has been shown to be protective against the spread of the disease in Africa, in areas where education has not been as effective.[35] Similar to HIV, other sexually transmitted diseases seem to affect circumcised men less frequently than men who remain intact.[36] The behavior of these men has much to do with these infections. Critics of circumcision argue that perhaps greater attempts could be made to alter these adult behaviors or, failing that, circumcision could be performed on these adult men in lieu of condoning the removal of the foreskin of a baby.

TECHNIQUES

Although there is considerable discussion about whether circumcision should be performed, there is little controversy as to how. The 3 main methods of circumcision performed in the United States, namely Plastibell, Gomco, and Mogen, all have their proponents. Each method, by a competent operator, has an acceptably low complication rate. The last controversy over technique is the use of anesthesia. There was a belief, now disproven and abandoned, that newborns did not feel pain and that it was inconsequential to them. Circumcision, by whatever device, should be performed with local anesthesia.[2,37]

CONSENT

There is an honest disagreement in the medical community about the medical risks and benefits of circumcision, and there is accumulating evidence that circumcision may benefit the individual over their life time. This growing surety must be tempered by the fact that, barely a century ago, physicians were sure that this same procedure was a cure for a variety of postulated ills, such as masturbation and bedwetting. These views have been discredited. Even in those instances in which contemporary wisdom says that circumcision is helpful, there is little incontrovertible evidence that circumcision needs to be done on newborns. No medical association in the western world condones routine neonatal circumcision.[38]

The medical merits of circumcision are not the only argument surrounding this procedure. Ethicists, lawyers, philosophers, and members of anti-circumcision groups also have concerns about the legal and moral issues surrounding the operation. The question of what informed consent is for newborn circumcision, and who, if anyone, is truly capable of consenting for the child when no real medical issue exists are matters of significant disagreement.

In any operation, the consent of the patient is paramount. In the Unites States the performance of a medical procedure (absent a life-threatening emergency) without the patient's consent, is battery. Informed consent includes the physician's duty to disclose to the patient what reasonable people would need to know about a procedure to make an informed decision, the patient's understanding of the information being presented, and the patient's freedom to come to a decision without undue external influence.[38]

PARENTAL ROLE

A newborn does not understand the complexities of any procedure and so, as in many decisions that involve children, the duty falls to the parents. There are no valid arguments against a parent's rights to consent to procedures if the operation is life saving, life sustaining, or of undeniable benefit to the patient.[39,40] Parents who make medical decisions for their children are doing so under the concept of substituted judgment; the idea that the person making the decision for the patient will do so as the incompetent patient would have, were they able. In cases of circumcision, the parent is consenting to the procedure because they conclude it is what the boy would want faced with the same decision. There is case law, however, that says that children are not simply the chattel of their parents. Courts have stopped parents from unfettered consent on the behalf of the child in other medical scenarios: children have been forbidden from being tissue donors for their siblings because the procedure was of no medical benefit to them personally. Further, men who are medically competent rarely volunteer for elective circumcision, suggesting that most American parents may be coming to the wrong conclusion about their boy's future wishes about his foreskin.[38]

There are serious questions as to whether parents even have any standing here. If newborn circumcision is a cosmetic procedure, mutilative or psychologically harmful, and not the beneficent safe procedure advocates claim, are the parents acting in the best interest of the child?[41] Parents can consent for immunizations, so there is precedence for allowing invasive procedures based on future benefits. The benefits of immunizations are less controversial than those of circumcision, however. An evenhanded presentation by the clinician actually has been shown to have little effect on the parents' ultimate decision. Despite this frustration, practitioners should not dismiss the cultural and social reasons that parents cite in their decision. These beliefs are often as important than any list of complications a practitioner provides.[22,42,43] The solution to these legal and moral questions is mired in the deadlocked medical opinions of the worth of this operation. If there were unanimity, these other issues could be more easily resolved.

HEALTH CARE PROVIDER'S ROLE

As the technique of circumcision has been refined and made safer, acquiring an informed consent may be the most difficult role for the practitioner in this process.

The doctor has to ensure that the parents of the patient understand the reasons why their child should or should not be circumcised, how the procedure will be performed, and what the short-term and long-term consequences might be. Physicians are obligated to ensure that this information is presented in a way the parents can comprehend, and then be sure the parents are not pressured toward any decision.[38]

Proponents of circumcision argue that this consultation should include a discussion of how removal of the foreskin in the infant provides the boy with life-long protection against UTI's, sexually transmitted diseases (including HIV), and penile cancer. Further, they believe neonatal circumcision benefits society as a whole not simply because it curbs these ills,but because when done at this young age, it is without significant morbidity, has negligible mortality, and is cheaper than doing the same procedure on older boys.[44,45]

Opponents of newborn circumcision argue that the loss of foreskin during circumcision, in itself, is an irreversible and unnecessary harm and that parents cannot consent to procedures that do not benefit their child. They say that most of the purported medical benefits of circumcision can be mitigated by other methods (eg, antibiotics for infections) that don't require circumcision. They believe circumcision should be performed under similar circumstances to other invasive procedures, at the time of demonstrable pathologic conditions. In their view, elective circumcision should be done only with the consent of the patient and that this later circumcision, if it is performed at all, provides the same health benefits without the ugsome assault on a helpless newborn. The circumcised child, they say, has a normal penis at birth and is potentially exposed to complications and possible lifelong deformities from these complications without medical or moral justification. The costs, detractors say, are not only monetary.[38]

In most instances of surgery on children, the physician presents to the family what is believed to be the medical truth based on the facts at hand and the accumulated medical knowledge of what is prudent in these circumstances. The lack of consensus in the medical community about circumcision places practitioners in a precarious position. If a clinician sincerely feels as though circumcision isn't indicated, should they perform it at the parent's behest? Conversely, if a clinician feels neonatal circumcision is indicated, should they pursue legal action against parent who decline circumcision? Finally, and most probably, if a physician is truly ambivalent about the necessity of circumcision is it disingenuous or greedy for them to perform a procedure they do not recommend?

SUMMARY

The ultimate fate of neonatal circumcision is as obscure as its origin. Despite the exhaustive research on this fascinating subject, the lack of consensus calls for even more unbiased study. If medical research does not answer the outstanding questions about circumcision, clinicians should be aware of the sobering reality that there are legal and socioeconomic forces marshaling eager to answer these questions for us. Competent provision of neonatal circumcision behooves individual clinicians to be knowledgeable of the history of the procedure, to be aware of the details of the procedure, to keep abreast of new findings on the subject, to safely perform the operation and to decide for themselves a defensible opinion (pro, con, or neutral), so that they can provide honest, and most importantly, competent care of their patients. No matter the ultimate outcome of this debate, there can be no arguing with physicians who are earnestly trying to do the best for their patients.

REFERENCES

1. Random house unabridged dictionary. 2nd edition. New York: Random House; 1993.
2. American Academy of Pediatrics, Task force on circumcision. Circumcision Policy Statement. Pediatrics 1999;103:686–93.
3. Dunsmuir WD, Gordon EM. The history of circumcision. BJU Int 1999;83(Suppl 1):1–12.
4. Gollaher DL. Circumcision: a history of the world's most controversial surgery. New York: Basic Books; 2000.
5. Goodman J. Jewish circumcision: an alternative perspective. BJU Int 1999; 83(Suppl 1):22–7.
6. Cohen A. San Francisco circumcision ban: an attack on religious freedom? In: time, 2011. Available at: http://www.time.com/time/nation/article/0.8599.2077240.html. Accessed December 17, 2011.
7. United States Crimes and criminal procedure code 1996 - Pub. L. 104-208, div. C, title VI, Sec. 645(b)(2), Sept. 30, 1996, 110 Stat. 3009-709, item 116. Available at: http://uscode.house.gov/download/pls/18C7.txt. Accessed January 3, 2012.
8. Merrill CT, Nagamine M, Steiner C. Circumcisions performed in U.S. Community hospitals, 2005. HCUP statistical brief #45. Rockville (MD): Agency for Healthcare Research and Quality; 2008. Available at: http://www.hcup-us.ahrq.gov/reports/statbriefs/sb45.pdf. Accessed January 8, 2012.
9. Martin E, Thomas BA, Moorhead SW. Surgery of the penis. Chapter 9. In: White and Martin's Genitourinary Surgery and Venereal Disease. 10th edition. London: J.B. Lippincott; 1917. p. 99–102.
10. Remondino PC. General systemic diseases induced by the prepuce. Chapter XXV. In: History of circumcision from the earliest times to the present. Philadelphia: F. Davies Co; 1900. p. 284–301.
11. Rickwood AM. Medical indications for circumcision. BJU Int 1999;83(Suppl 1):45–51.
12. Webster TM, Leonard MP. Topical steroid therapy for phimosis. Can J Urol 2002; 9(2):1492–5.
13. Wiswell TE, Geschke D. Risk from circumcision during the first month of life compared to uncircumcised boys. Pediatrics 1989;83:1011–5.
14. Spach DH, Stapleton AE, Stam WE. Lack of circumcision increases the risk of urinary tract infection in young men. JAMA 1992;267:569–81.
15. Enzenauer RW. Circumcision: needless risks, no medical benefits. RN 1983;46: 99–100.
16. Harkavy KL. The circumcision debate (letters to the editor). Pediatrics 1987;79: 649–50.
17. Schoen EJ, Colby CJ, To TT. Cost analysis of neonatal circumcision in a large health maintenance organization. J Urol 2006;175:1111–5.
18. Leibowitz AA, Desmond K, Belin T. Determinants and policy implications of male circumcision in the United States. Am J Public Health 2009;99:138–45.
19. Quayle SS, Coplen DE, Austin PF. The effect of health care coverage on circumcision rates among newborns. J Urol 2003;170:1533–6.
20. Centers for Disease Control and Prevention. "Trends in in-hospital newborn male circumcision –– United States, 1999–2010." Morbidity and mortality weekly report. Available at: http://www.cdc.gov/mmwr/preview/mmwrhtml/mm6034a4.htm?s_cid=mm6034a4_w. Accessed January 5, 2012.
21. StateMaster.com, iBrths financed by medicaid as percent of state births (most recent) by state. 2011. Available at: http://www.statemaster.com/graph/hea_as_per_of_sta_bir-births-financed-medicaid-percent-state. Accessed January 7, 2012.

22. Bailey RC, Moses S, Parker CB, et al. Male circumcision for HIV prevention in young men in Kisumu, Kenya: a randomized controlled trial. Lancet 2007;369: 643–56.

23. Tobian A, Gray RH, Quinn TC. Male circumcision for the prevention of acquisition and transmission of sexually transmitted infections: the case for neonatal circumcision. Arch Pediatr Adolesc Med 2010;164:78–84.

24. Morris BJ, Bailis SA, Waskett AH, et al. Medicaid coverage of newborn circumcision: a health parity right of the poor. Am J Public Health 2009; 99(6):969–71.

25. Green LW, McAllister RG, Peterson KW, et al. Medicaid coverage of circumcision spreads harm to the poor. Am J Public Health 2009;99:584.

26. Bean G, Egelhoff C. Neonatal circumcision; when is the decision made? J Fam Pract 1984;18:883–7.

27. Riser JM, Wiser WL, Eissa MA, et al. Self-assessment of circumcision status by adolescents. Am J Epidemiol 2004;159:1095–7.

28. Hammond T. A preliminary poll of men circumcised in infancy or childhood. BJU Int 1999;83(Suppl 1):85–92.

29. Williamson ML, Williamson PS. Women's preferences for penile circumcision in sexual partners. J Sex Educ Ther 1988;14:8–12.

30. Tiemstra JD. Factors affecting the circumcision decision. J Am Board Fam Pract 1999;12:16–20.

31. American Cancer Society. Estimated new cancer cases and deaths by site for all sites. US 2011-Cancer facts and figures. 2011. Available at: http://www.cancer. org/acs/groups/content/@epidemiologysurveilance/documents/document/acspc-029771.pdf. Accessed January 8, 2012.

32. Wisewell TE. Routine neonatal circumcision: a reappraisal. Am Fam Physician 1990;41:859–63.

33. Morris BJ, Gray RH, Castellsague X, et al. The strong protective effect of circumcision against cancer of the penis. In: Advances in urology. Avaiable at: http://www.hindawi.com/journals/au/2011/812368/cta/. Accessed January 8, 2012.

34. Frisch M, Friis S, Kruger KS, et al. Falling incidence of penis cancer in an uncircumcised population (Denmark 1943–1990). Br Med J 1995;311:1471.

35. Wamai RG, Weiss HA, Hankins C, et al. Male circumcision is an efficacious, lasting and cost-effective strategy for combating HIV in high-prevalence AIDS epidemics. Futur HIV Ther 2008;2:399–405.

36. Weiss HA, Thomas SL, Munabi SK, et al. Male circumcision and risk of syphilis, chancroid and genital herpes: a systemic review and meta-analysis. Sex Transm Infect 2006;82:101.

37. Taddi A, Katz J, Ilersich AL, et al. Effect of neonatal circumcision on pain response during subsequent routine vaccination. Lancet 1997;349:599–603.

38. Svoboda JS, Van Howe RS, Dwyer JG. Informed consent for neonatal circumcision: an ethical and legal conundrum. J Contemp Health Law Policy 2000;17:61–133.

39. Benatar M, Benatar D. Between prophylaxis and child abuse: the ethics of neonatal male circumcision. Am J Bioeth 2003;3:35–48.

40. Benatr D, Benatar M. How not to argue about circumcision. Am J Bioeth 2003;3: W1–9.

41. Jones CM. Neonatal male circumcision: ethical issues and physician responsibility. Am J Bioeth 2003;3:59–60.

42. Herrera AJ, Hsu AS, Salcedo UT, et al. The role of parental information in the incidence of circumcision. Pediatrics 1982;70:597–8.

43. Stein M, Marx M, Taggert S, et al. Routine neonatal circumcision: the gap between contemporary policy and practice. J Fam Pract 1982;83(Suppl 1):93.
44. Diekema D. Boldt v. Boldt: a pediatric ethics perspective. J Clin Ethics 2009;20: 251–7.
45. Schoen EJ. Rebuttal: should newborns be circumcised? yes. Can Fam Physician 2008;54(1):22.

Index

Note: Page numbers of article titles are in **boldface** type.

A

Abdomen, acute pain in, 966

Adrenal hyperplasia, congenital, 858–860, 863–864, 874

AGXT gene mutations, hyperoxaluria in, 885

Alfuzosin, for bladder dysfunction, 809

Alkali agents, for urolithiasis, 892–893

Allopurinol, for urolithiasis, 893

Alpha blockers, for bladder dysfunction, 809–810

5-Alpha reductase gene defects, in partial androgen insensitivity syndrome, 861, 864

Alpha-fetoprotein, for testicular tumors, 954

American Academy of Pediatrics guidelines, for urinary tract infections, 910–912, 915

American Urological Association guidelines, for urinary tract infections, 910–912, 934

Amiloride, for urolithiasis, 892

Amitriptyline, for bladder dysfunction, 810

Amoxicillin, for vesicoureteral reflux, 820–821

Androgen insensitivity syndrome

    complete, 862–863

    partial, 861–863

Anomalies. *See also specific organs and anomalies.*

    genital, 773–779

    hydronephrosis in, **839–851**

    in neonates, 973

    inguinal, 769–773

    penile, 778–779

    prenatal ultrasound for, **739–756**

    sex developmental, **853–869, 871–880**

    surgical management for, **927–941**

    vesicoureteral reflux, **819–838**

Antegrade continence enema, for neurogenic bladder, 763–764

Anterior posterior diameter, of kidney, in hydronephrosis, 741–744

Antibiotics

    for urinary tract infections, 912–914

    for vesicoureteral reflux, 820–821

Anticholinergics, for bladder dysfunction, 808–809

Antimuscarinics, for bladder dysfunction, 808–809

Appendicovesicostomy, for neurogenic bladder, 763

Appendix testis, torsion of, 968

ATP6V mutations, hypercalciuria in, 885

Attention-deficit hyperactivity disorder, in bladder dysfunction, 791–792

Australian Prevention of Recurrent Urinary Tract Infections in Children with Vesicoureteric Reflux and Normal Renal Tracts (PRIVENT) study, 913

Pediatr Clin N Am 59 (2012) 987–1000

http://dx.doi.org/10.1016/S0031-3955(12)00103-4

pediatric.theclinics.com

0031-3955/12/$ – see front matter © 2012 Elsevier Inc. All rights reserved.

Moving?

Make sure your subscription moves with you!

To notify us of your new address, find your **Clinics Account Number** (located on your mailing label above your name), and contact customer service at:

Email: journalscustomerservice-usa@elsevier.com

800-654-2452 (subscribers in the U.S. & Canada)
314-447-8871 (subscribers outside of the U.S. & Canada)

Fax number: 314-447-8029

Elsevier Health Sciences Division
Subscription Customer Service
3251 Riverport Lane
Maryland Heights, MO 63043

*To ensure uninterrupted delivery of your subscription, please notify us at least 4 weeks in advance of move.